Editors

ASIF M. ILYAS
SHITAL N. PARIKH
SAQIB REHMAN
GILES R. SCUDERI

ORTHOPEDIC CLINICS OF NORTH AMERICA

www.orthopedic.theclinics.com

October 2014 • Volume 45 • Number 4

ELSEVIER

1600 John F. Kennedy Boulevard • Suite 1800 • Philadelphia, Pennsylvania, 19103-2899.

http://www.orthopedic.theclinics.com

ORTHOPEDIC CLINICS OF NORTH AMERICA Volume 45, Number 4
October 2014 ISSN 0030-5898, ISBN-13: 978-0-323-32620-9

Editor: Jennifer Flynn-Briggs
Developmental Editor: Stephanie Carter

Orthopedic Clinics of North America (ISSN 0030-5898) is published quarterly by Elsevier Inc., 360 Park Avenue South, New York, NY 10010-1710. Months of issue are January, April, July, and October. Business and Editorial Offices: 1600 John F. Kennedy Blvd., Suite 1800, Philadelphia, PA 19103-2899. Customer Service Office: 3251 Riverport Lane, Maryland Heights, MO 63043. Periodicals postage paid at New York, NY and additional mailing offices. Subscription prices are $310.00 per year for (US individuals), $596.00 per year for (US institutions), $365.00 per year (Canadian individuals), $727.00 per year (Canadian institutions), $450.00 per year (international individuals), $727.00 per year (international institutions), $150.00 per year (US students), $220.00 per year (Canadian and international students). Foreign air speed delivery is included in all *Clinics* subscription prices. All prices are subject to change without notice. **POSTMASTER:** Send change of address to *Orthopedic Clinics of North America*, **Elsevier Health Sciences Division, Subscription Customer Service, 3251 Riverport Lane, Maryland Heights, MO 63043. Customer Service (orders, claims, online, change of address): Elsevier Health Sciences Division, Subscription Customer Service, 3251 Riverport Lane, Maryland Heights, MO 63043. Tel: 1-800-654-2452 (U.S. and Canada); 314-447-8871 (outside U.S. and Canada). Fax: 314-447-8029. E-mail: journalscustomerservice-usa@elsevier.com (for print support); journalsonlinesupport-usa@elsevier.com (for online support).**

Reprints. For copies of 100 or more, of articles in this publication, please contact the Commercial Reprints Department, Elsevier Inc., 360 Park Avenue South, New York, NY 10010-1710. Tel.: 212-633-3874; Fax: 212-633-3820; E-mail: reprints@elsevier.com.

Orthopedic Clinics of North America is covered in *MEDLINE/PubMed* (*Index Medicus*), *Cinahl, Excerpta Medica,* and *Cumulative Index to Nursing and Allied Health Literature.*

PROGRAM OBJECTIVE

Orthopedic Clinics of North America offers clinical review articles on the most cutting-edge technologies and techniques in the field, including adult reconstruction, the upper extremity, pediatrics, trauma, oncology, and sports medicine.

TARGET AUDIENCE

Practicing orthopedic surgeons, orthopedic residents, and other healthcare professionals who specialize in orthopedic technologies and techniques for adult reconstruction, the upper extremity, pediatrics, trauma, oncology, and sports medicine.

LEARNING OBJECTIVES

Upon completion of this activity, participants will be able to:

1. Discuss orthopedic considerations of the upper extremities including injuries of the throwing athletes, oncologic surgery, and infections of shoulder surgery.
2. Review recent advances in the management of early onset scoliosis.
3. Discuss orthopedic considerations for adult reconstructive surgery and treatment and management of traumatic injury.

ACCREDITATION

The Elsevier Office of Continuing Medical Education (EOCME) is accredited by the Accreditation Council for Continuing Medical Education (ACCME) to provide continuing medical education for physicians.

The EOCME designates this enduring material for a maximum of 15 *AMA PRA Category 1 Credit*(s)™. Physicians should claim only the credit commensurate with the extent of their participation in the activity.

All other health care professionals requesting continuing education credit for this enduring material will be issued a certificate of participation.

DISCLOSURE OF CONFLICTS OF INTEREST

The EOCME assesses conflict of interest with its instructors, faculty, planners, and other individuals who are in a position to control the content of CME activities. All relevant conflicts of interest that are identified are thoroughly vetted by EOCME for fair balance, scientific objectivity, and patient care recommendations. EOCME is committed to providing its learners with CME activities that promote improvements or quality in healthcare and not a specific proprietary business or a commercial interest.

The planning committee, staff, authors and editors listed below have identified no financial relationships or relationships to products or devices they or their spouse/life partner have with commercial interest related to the content of this CME activity:

Matthew P. Abdel, MD; John A. Abraham, MD; Nirav H. Amin, MD; Louis F. Amorosa, MD; Jennifer M. Anadio, MA; Nicholas M. Caggiano, MD; Stephanie Carter; Ozgur Dede, MD; Christopher C. Dodson, MD; Mark P. Figgie, MD; Jennifer Flynn-Briggs; David L. Helfet, MD; Kristen Helm; John G. Horneff, MD; Jason E. Hsu, MD; G. Russell Huffman, MD, MPH; Brynne Hunter; Asif M. Ilyas, MD; Vamsi K. Kancherla, MD; Peter Kloen, MD, PhD; Sandy Lavery; T. Sean Lynch, MD; Kristofer S. Matullo, MD; Jill McNair; Andrew Miller, MD; Chinenye O. Nwachuku, MD; Shital N. Parikh, MD; Lindsay Parnell; Ronak M. Patel, MD; Paul S. Pipitone, DO; Santha Priya; Justin C. Wong, MD.

The planning committee, staff, authors and editors listed below have identified financial relationships or relationships to products or devices they or their spouse/life partner have with commercial interest related to the content of this CME activity:

Matthew S. Hepinstall, MD is a consultant/advisor for Smith and Nephew Orthopaedics.

Anthony Miniaci, MD has stock ownership and royalties/patents with Arthrosurface; has royalties/patents with Zimmer, Inc.; is on speakers bureau for Smith and Nephew and his spouse/partner has stock ownership with Smith and Nephew; is a consultant/advisor and has a research grant from Stryker, and his spouse/partner has stock ownership with Stryker.

Saqib Rehman, MD is a consultant/advisor for Depuy Synthes Companies; and has royalties/patents with Jaypee Brothers Medical Publishing Ltd.

Giles R. Scuderi, MD is on speakers bureau for Zimmer, Inc., ConvaTec, Inc., and Medtronic, Inc.; is a consultant/advisor for Zimmer, Inc., Pacira Pharmaceuticals and Medtronic, Inc.; has a research grant from Pacira Pharmaceuticals; and has royalties/patents from Zimmer, Inc.

Peter F. Sturm, MD; is a consultant/advisor for Depuy Spine and Orthopediatrics; has stock ownership in Pioneer Surgical; and has a research grant from Depuy Spine.

Felasfa M. Wodajo, MD has royalties/patents with Stryker and Elsevier B.V.

UNAPPROVED/OFF-LABEL USE DISCLOSURE

The EOCME requires CME faculty to disclose to the participants:

1. When products or procedures being discussed are off-label, unlabelled, experimental, and/or investigational (not US Food and Drug Administration (FDA) approved); and
2. Any limitations on the information presented, such as data that are preliminary or that represent ongoing research, interim analyses, and/or unsupported opinions. Faculty may discuss information about pharmaceutical agents that is outside of FDA-approved labelling. This information is intended solely for CME and is not intended to promote off-label use of these medications. If you have any questions, contact the medical affairs department of the manufacturer for the most recent prescribing information.

TO ENROLL

To enroll in the *Orthopedic Clinics of North America* Continuing Medical Education program, call customer service at 1-800-654-2452 or sign up online at http://www.theclinics.com/home/cme. The CME program is available to subscribers for an additional annual fee of USD $310.

METHOD OF PARTICIPATION

In order to claim credit, participants must complete the following:

1. Complete enrolment as indicated above.
2. Read the activity.
3. Complete the CME Test and Evaluation. Participants must achieve a score of 70% on the test. All CME Tests and Evaluations must be completed online.

CME INQUIRIES/SPECIAL NEEDS

For all CME inquiries or special needs, please contact elsevierCME@elsevier.com.

Contributors

EDITORS

ASIF M. ILYAS, MD - *Upper Extremity*
Program Fellowship Director of Hand and
Upper Extremity Surgery, Rothman Institute;
Associate Professor of Orthopaedic Sugery,
Thomas Jefferson University, Philadelphia,
Pennsylvania

SHITAL N. PARIKH, MD - *Pediatric
Orthopaedics*
Pediatric Orthopaedic Sports Medicine,
Associate Professor of Orthopaedic Sugery,
Cincinnati Children's Hospital Medical Center,
University of Cincinnati School of Medicine,
Cincinnati, Ohio

SAQIB REHMAN, MD - *Trauma*
Director of Orthopaedic Trauma, Associate
Professor of Orthopaedic Surgery and Sports
Medicine, School of Medicine, Temple
University Hospital, Temple University,
Philadelphia, Pennsylvania

GILES R. SCUDERI, MD - *Adult
Reconstruction*
Vice President, Orthopedic Service Line,
Northshore Long Island Jewish Health System;
Director, Insall Scott Kelly Institute, New York,
New York

AUTHORS

MATTHEW P. ABDEL, MD
Assistant Professor, Department of Orthopedic
Surgery, Mayo Clinic, Rochester, Minnesota

JOHN A. ABRAHAM, MD
Assistant Professor, The Rothman Institute of
Orthopaedics, Thomas Jefferson University
Hospital, Philadelphia, Pennsylvania

NIRAV H. AMIN, MD
Fellow in Sports Medicine, Sports Health,
Department of Orthopaedic Surgery, Cleveland
Clinic Foundation, Cleveland, Ohio

LOUIS F. AMOROSA, MD
Clinical Instructor, Department of
Orthopaedic Surgery, New York Medical
College, Westchester Medical Center,
Valhalla, New York

JENNIFER M. ANADIO, MA
Department of Pediatric Orthopaedic Surgery,
Cincinnati Children's Hospital Medical Center,
Cincinnati, Ohio

NICHOLAS M. CAGGIANO, MD
Department of Orthopaedic Surgery,
St. Luke's University Hospital, Bethlehem,
Pennsylvania

OZGUR DEDE, MD
Department of Pediatric Orthopaedic
Surgery, Cincinnati Children's Hospital
Medical Center, Cincinnati, Ohio;
Department of Orthopaedic Surgery,
Children's Hospital of Pittsburgh of
University of Pittsburgh Medical Center,
Pittsburgh, Pennsylvania

CHRISTOPHER C. DODSON, MD
Rothman Institute, Thomas Jefferson
University, Philadelphia, Pennsylvania

MARK P. FIGGIE, MD
Professor of Clinical Orthopaedic Surgery,
Division of Adult Reconstruction and Joint
Replacement, Hospital for Special Surgery,
New York, New York

DAVID L. HELFET, MD
Chief of Orthopaedic Trauma and Professor of
Orthopaedics, Orthopaedic Trauma Service,
Hospital for Special Surgery, New York,
New York

MATTHEW S. HEPINSTALL, MD
Assistant Attending and Basic Science
Coordinator, Department of Orthopaedic
Surgery, Lenox Hill Hospital, New York, New
York; Attending, Department of Orthopaedic
Surgery, Franklin Hospital, Valley Stream,
New York

JOHN G. HORNEFF, MD
Resident, Department of Orthopedic Surgery,
Hospital of University of Pennsylvania,
Philadelphia, Pennsylvania

JASON E. HSU, MD
Resident, Department of Orthopedic Surgery,
Hospital of University of Pennsylvania,
Philadelphia, Pennsylvania

G. RUSSELL HUFFMAN, MD, MPH
Assistant Professor, Department of Orthopedic
Surgery, Hospital of University of Pennsylvania,
Philadelphia, Pennsylvania

ASIF M. ILYAS, MD
Program Fellowship Director of Hand and
Upper Extremity Surgery, Rothman Institute;
Associate Professor of Orthopaedic Sugery,
Thomas Jefferson University, Philadelphia,
Pennsylvania

VAMSI K. KANCHERLA, MD
Department of Orthopaedic Surgery, St. Luke's
University Health Network, Bethlehem,
Pennsylvania

PETER KLOEN, MD, PhD
Department of Orthopaedic Surgery,
Academic Medical Center, Amsterdam,
The Netherlands

T. SEAN LYNCH, MD
Fellow in Sports Medicine, Sports Health,
Department of Orthopaedic Surgery, Cleveland
Clinic Foundation, Cleveland, Ohio

KRISTOFER S. MATULLO, MD
Chief of Hand Surgery, Department of
Orthopaedic Surgery, St. Luke's University
Hospital, Bethlehem, Pennsylvania

ANDREW MILLER, MD
Department of Orthopaedic Surgery, Thomas
Jefferson University, Philadelphia,
Pennsylvania

ANTHONY MINIACI, MD
Professor of Orthopaedic Surgery, Sports
Health, Department of Orthopaedic Surgery,
Cleveland Clinic Foundation, Cleveland, Ohio

CHINENYE O. NWACHUKU, MD
Department of Orthopaedic Surgery, St. Luke's
University Health Network, Bethlehem,
Pennsylvania

RONAK M. PATEL, MD
Fellow in Sports Medicine, Sports Health,
Department of Orthopaedic Surgery, Cleveland
Clinic Foundation, Cleveland, Ohio

PAUL S. PIPITONE, DO
Department of Orthopaedic Surgery and
Sports Medicine, Temple University School
of Medicine, Philadelphia, Pennsylvania

SAQIB REHMAN, MD
Director of Orthopaedic Trauma, Associate
Professor of Orthopaedic Surgery and
Sports Medicine, School of Medicine,
Temple University Hospital, Temple
University, Philadelphia, Pennsylvania

PETER F. STURM, MD
Alvin H. Crawford Chair of Spine Surgery;
Director Crawford Spine Center; Professor
Pediatric Orthopaedic Surgery, Department
of Pediatric Orthopaedic Surgery, Cincinnati
Children's Hospital Medical Center,
Cincinnati, Ohio

JUSTIN C. WONG, MD
Department of Orthopaedic Surgery, Thomas
Jefferson University, Philadelphia,
Pennsylvania

Contents

Adult Reconstruction

> Juvenile idiopathic arthritis (JIA) is recognized as a heterogenous group of disorders in which the common factor is persistent arthritis in at least 1 joint occurring before the age of 16 years. Although conservative management with nonsteroidal anti-inflammatory drugs and disease-modifying antirheumatic drugs can be effective, approximately 10% of JIA patients have end-stage degenerative changes requiring total hip arthroplasties (THAs) and total knee arthroplasties (TKAs). This article discusses the overall epidemiology, coordination of care, and medical and surgical management of JIA patients undergoing THA and TKA.

> Modern total hip replacement is typically effective and durable, but early failures do occur. Component position influences functional outcome, durability, and risk of complications. Surgical robotics provides the detail-oriented surgeon with a robust tool to optimize the accuracy and precision of total hip arthroplasty, with the potential to minimize risk of mechanical failure. This article describes efficient workflows for using surgical robotics to optimize surgical precision without increasing surgical complexity.

Trauma

> Periprosthetic femur fractures after total knee arthroplasty are a rising concern; however, when properly diagnosed, they can be managed nonoperatively or operatively in the form of locking plate fixation, intramedullary nailing, and arthroplasty. The degree of osteoporosis, stability of the femoral implant, and goals of the patient are a few critical variables in determining the ideal treatment. Despite excellent outcomes from each of these operative choices, the risk of nonunion, malunion, instability, and refracture cannot be ignored.

> Segmental bone loss represents a difficult clinical entity for the treating orthopedic surgeon. This article discusses the various treatment modalities available for limb

Pediatric Orthopaedics

Upper Extremity

associated with traumatic injury or through repetitive atraumatic events. Nearly 62% of cases with recurrent dislocation have both Hill-Sachs and bony Bankart defects. Treatment of unstable bone defects may require soft-tissue repair, bone grafting, or both, depending on the size and nature of the defects. The most common treatment is isolated soft-tissue repair, leaving the bone defects untreated, although emerging evidence supports directly addressing these bony defects.

It was estimated that more than 3000 people would be diagnosed with a primary bone or joint malignancy and more than 11,000 people would be diagnosed with a soft tissue sarcoma in 2013. Although primary bone and soft tissue tumors of the upper extremity are infrequent, it is imperative that the clinician be familiar with a systematic approach to the diagnosis and treatment of these conditions to prevent inadvertently compromising patient outcome. With advances in chemotherapy, radiotherapy, tumor imaging, and surgical reconstructive options, limb salvage surgery is estimated to be feasible in 95% of extremity bone or soft tissue sarcomas.

Thrower's fractures are spiral fractures of the humerus caused by forceful throwing of a ball. Although these fractures have been cited in the literature, little research exists regarding the significance of stress fractures and fatigue injuries that may precede these injuries. This article presents 3 cases of middle-aged recreational baseball pitchers who sustained mid to distal third spiral humerus fractures, reviews the biomechanics of a thrower's fracture, and provides a detailed review of the literature to help better understand this condition and guide treatment.

High valgus and extension loads imparted to the athlete's elbow during repetitive overhead throwing can lead to acute and chronic pathology. Over time, normal soft tissue and bony stabilizing structures of the elbow undergo progressive structural changes and can succumb to injury. Modern diagnostic modalities, including plain radiographs, computed tomography, and magnetic resonance imaging, in addition to arthroscopy, can aid in diagnosis. Although nonoperative management is often successful, surgical intervention may be necessary before allowing return to play.

ORTHOPEDIC CLINICS OF NORTH AMERICA

FORTHCOMING ISSUES

Beginning with the July 2013 issue, *Orthopedic Clinics of North America* began to appear in this new format. Rather than focusing on a single topic, each issue contains articles on key areas in orthopedics—adult reconstruction, upper extremity, trauma, pediatrics and oncology. Articles on sports medicine and foot and ankle will also be included on a regular basis. As the practice of orthopedics has become more specialized, the format of one topic per issue is no longer fulfilling our readers' needs. The new format is intended to address these changing needs.

Orthopedic Clinics of North America continues to publish a print issue four times a year, in January, April, July, and October. However, this series also includes online-only articles that will be published on a rolling basis (not in accordance with our quarterly publication dates). These articles, along with articles from our print issues, are available on http://www.orthopedic.theclinics.com/.

YOUR iPhone and iPad

Call for Papers

Orthopedic Clinics of North America is issuing a call for clinical review articles. Listed below are the areas of specialization of which we are currently accepting proposals:

UPPER EXTREMITY
ADULT RECONSTRUCTION
TRAUMA
ONCOLOGY
PEDIATRICS
LOWER EXTREMITY (including Foot and Ankle)
SPORTS MEDICINE

Please keep proposals to less than two pages in length, including title, author names and affiliations, disclosures, and brief abstract and/or outline of your proposed paper. Original research, editorials, and book reviews will not be accepted. If your paper is accepted, a publication date will be determined at that time.

For consideration, please email proposals to:

Senior Clinics Editor, Jennifer Flynn-Briggs, at
j.flynn-briggs@elsevier.com
To learn more about the *Clinics,* visit http://orthopedic.theclinics.com/

Jennifer Flynn-Briggs
Senior Clinics Editor

Orthop Clin N Am 45 (2014) xi
http://dx.doi.org/10.1016/j.ocl.2014.08.001
0030-5898/14/$ – see front matter © 2014 Published by Elsevier Inc.

orthopedic.theclinics.com

Adult Reconstruction

Preface
Adult Reconstruction

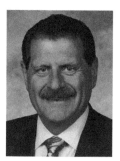

Giles R. Scuderi, MD
Editor

In this issue of *Orthopedic Clinics of North America,* we focus on two interesting topics. In the first article, on juvenile idiopathic arthritis (JIA), Figgie and Abdel discuss the epidemiology and coordination of care, including medical and surgical management for patients with JIA undergoing total hip arthroplasty (THA) and total knee arthroplasty. This select group of patients has persistent arthritis in one or more joints occurring before the age of 16 years. Although medical management can be effective, approximately 10% have end-stage arthritis requiring joint arthroplasty. The surgical management of these patients requires a multidisciplinary team approach and the authors clearly describe the challenges that may be present.

In the second article, Hepinstall reports the recent advances in robotic total hip arthroplasty. It has been well established that component position in total hip arthroplasty influences the functional outcome, durability of the implant, and risk of complications. With the introduction of robots into the surgical arena, the author suggests that surgeons may be able to optimize the accuracy and precision of THA. This well-written review article describes the utility of robots in the surgical workflow with optimization of surgical precision without increasing this surgical complexity.

Giles R. Scuderi, MD
Orthopedic Service Line
Northshore Long Island Jewish Health System
New York, NY, USA

Insall Scott Kelly Institute
New York, NY, USA

E-mail address:
gscuderi@nshs.edu

orthopedic.theclinics.com

Orthop Clin N Am 45 (2014) xiii
http://dx.doi.org/10.1016/j.ocl.2014.07.001
0030-5898/14/$ – see front matter © 2014 Elsevier Inc. All rights reserved.

Surgical Management of the Juvenile Idiopathic Arthritis Patient with Multiple Joint Involvement

Matthew P. Abdel, MD[a],*, Mark P. Figgie, MD[b]

KEYWORDS

- Juvenile idiopathic arthritis • Juvenile rheumatoid arthritis • Total hip arthroplasty
- Total knee arthroplasty

KEY POINTS

- Juvenile idiopathic arthritis (JIA) is recognized as a heterogenous group of disorders in which the common factor is persistent arthritis in at least 1 joint occurring before the age of 16 years.
- Although conservative management with nonsteroidal anti-inflammatory drugs and disease-modifying antirheumatic drugs (DMARDs) can be effective, approximately 10% of JIA patients have end-stage degenerative changes requiring total hip arthroplasties and total knee arthroplasties. Such procedures can provide significant pain relief and functional improvements.
- The surgical management of patients with JIA includes a multidisciplinary team approach, and the overall status of the patient, including other joints, must be taken into consideration.

INTRODUCTION

Juvenile idiopathic arthritis (JIA) is recognized as a heterogenous group of disorders in which the common factor is persistent arthritis in at least 1 joint occurring before the age of 16 years.[1] It commonly occurs in children between the ages of 7 and 12 years.[2] The incidence of JIA is approximately 6 cases per 10,000 children,[3] and it affects an estimated 294,000 children in the United States.[4] It is the leading cause of childhood disability, with the knee involved in approximately two-thirds of patients,[3] and the hip in one-third of cases.[1] However, hip joint involvement in JIA is the most significant factor affecting mobility and independence of these patients.[5,6]

Approximately 10% of JIA patients will have disabling knee and hip arthritis.[7] Total knee arthroplasty (TKA) and total hip arthroplasty (THA) in JIA patients are challenging given their young age, small abnormally shaped bones, complex deformities, and longer life span.[8] When considering a TKA in a JIA patient, premature growth plate closures resulting in trumpet-shaped femurs and tibias, complex deformities including valgus alignment, flexion contractures, and external tibial torsion and poor bone quality must be considered (**Fig. 1**).[2] For the hip, JIA patients often have smaller pelvises, thinner femoral cortices, smaller femoral canals, and excessive femoral and acetabular anteversion.[8] Regardless, TKA and THA in JIA

The authors have nothing to disclose.
Investigation performed at the Hospital for Special Surgery, Weill Cornell Medical College, Cornell University, New York, NY, USA.
[a] Department of Orthopedic Surgery, Mayo Clinic, 200 First Street Southwest, Rochester, MN 55905, USA;
[b] Division of Adult Reconstruction and Joint Replacement, Hospital for Special Surgery, 535 East 70th Street, New York, NY 10021, USA
* Corresponding author.
E-mail address: abdel.matthew@mayo.edu

Orthop Clin N Am 45 (2014) 435–442
http://dx.doi.org/10.1016/j.ocl.2014.06.002
0030-5898/14/$ – see front matter © 2014 Elsevier Inc. All rights reserved.

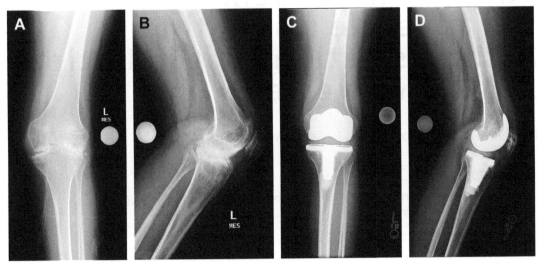

Fig. 1. (*A*) Anteroposterior (AP) view of a 24-year-old patient with advanced JIA. She has a fixed valgus deformity with a flexion contracture and external tibial rotation. (*B*) Lateral view. (*C*) AP view after total knee replacement. (*D*) Lateral view.

patients can provide relief of pain and improved function if the appropriate preoperative assessment and perioperative management are enacted.[1,2,7–18]

COORDINATION OF MEDICAL CARE AND MEDICATIONS

JIA patients have multiple musculoskeletal and nonmusculoskeletal manifestations that must be managed by a comprehensive medical and surgical team. Careful evaluation of all joints, including the spine, is mandatory. Assessment of cervical spine involvement is necessary to permit safe airway management, which may be challenging due to neck instability.[19] Patients with basilar invagination, C1-2 or subaxial instability with a space available for the cord of no more than 13 mm, or myelopathy should first be evaluated by a spine surgeon. Mandibular hypoplasia is also important to identify, as it may make intubation difficult. A thorough evaluation by the patient's rheumatologist prior to surgery is essential to evaluate for associated systemic involvement of the pericardium, respiratory system, and clotting cascade.[19] Occasionally, evaluation by a specialist to evaluate cardiac and pulmonary status of JIA patients undergoing TKA or THA is warranted.

Perioperative management of medications used to manage inflammatory arthritis is essential, as such medications may place JIA patients at increased risk of delayed wound healing and perioperative infections. However, withholding such medications places patients at risk for a flare, thereby compromising rehabilitation. The most

commonly used medications are synthetic DMARDs (such as methotrexate, hydroxychloroquine, and leflunomide), corticosteroids, and biologic agents (such as tumor necrosis factor [TNF]-blocking agents).[19]

In regards to methotrexate, the international task force recommends that it should be continued through the perioperative period.[19,20] It is also recommended that hydroxychloroquine be continued through the perioperative period given that it is not an immunosuppressant, and it may confer some protections against postoperative thromboembolism.[19] However, corticosteroids are a potent anti-inflammatory and immunosuppressant. There are data showing that the risk of infection increases with corticosteroid dose.[21,22] An increased risk of infection persists with doses of less than 5 mg/d, and the risk increases with duration of therapy.[19] However, when more extensive surgeries such as arthroplasty are undertaken, stress dose steroids including an intraoperative supplemental dose of hydrocortisone should be given.[19]

The risk of infection with anti-TNF agents is well recognized, with multiple series documenting an increased risk of infection, including surgical site infection.[23,24] The infection risk is highest in the first 6 months of therapy.[25,26] Given the variety of currently utilized anti-TNF medications, there are various times when they should be discontinued prior to surgery. The authors usually stop these agents at a half-life of the drug before surgery, but no more than a month before if they have a longer half-life. These drugs typically can be started after the sutures are out and the wound is healing well, typically 2 weeks after surgery.

STAGING OF SURGICAL INTERVENTIONS

JIA patients often present with multiple joint involvement. Because upper extremity involvement has a direct impact on the ability to utilize gait aids after lower extremity surgery, these joints must be taken into consideration.[19] If a patient is able to utilize ambulatory aids, then lower extremity surgery is preferred. This allows patients to be free from gait aids prior to total elbow arthroplasties and total shoulder arthroplasties. However, in cases in which the upper extremities are so painful or debilitating, it is reasonable to proceed with upper extremity surgery first.

In general, it is best to perform surgery on the most painful joint first. However, in JIA patients who have multiple lower extremity joints that are affected, the authors prefer to operate on the involved foot first so that the foot is free of pain and plantigrade. This will help facilitate proper rehabilitation after TKA and THA. Next, with all other factors being equal, the authors prefer to perform a THA prior to TKA. It is difficult to rehabilitate the knee if the hip is stiff and painful. Also, if there is a flexion contracture of the hip, it is difficult to maintain full extension in the knee. Replacing the hip first should also eliminate any referred pain to the knee. Of note, bilateral THAs or TKAs are performed when possible, especially in patients with flexion contractures. Rehabilitation is facilitated when both legs can be fully extended.

OVERVIEW OF LOWER EXTREMITY JOINT REPLACEMENTS
Total Hip Arthroplasty

THA in JIA can provide relief of pain and improved function even if skeletal maturity has not yet occurred.[1,8–13,15,27,28] Given their small size and weight and relatively low activity level, JIA patients are less vulnerable to wear from joint surfaces.[1] As previously noted, there are several factors to consider prior to completing a THA in a JIA patient, including the small and abnormal anatomic structures of the femur and acetabulum, growth and remodeling of bone in young patients, osteoporosis from disuse and steroids, and soft tissue contractures (**Fig. 2**).

THA in JIA patients can either be cemented or cementless. Primary cemented THA in JIA patients has demonstrated aseptic loosening rates of 19% to 57% at 5 to 10 years of follow-up.[1,29–31] However, the survivorship of cementless primary THA in patients with JIA is 96% to 100% for the femoral stem and 88% to 90% for the acetabular cup at 5 to 13 years of follow-up.[1,13,32] Daurka and colleagues[9] reported on 52 consecutive uncemented THAs in JIA patients with a mean age of 14.4 years, and a median follow-up of 10.5 years. They found 94% survivorship of the femoral component and 62% survivorship of the acetabular component. However, there was 100% survivorship of the ceramic-on-ceramic THAs, but only 55% survivorship with metal- or ceramic-on-polyethylene. Similarly, Odent and colleagues[13] reported on 62 uncemented THAs in 34 JIA patients after an average follow-up of 6 years. At 13 years, the survivorship was 100% for the femoral component and 90% for the acetabular component. Witt and colleagues[18] reported on 96 cemented THAs in patients with JIA with a mean follow-up of 11.5 years and a mean age of 16.7 years. Revision was required in 25% of patients and a further 18% had radiological signs of loosening.

Both hybrid and cemented THAs have also been completed in JIA patients. Kitsoulis and colleagues[11] reported on 20 THAs of which all

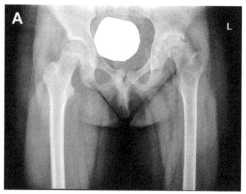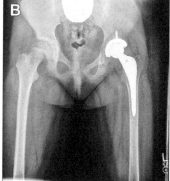

Fig. 2. (A) AP view of the pelvis of an 8-year-old patient with advanced destruction of the left hip. Note that the growth plates are still open. (B) Noncemented total hip replacement was performed with closure of the triradiate cartilage.

acetabular cups were uncemented, and 50% of all femoral stems were uncemented. All patients experienced excellent pain relief, and there were no failures for the femoral stems at a mean 10-year follow-up. Two acetabular cups (10%) required revision because of aseptic loosening. In 50 patients between the ages of 11 and 19 years, Torchia and colleagues[17] found 73% survival of cemented THAs at 10 years. Similarly, De Ranieri and colleagues[8] described the outcomes of 37 primary THAs in Charnley class C JIA patients. They noted good pain relief and functional improvements, but had 12 failures. Lachiewicz and colleagues[12] reported 100% survival in 10 patients at 4.5 years, with a mean postoperative Harris hip score of 78. On the other hand, Wroblewski and colleagues[33] reviewed 195 Charnley low friction arthroplasties at a mean 15-year follow-up and found that 22% of acetabular components and 8% of femoral stems were loose. The results of cemented THA seem to be better in older patients. Lehtimaki and colleagues[34] reviewed 186 cemented THAs in 116 patients with JIA. The overall survival was 91.9% at 10 years.

The authors' current approach to THA is to utilize cementless fixation with either a metal-on-polyethylene or ceramic-on-polyethylene articulation. We frequently obtain preoperative computed tomography (CT) scans to evaluate femoral anteversion and the need for custom-fit components (**Fig. 3**).

Revision hip surgery in patients with JIA is even more challenging. This is secondary to the small proportions with narrow femoral canals, numerous contractures, and compromised bone stock.[19] Goodman and Figgie[19] recently reported high complication rates in revision THA for JIA. In their series of 24 revision THAs in 15 patients, 29% of patients required reoperation. The authors noted high intraoperative and postoperative complications, with a guarded prognosis for long-term survivorship.

Surgeons should be aware that a wide exposure with extensive capsulotomy is often required. Oftentimes, both anterior and posterior soft tissue releases are required. Moreover, an in situ femoral neck osteotomy for bony ankylosis or protrusio deformities may be required. Occasionally, an adductor tenotomy may be required at the time of THA to improve abduction and decrease the risk of posterior instability. On the acetabular side, challenges are either related to the shallow, dysplastic socket that appears similar to developmental dysplasia of the hip, or protrusio (**Fig. 4**). These problems can often be addressed with autogenous femoral head graft, combined with an uncemented socket and supplemental screw fixation (**Fig. 5**).

Total Knee Arthroplasty

TKA is a successful procedure for the treatment of end-stage arthritis, with national registries reporting survival rates in patients with osteoarthritis of nearly 95% at 10 years, and just below 90% at 20 years.[2,35,36] Survival rates of TKA in patients with rheumatoid arthritis are less favorable, with rates of 93% at 10 years and 85% at 20 years.[2,35,37] However, few studies have reported their results with TKAs in JIA patients.[2,7,14]

In the largest series to date, Heyse and colleagues[2] reported on 349 TKAs completed in JIA patients in their multicenter study. The 10-year survivorship was 95%, decreasing to 82% at 20 years. Palmer and colleagues[14] described 8 consecutive patients (15 knees) with JIA who

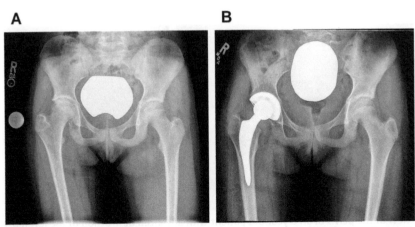

A   **B**

Fig. 3. (*A*) AP view of the pelvis of a 12-year-old girl with JIA. (*B*) Custom total hip was performed because of the patient's size and excessive femoral anteversion.

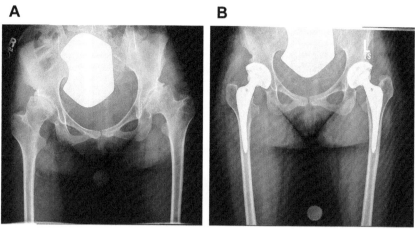

Fig. 4. (*A*) AP view of the pelvis of a 24-year-old patient with JIA and dysplastic hips. (*B*) Non-cemented total hip replacements were performed.

underwent TKA at an average age of 16.8 years. With a mean follow-up of 15.5 years, all patients had substantial pain and functional improvements. Failure occurred in 3 patients. Likewise, Parvizi and colleagues[7] reviewed the results of 25 consecutive TKAs (13 patients) that were performed between 1982 and 1997. While the Knee Society pain and function scores improved, there were several postoperative complications. Thomas and colleagues[38] reported a 5.9% failure rate at an average follow-up of 6 months for 17 TKAs completed in 10 JIA patients. Moreover, Jolles and Bogoch[39] described 22 TKAs in 14 patients and found no revisions at a mean follow-up of 8 years. On the other hand, Malviya and colleagues[40] found a 41.5% failure rate at 20 years of 34 TKAs completed in 20 JIA patients.

TKA survivorship in JIA patients is likely influenced by the poor bone quality, joint deformities, and contractures with which these patients present. In addition, the immunosuppressive medications utilized to treat the disease play a role in the process. Patients with JIA have some of the most challenging deformities and bone abnormalities. In addition, they are typically very young in age.

The authors' current management is to optimize medial management preoperatively, while also maximizing physical therapy to maintain range of motion. When patients have contractures in both knees, the authors prefer to perform simultaneous bilateral TKAs to correct deformities as long as the patients are healthy enough for such a procedure. The surgical exposure can be difficult due to the severe deformities, and occasionally the patella is ankylosed to the femur. More extensive exposures are sometimes required, but tibial tubercle osteotomies are avoided, especially if the tibia is small and osteopenic. In addition, the

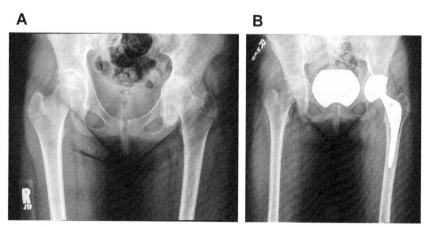

Fig. 5. (*A*) AP view of the pelvis of a 19-year-old patient with JIA and protrusion. (*B*) Bone grafting was performed using the autogenous femoral head.

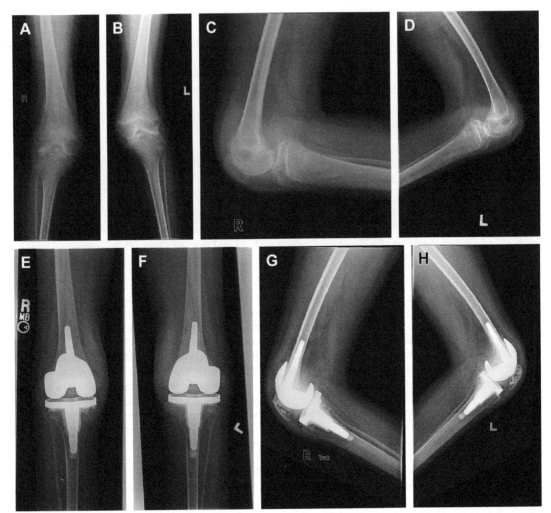

Fig. 6. (*A, B*) AP views of a 12 year old with JIA that had stopped walking. (*C, D*) Lateral views. (*E, F*) Views after bilateral TKAs; custom implants were used because of size. (*G, H*) Postoperative lateral views.

proximal part of the tibia is frequently dysplastic with rapid tapering of the metaphysis. Gentle retractor placement is essential to avoid compression fractures. Moreover, resurfacing of the patella is recommended in all JIA patients.[7] Although the authors attempt to utilize the least constraint possible, often the extensive releases necessitate the use of a more constrained articulation. Finally, preoperative planning with a CT scan can be helpful if custom implants are considered (**Fig. 6**).

COMPLICATIONS

As previously noted, hip and knee arthroplasties in JIA patients present unique surgical situations, along with a distinctive set of complications. Intraoperative and postoperative fractures are more frequent given the narrow femoral canals and compromised bone. In addition, preoperative contractures predispose JIA patients to postoperative arthrofibrosis. In addition, there is an increased incidence of sciatic nerve injury and deep periprosthetic infection.[1,19]

SUMMARY

The surgical management of patients with JIA includes a multidisciplinary team approach. Conservative management with NSAIDs and DMARDs can be effective. However, when end-stage degenerative changes occur in the hip and knee, THA and TKA are indicated, respectively. Surgical considerations include perioperative medical management (including medications), as well as intraoperative management of the dysplasia and bone stock deficiencies. Further long-term studies with strict inclusions criteria and validated outcome measures are needed, particularly with uncemented fixation in the hip and knee.

REFERENCES

1. Goodman SB, Hwang K, Imrie S. High complication rate in revision total hip arthroplasty in juvenile idiopathic arthritis. Clin Orthop Relat Res 2014;472(2): 637–44.

2. Heyse TJ, Ries MD, Bellemans J, et al. Total knee arthroplasty in patients with juvenile idiopathic arthritis. Clin Orthop Relat Res 2014; 472(1):147–54.

3. Behrens EM, Beukelman T, Gallo L, et al. Evaluation of the presentation of systemic onset juvenile rheumatoid arthritis: data from the Pennsylvania Systemic Onset Juvenile Arthritis Registry (PASOJAR). J Rheumatol 2008;35(2):343–8.

4. Iesaka K, Kubiak EN, Bong MR, et al. Orthopedic surgical management of hip and knee involvement in patients with juvenile rheumatoid arthritis. Am J Orthop 2006;35(2):67–73.

5. Albright JA, Ablright JP, Ogden JA. Synovectomy of the hip in juvenile rheumatoid arthritis. Clin Orthop Relat Res 1975;(106):48–55.

6. Isdale IC. Hip disease in juvenile rheumatoid arthritis. Ann Rheum Dis 1970;29(6):603–8.

7. Parvizi J, Lajam CM, Trousdale RT, et al. Total knee arthroplasty in young patients with juvenile rheumatoid arthritis. J Bone Joint Surg Am 2003;85-A(6): 1090–4.

8. De Ranieri A, Wagner N, Imrie SN, et al. Outcome of primary total hip arthroplasty in Charnley class C patients with juvenile idiopathic arthritis: a case series. J Arthroplasty 2011;26(8):1182–8.

9. Daurka JS, Malik AK, Robin DA, et al. The results of uncemented total hip replacement in children with juvenile idiopathic arthritis at ten years. J Bone Joint Surg Br 2012;94(12):1618–24.

10. Goodman SB, Oh KJ, Imrie S, et al. Revision total hip arthroplasty in juvenile chronic arthritis: 17 revisions in 11 patients followed for 4-12 years. Acta Orthop 2006;77(2):242–50.

11. Kitsoulis PB, Stafilas KS, Siamopoulou A, et al. Total hip arthroplasty in children with juvenile chronic arthritis: long-term results. J Pediatr Orthop 2006; 26(1):8–12.

12. Lachiewicz PF, McCaskill B, Inglis A, et al. Total hip arthroplasty in juvenile rheumatoid arthritis. Two to eleven-year results. J Bone Joint Surg Am 1986; 68(4):502–8.

13. Odent T, Journeau P, Prieur AM, et al. Cementless hip arthroplasty in juvenile idiopathic arthritis. J Pediatr Orthop 2005;25(4):465–70.

14. Palmer DH, Mulhall KJ, Thompson CA, et al. Total knee arthroplasty in juvenile rheumatoid arthritis. J Bone Joint Surg Am 2005;87(7):1510–4.

15. Scott RD. Total hip and knee arthroplasty in juvenile rheumatoid arthritis. Clin Orthop Relat Res 1990;(259):83–91.

16. Scott RD, Sarokhan AJ, Dalziel R. Total hip and total knee arthroplasty in juvenile rheumatoid arthritis. Clin Orthop Relat Res 1984;(182):90–8.

17. Torchia ME, Klassen RA, Bianco AJ. Total hip arthroplasty with cement in patients less than twenty years old. Long-term results. J Bone Joint Surg Am 1996; 78(7):995–1003.

18. Witt JD, Swann M, Ansell BM. Total hip replacement for juvenile chronic arthritis. J Bone Joint Surg Br 1991;73(5):770–3.

19. Goodman SM, Figgie M. Lower extremity arthroplasty in patients with inflammatory arthritis: preoperative and perioperative management. J Am Acad Orthop Surg 2013;21(6):355–63.

20. Visser K, Katchamart W, Loza E, et al. Multinational evidence-based recommendations for the use of methotrexate in rheumatic disorders with a focus on rheumatoid arthritis: integrating systematic literature research and expert opinion of a broad international panel of rheumatologists in the 3E Initiative. Ann Rheum Dis 2009;68(7):1086–93.

21. Dixon WG, Suissa S, Hudson M. The association between systemic glucocorticoid therapy and the risk of infection in patients with rheumatoid arthritis: systematic review and meta-analyses. Arthritis Res Ther 2011;13(4):R139.

22. Grijalva CG, Chen L, Delzell E, et al. Initiation of tumor necrosis factor-alpha antagonists and the risk of hospitalization for infection in patients with autoimmune diseases. JAMA 2011;306(21): 2331–9.

23. Giles JT, Bartlett SJ, Gelber AC, et al. Tumor necrosis factor inhibitor therapy and risk of serious postoperative orthopedic infection in rheumatoid arthritis. Arthritis Rheum 2006;55(2):333–7.

24. den Broeder AA, Creemers MC, Fransen J, et al. Risk factors for surgical site infections and other complications in elective surgery in patients with rheumatoid arthritis with special attention for anti-tumor necrosis factor: a large retrospective study. J Rheumatol 2007;34(4):689–95.

25. Curtis JR, Xi J, Patkar N, et al. Drug-specific and time-dependent risks of bacterial infection among patients with rheumatoid arthritis who were exposed to tumor necrosis factor alpha antagonists. Arthritis Rheum 2007;56(12):4226–7.

26. Galloway JB, Hyrich KL, Mercer LK, et al. Anti-TNF therapy is associated with an increased risk of serious infections in patients with rheumatoid arthritis especially in the first 6 months of treatment: updated results from the British Society for Rheumatology Biologics Register with special emphasis on risks in the elderly. Rheumatology 2011;50(1): 124–31.

27. Ruddlesdin C, Ansell BM, Arden GP, et al. Total hip replacement in children with juvenile chronic arthritis. J Bone Joint Surg Br 1986;68(2):218–22.

28. Oen K, Malleson PN, Cabral DA, et al. Disease course and outcome of juvenile rheumatoid arthritis in a multicenter cohort. J Rheumatol 2002;29(9):1989–99.

29. Chmell MJ, Scott RD, Thomas WH, et al. Total hip arthroplasty with cement for juvenile rheumatoid arthritis. Results at a minimum of ten years in patients less than thirty years old. J Bone Joint Surg Am 1997;79(1):44–52.

30. Mogensen B, Brattstrom H, Ekelund L, et al. Synovectomy of the hip in juvenile chronic arthritis. J Bone Joint Surg Br 1982;64(3):295–9.

31. Williams WW, McCullough CJ. Results of cemented total hip replacement in juvenile chronic arthritis. A radiological review. J Bone Joint Surg Br 1993; 75(6):872–4.

32. Kumar MN, Swann M. Uncemented total hip arthroplasty in young patients with juvenile chronic arthritis. Ann R Coll Surg Engl 1998;80(3):203–9.

33. Wroblewski BM, Siney PD, Fleming PA. Charnley low-frictional torque arthroplasty in young rheumatoid and juvenile rheumatoid arthritis: 292 hips followed for an average of 15 years. Acta Orthop 2007;78(2):206–10.

34. Lehtimaki MY, Lehto MU, Kautiainen H, et al. Survivorship of the Charnley total hip arthroplasty in juvenile chronic arthritis. A follow-up of 186 cases for 22 years. J Bone Joint Surg Br 1997;79(5): 792–5.

35. Knutson K, Robertsson O. The Swedish knee arthroplasty register (www.knee.se). Acta Orthop 2010; 81(1):5–7.

36. Paxton EW, Furnes O, Namba RS, et al. Comparison of the Norwegian knee arthroplasty register and a United States arthroplasty registry. J Bone Joint Surg Am 2011;93(Suppl 3):20–30.

37. Schrama JC, Espehaug B, Hallan G, et al. Risk of revision for infection in primary total hip and knee arthroplasty in patients with rheumatoid arthritis compared with osteoarthritis: a prospective, population-based study on 108,786 hip and knee joint arthroplasties from the Norwegian arthroplasty register. Arthritis Care Res 2010;62(4):473–9.

38. Thomas A, Rojer D, Imrie S, et al. Cemented total knee arthroplasty in patients with juvenile rheumatoid arthritis. Clin Orthop Relat Res 2005;(433): 140–6.

39. Jolles BM, Bogoch ER. Quality of life after TKA for patients with juvenile rheumatoid arthritis. Clin Orthop Relat Res 2008;466(1):167–78.

40. Malviya A, Foster HE, Avery P, et al. Long term outcome following knee replacement in patients with juvenile idiopathic arthritis. Knee 2010;17(5): 340–4.

Robotic Total Hip Arthroplasty

Matthew S. Hepinstall, MD[a,b],*

KEYWORDS

- Hip • Arthritis • Joint replacement • Arthroplasty • Robotic • Navigation

KEY POINTS

- Component position influences functional outcome, durability, and risk of complications after total hip arthroplasty.
- Optimal component position requires meticulous planning based on reliable information, followed by accurate and precise execution of the plan.
- Surgical robotics provides the detail-oriented surgeon with a robust tool to optimize the accuracy and precision of total hip arthroplasty.

INTRODUCTION

Total hip replacement (THR) was described as the "operation of the [twentieth] century."[1] Although highly cross-linked polyethylene has reduced wear at the bearing surface and cementless fixation has reduced mechanical failure at the fixation interface, several attempts to improve on John Charnley's innovation in the early twenty-first century have proved less rewarding.[2] A trend toward cementless tapered femoral implants, cementless hemispherical acetabular implants, and cobalt-chromium or ceramic on highly cross-linked polyethylene articulations is emerging.[3] When proven implants are used, high rates of patient satisfaction are experienced and durability longer than 20 years is anticipated.[4]

Is there room for improvement in modern THR? Patients and payers are no longer willing to tolerate early failure after THR,[5] but infection, dislocation, leg length discrepancy, and periprosthetic fracture continue to occur. Furthermore, edge loading, impingement, and other mechanical consequences of imprecise implant positioning continue to adversely affect implant durability for many patients.[6–9] Recent Medicare data show that 10% of patients age 65 to 74 years at the time of hip replacement undergo revision surgery within the first 10 years,[10] and recent European registry data show a 17% revision rate at 10 years for patients less than 50 years old at the time of surgery.[11]

As surgeons try to meet ever-higher expectations, they must endeavor to embrace improvements without subjecting patients to the safety concerns that come with unproven technologies.[2] The last 10 years have provided ample opportunity to reflect with humility on the consequences of supposedly improving THR. Nevertheless, avoidance of mechanical failure requires improvements in surgical implants and/or technique.

With surgeons, regulators, and patients now more skeptical of new THR implants, the greatest opportunities for improvement may be at the level of surgical technique. Imprecision of acetabular component position, a major source of variability in THR outcomes,[6,7,9,12–16] presents such an opportunity.

Funding Sources: None.

Conflict of Interest: Dr M.S. Hepinstall is a paid consultant for Smith & Nephew Orthopaedics.

[a] Department of Orthopaedic Surgery, Lenox Hill Hospital, 100 East 77th Street, New York, NY 10075, USA;
[b] Department of Orthopaedic Surgery, Franklin Hospital, 900 Franklin Avenue, Valley Stream, NY 11580, USA
* Center for Joint Preservation & Reconstruction, Department of Orthopaedic Surgery, Lenox Hill Hospital, 130 East 77th Street, 11th Floor, New York, NY 10075.
E-mail address: mhepinstall@nshs.edu

Surgeons embarking on THR, whether simple or complex, must first establish targets for component position and then endeavor to reproduce the plan within accepted tolerances.[17] Several investigators have proposed ranges of acceptable component acetabular position.[12,13,18–20] Femoral offset and length must be informed by both femoral anatomy and the selected acetabular position so as to optimize limb length reconstruction, abductor function, joint stability, and impingement-free range of motion.[21] Ideal implant position for a given patient may also be affected by surgical approach, soft tissue constraints, functional requirements, and extra-articular deformities such as fixed pelvic obliquity or tilt.

Planning based on plain radiographs remains limited by inability to (1) consistently control or assess magnification and (2) obtain simultaneous perfect anteroposterior (AP) images of the pelvis and proximal femur in patients with joint contractures. The imprecision of manual component positioning is well documented, and rigorous assessment of radiographic outcomes reveals that a large percentage of acetabular prostheses are implanted outside accepted parameters for optimal position.[19]

Computer navigation was developed to improve on manual techniques and can be image guided or imageless. Although imageless navigation can improve intraoperative assessment of component position and limb length change, only image-based systems can improve surgical planning. Preoperative planning based on three-dimensional (3D) patient anatomy facilitates restoration of acetabular center of rotation and allows the ideal acetabular abduction and anteversion angle to be informed by relationships with bone anatomy. For example, patients with anteverted dysplastic acetabulae are at risk for psoas tendon impingement if the acetabular implant is not positioned within the anterior lip of the acetabular bone. Preoperative 3D planning allows the surgeon to select a position that avoids implant prominence but also avoids excessive anteversion or reaming through the medial wall of the acetabulum, technical errors that can easily occur in the service of a well-covered implant in a dysplastic acetabulum. However, navigation alone inadequately facilitates this precision because depth and location of acetabular reaming are not precisely controlled.

Surgical robotics allows the coupling of 3D planning with precision bone preparation and implant insertion. Robots have been investigated for use in joint replacement since the 1980s and used clinically since 1992. ROBODOC (Curexo Technology Corporation, Fremont, CA) was the first surgical robot developed and commercialized for THR.[22]

Although initially developed domestically by IBM, the ROBODOC active robotic system has had limited popularity in the United States and much of the published experience is from Europe and Asia.[23–25] The system is approved by the US Food and Drug Administration (FDA) for THR, but has not yet been widely accepted by the domestic orthopedic community.

Widespread interest in robotic joint replacement surgery began with the commercialization of the RIO Robotic Arm Interactive Orthopedic System (Stryker Mako Surgical Corporation, Fort Lauderdale, FL) for partial knee replacement. The device has been shown to improve the precision of limb and implant alignment compared with manual techniques,[26–28] but does not remove the necessity of attention to details such as cement technique.[29] Short-term clinical outcomes have been favorable, but long-term results are not available. Software and hardware to facilitate THR were recently introduced.[30] The robot assists with reaming of the acetabular cavity and positioning the acetabular implant using haptics, and its software package allows navigation of the femoral neck cut, leg length, and offset. The remainder of this article describes techniques for leveraging surgical robotics to optimize implant positioning for hip reconstruction, with figures to clarify the technique and illustrate the capacity of the robot to simplify complex reconstructions. The details described are specific to the widely available Mako RIO robot, but the concepts are generally applicable to other robotic platforms using image-based navigation and haptic control.

SURGICAL TECHNIQUE

The design of a surgical robot could theoretically limit the surgeon's choice of surgical approaches. The Mako RIO robot has software packages to facilitate THR through posterior, lateral, anterolateral, and direct anterior approaches. The posterior approach is emphasized in this review, followed by changes in the workflow for the direct anterior approach.

Preoperative Planning

Segmentation

Surgical planning software accompanies the Mako RIO surgical robot. A computed tomography (CT) scan of the pelvis and both femora is performed according to a specific protocol. CT images are segmented and 3D reconstruction is performed. Bony landmarks such as the anterior superior iliac spines and the medial tips of the lesser trochanters are identified. This process is performed by engineers but can be verified by the surgeon.

Establishing reference planes and quantifying preoperative deformity

In the current Mako software (THA version 2.1), the anterior pelvic plane is determined using the tilt of the pelvis while the patient is supine in the CT scanner, and the medial-lateral axis is defined as the line connecting the anterior superior iliac spines. Acetabular anteversion is thus calculated in a functional plane. The surgeon must decide how best to use this information, because pelvic tilt can change between sitting and standing positions and between preoperative and postoperative states,[31] but use of a functional reference is important. When anatomic planes alone are used to guide acetabular positioning, excessive functional abduction and anteversion can occur in the patient with decreased pelvic tilt, whereas functional retroversion can occur in the patient with increased pelvic tilt.

The software transforms the 3D models of the pelvis and femora into a two-dimensional image that mimics an idealized AP pelvis radiograph in the functional plane. If there is no pelvic deformity, this should result in an image with symmetric obturator foramina and the midline of the sacrum should align with the pubic symphysis. The femora are aligned so that the long axis of each femur is oriented parallel to the frontal plane, as is the maximum femoral offset. The virtual AP radiograph thus eliminates any distortion from flexion contracture and shows true femoral offset.

The software measures preoperative differences in leg length and combined offset (defined as the distance between the midsagittal plane of the pelvis and the diaphyseal axis of the femur). Measurements assume no pelvic obliquity and no length discrepancy below the lesser trochanters. The surgeon retains responsibility for determining the clinical leg length difference. Planned deformity correction should compromise between radiographic and clinical leg length discrepancy, informed by patient perceptions and clinician judgment.

Misidentification of bone landmarks can distort the image and resultant measurements (leg length, offset and acetabular version), so the surgeon must visually confirm that the reconstructed preoperative AP pelvis radiograph appears optimized. If the obturator foramina are not symmetric, the interteardrop line is not parallel to the horizontal reference line, or the sacrum is not centered on the pubic symphysis, the surgeon can identify the bone deformity or error in segmentation that distorted the image and change the landmarks if appropriate. This process can be done in the operating room and does not require the surgeon to review the plan days or hours in advance.

Acetabular templating

The procedure starts with the virtual acetabular template positioned in 40° abduction and 20° of anteversion, with the medial aspect of the template at the lateral edge of the acetabular teardrop. Size is selected to remove cartilage and sclerotic bone but preserve as much bone as possible for fixation, and to restore the center of rotation at or medial to the anatomic location. AP position is selected to remove similar amounts of subchondral bone from the anterior and posterior walls of the acetabulum. Proximal-distal position is selected to match the location of the contralateral center of rotation (when normal), and to penetrate but not remove the subchondral bone of the acetabular sourcil. The surgeon can view the planned reaming of the acetabulum on the 3D model and the planned 3D appearance of the implant within the bone, in addition to cross sections of the planned position in the axial, coronal, and sagittal planes. This technique allows identification of problems such as exposed implant at the psoas recess. Acetabular version references the functional plane, so the initial plan does not always optimally match the local anatomy. Minor alterations of component size, orientation, and position can and should be made to compromise between competing goals (**Fig. 1**).

Templating in 3D on CT images is helpful with complex anatomy (**Fig. 2**) but initially unfamiliar. The planning software allows the surgeon to visualize how the planned cup position will appear on the postoperative AP pelvis radiograph. This perspective is familiar and allows additional adjustments to the plan as desired.

Femoral templating

A femoral implant is chosen that will wedge within the bony confines of the proximal femur in a location that allows reconstruction of limb length and offset with the available neck and head options (**Fig. 3**). Three-dimensional femoral planning allows accurate assessment of femoral offset and length. When coupled with 3D acetabular planning, it also allows anticipation of the changes in femoral anatomy that are necessary to compensate for changes in the acetabular center of rotation. If the acetabular center of rotation is shifted medially in accordance with Charnley principles,[32] increased femoral offset is required to restore combined offset, optimizing stability, abductor function, and impingement-free range of motion.[21]

For any combination of selected implant sizes and positions, the software measures the change in limb length and combined offset relative to (1) the preoperative status and (2) the contralateral hip. The surgeon must decide which of these measurements

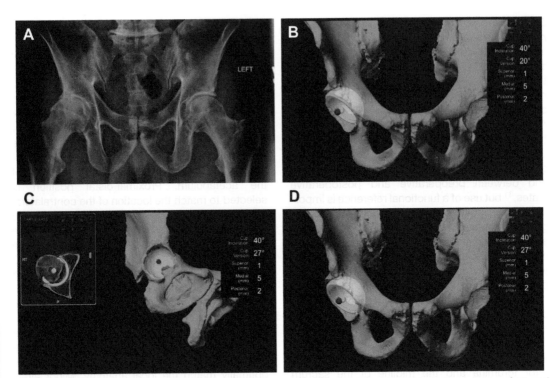

Fig. 1. Acetabular position is planned in 3 dimensions and adjustments are possible in increments of 1° and 0.3 mm. In this patient with abnormal pelvic tilt secondary to loss of lumbar lordosis (*A*) functional anteversion of 20° would have resulted in implant prominence at the psoas recess (*B*). This outcome was avoided by increasing planned anteversion to 27° (*C*), which eliminated the prominence (*D*).

to prioritize. If the contralateral hip is normal, clinical and radiographic leg length discrepancies are equal, and the virtual AP pelvis appears optimized, it is simplest to match the contralateral side. When these variables are not aligned, the author makes a clinical assessment of desired change in limb length and combined offset and then references off the preoperative position for the surgical hip.

The software measures native femoral anteversion. When mild to moderate version abnormalities are encountered, the surgeon can compensate with small adjustments in acetabular version[33,34] and/or use of an elevated rim liner. When femoral version is markedly abnormal, the surgeon can plan to use a femoral stem that allows version to be decoupled from bone morphology (eg, Wagner-style, modular, or cemented stems).

Although not part of the manufacturer's recommended workflow, the software can be used to measure (1) the lesser-to-center distance (LTC) from the proximal aspect of the lesser trochanter to the center of the femoral head, and (2) the distance of the neck cut from the top of lesser trochanter. The preoperative LTC will be different from the planned LTC after reconstruction when the selected acetabular position does not restore the prearthritic center of rotation. Both the preoperative and anticipated

postreconstruction LTC values should be measured during preoperative planning.

Preparation and Patient Positioning

For the posterior approach, the patient is positioned in the lateral decubitus position on a pegboard. The navigation tower and robotic arm are positioned anterior to the patient and opposite the surgeon, who stands behind the patient. Mobility of the robotic arm is optimal at its ideal working height. The surgical table can be lowered for the obese patient with a wide pelvis, and tilted away from the robot to facilitate acetabular reaming in adequate anteversion.

The limb is prepped and draped free, including the iliac crest and the proximal half of the femur in the sterile field. The robot is kept well away from the surgical field during exposure. This technique allows access to the patient and allows the robot to be draped and registered by the surgical technician during exposure. Standardized steps are performed, taking less than 3 minutes. This task can safely be delegated, because the software does not allow required steps to be bypassed and a 5-second final check by the surgeon is required before reaming.

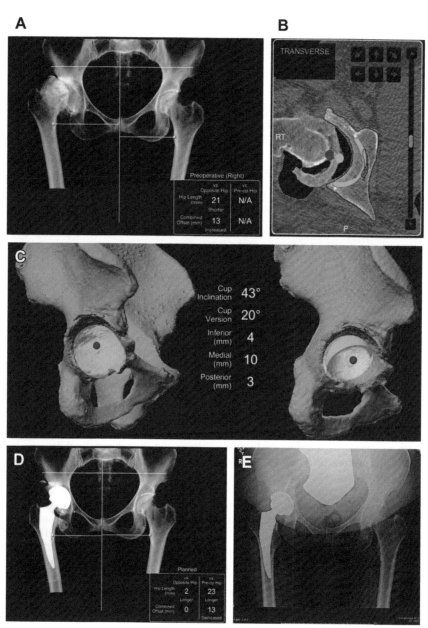

Fig. 2. Three-dimensional planning is particularly helpful in cases in which acetabular bone loss distorts the anatomic center of rotation (*A*) allowing the plan to compromise between achieving adequate bone coverage for fixation (*B, C*) and restoration of a near-anatomic center of rotation (*D*). Previewing the anticipated postoperative radiograph allows the surgeon to understand the consequences of the 3D plan in a familiar format. Impaction grafting was used to restore acetabular bone stock in this young patient (*E*).

Surgical Approach

For the posterior approach, a gently curved skin incision of 8 to 12 cm is made just anterior to the posterior margin of the femur. The length of the incision has little effect on patient outcome and should not be a higher priority than adequate femoral mobility to accurately prepare the acetabulum.

The distal portion of the fascial incision should be anterior to the insertion of the gluteal sling at the linea aspera to avoid tethering the surgical window. In morbidly obese patients, muscular men, and patients with severe stiffness or shortening at the hip, partial or complete release of the gluteal sling is considered.

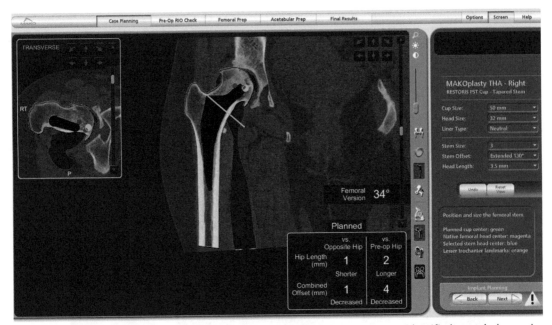

Fig. 3. Femoral position is planned in 3 dimensions. If abnormal femoral version is identified, acetabular version can be adjusted, or a stem design allowing version control independent of bone geometry can be selected. In this patient, a slightly anterior entry point was used for femoral preparation, allowing the surgeon to dial out anteversion with a blade stem.

The quadratus femoris is released from the femur along with the overlying bursa, leaving a small cuff to facilitate anatomic repair. The piriformis, conjoint tendon, and obturator externus tendon are detached from their insertions on the greater trochanter and trochanteric fossa, along with the posterior capsule. A superior capsulotomy is performed along the posterior and inferior aspects of the gluteus minimus. A posterior-inferior capsulotomy is performed, with care to protect the obturator externus and associated branches of the medial femoral circumflex artery. If desired, a Steinman pin can be placed in the infracotyloid groove, perpendicular to the floor, and the location of the pin can be marked on the femur as a reference for leg length.[35] The availability of new technology does not mean the surgeon must neglect established techniques.

Surgical Procedure

At this point, the steps of the procedure depend on the extent to which the surgeon wishes to navigate femoral preparation, leg length, and offset. The current surgical software suggests one of 2 workflows: an express workflow with limited femoral registration in which the surgeon navigates leg length and offset, and an enhanced workflow with comprehensive femoral registration that allows the surgeon to also navigate femoral version

and neck cut. The express workflow is sufficient for most cases. The additional information gleaned from the enhanced workflow is helpful in the absence of easily identifiable femoral landmarks for planning the neck resection or measurement of the LTC distance.

Navigating the femur is helpful if the surgeon is unable to reliably measure the LTC or chooses a femoral implant not supported by the 3D templating software. It is preferred to navigate the femur in cases in which changes to the plan may be made during surgery, such as revisions, fused hips, and cases with acetabular bone loss. The standard express and enhanced workflows are described later, followed by an efficient cup-only workflow without femoral navigation, often used by the author for routine primary cases.

Express workflow

In the express workflow, no formal femoral registration is performed and no femoral array is required. An electrocardiogram (ECG) lead is placed at the superior aspect of the patella before skin preparation so that it is palpable through the drapes and a single checkpoint is placed on the greater trochanter. Percutaneous pins are used to secure the pelvic array to the iliac crest. Registration of limb length and offset is performed before dislocation by identifying the femoral checkpoint and ECG lead with the navigation probe. The pelvic array is used for reference, which requires that limb position be reproducible, and that the pelvic array be placed before dislocation.

The hip is dislocated posteriorly. The center of the femoral head is marked and a metal ruler is used to measure the LTC distance from the junction of the proximal aspect of the lesser trochanter to the center of the femoral head (**Fig. 4**). There is typically a vascular foramen along the intertrochanteric ridge. Measuring the distance between this foramen and the head center provides a second point of reference and reflects the femoral offset more than the limb length. The ruler is used to mark the location of the femoral neck cut relative to the lesser trochanter as planned before surgery. The femoral neck is cut manually with a power saw and the femoral head is removed from the wound.

Retractors are placed to optimize acetabular exposure. The femur is retracted anteriorly and the plane between the gluteus minimus and the superior capsule is developed. The superior capsule is released from the acetabular margin, permitting the femur to translate anterior to the acetabulum. If acetabular exposure is incomplete, femoral flexion and rotation typically allows access. If femoral mobility is inadequate, release of the reflected head of the rectus femoris and/or the gluteal sling may be required. The table is tilted toward the surgeon, improving visualization. Labrum and foveal soft tissues are excised. A pelvic checkpoint is placed, and its position is noted with the navigation probe. This checkpoint allows verification that the optical array has not moved if it is accidentally jostled after registration.

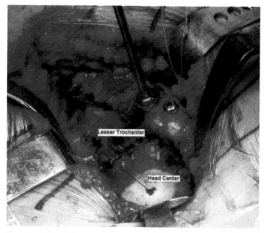

Fig. 4. LTC distance is measured and compared with the preoperative value obtained with 3D planning. Correspondence of these values suggests that similar landmarks have been identified, rendering the templated postreconstruction value useful during surgery.

Acetabular registration is performed (**Fig. 5**). Three initial points are taken for orientation, followed by 32 additional points in and around the acetabulum. For reproducible registration, the surgeon should choose points on firm sclerotic bone rather than within cysts or on osteophytes. The registration process is verified by moving the navigation probe along the bone surface to touch 8 points predicted to be on the bone surface. Verification is considered successful when the navigation predicts the bone surface within 1 mm of the probe tip.

The robot is positioned anterior to the patient, displacing an assistant. The navigation probe is used to confirm robotic registration (and thereby the location of the reamer). The reamer is assembled on the robotic arm and positioned within the acetabulum. Most surgeons use an anterior retractor to translate the femur anterior to the acetabulum during manual acetabular preparation. Once the reamer is placed within the acetabular concavity, no retraction of the femur is required if adequate soft tissue releases have been performed and limb position is optimized. Anteversion and abduction angle are set with navigation guidance. Haptics are engaged and the acetabulum is reamed (**Fig. 6**A). Only 1 reamer is typically required.

Overhanging anterior or inferior osteophyte occasionally interfere with central placement of the reamer within the acetabulum before initiating the reaming process. Obstructive osteophyte can be removed with a rongeur, or a smaller reamer can be used to ream away the osteophyte under robotic guidance. Once the final reamer is placed concentrically within the mouth of the acetabulum, haptic-guided reaming can proceed. The computer screen displays green bone that needs to be reamed (see **Fig. 6**B). Once the desired bone is removed, underlying bone appears white on the screen. This appearance occurs when the reamer is within 1 mm of the planned depth. If the reamer removes bone 1 mm beyond the surgical plan, the underlying bone appears red. Haptics resist reaming into the red and the power on the reamer turns off if the reamer deviates by 2.6 mm in any direction from the surgical plan.

After reaming is complete, the floor of the acetabulum is visualized and the blush of cancellous bone is identified in the pubis, ischium, and ilium. The reamer shaft is removed from the robot and replaced with the impaction shaft and acetabular implant. The acetabular implant is placed within the mouth of the acetabulum. Haptics are engaged, locking in the selected orientation. Impaction is performed with a mallet while the robot maintains orientation and gives real-time information about abduction and anteversion (**Fig. 7**). Depth of

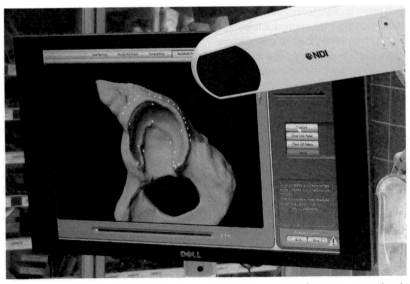

Fig. 5. Registration of bone landmarks is similar to traditional image-based computer navigation, in which a model of the bone surface constructed using the probe is merged with a model based on the preoperative imaging.

insertion is navigated relative to the depth of reaming. It is important to capture the final position of cup impaction with the navigation, because this point is used later for calculating leg length and offset.

Precision robotic control typically creates an excellent press fit with line-to-line reaming. Component seating can be difficult with under-reaming. In a flatter acetabulae, such as in cases of acetabular dysplasia, the reamer can skip slightly before engaging, compromising the peripheral fit. It may be preferred to initially under-ream by 1 to 2 mm in these cases, or to create the concavity with a small reamer and expand it with the final reamer. Under-reaming by 1 mm can also be considered in patients with soft bone.

In rare cases in which press fit is not optimal after reaming, the surgeon can select a reamer 1 to 2 mm smaller than the implant and ream slightly deeper. Bone appears red on the computer screen if the surgeon reams 1 mm deep to plan. The robot does not allow reaming more than 2.6 mm beyond plan and the deeper, smaller diameter ream can enhance press fit without compromising bone support.

Acetabular orientation is verified after impaction. The surgeon confirms visually that the implant is parallel to the transverse acetabular ligament and completely inside the anterior wall of the acetabulum. The implant may be partially exposed posteriorly and/or superiorly. The preoperative

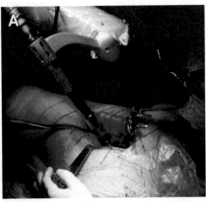
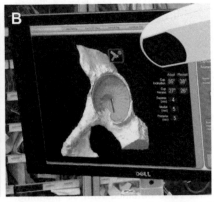

Fig. 6. Precision reaming of the acetabular concavity is performed using haptic robotic guidance (*A*) while the monitor gives feedback about inclination, anteversion, and reaming depth (*B*). Reaming continues until green bone is removed.

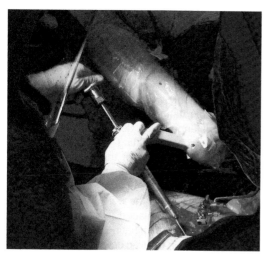

Fig. 7. Cup impaction is guided by haptics while the monitor gives numerical feedback about inclination, anteversion, and depth of impaction.

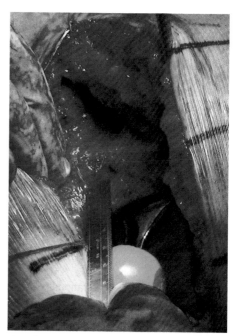

Fig. 8. When coupled with 3D planning and precision acetabular component placement, matching the goal LTC distance creates proper limb length and offset.

3D plan can be used to visually confirm the position of the implant relative to bone landmarks when osteophytes deform the apparent acetabular contours. The navigation probe can also be used to define 5 points around the rim of the implant to determine the cup position by navigation. In rare cases, the position can be altered if desired. Supplemental screw fixation is seldom required. The polyethylene insert is impacted, engaging the locking mechanism. Prominent acetabular osteophytes are removed manually. Osteophyte anatomy can be confirmed on the 3D plan, minimizing risk of accidental damage to the pubis when removing anteroinferior osteophytes.

The table is returned to the neutral position. Standard manual femoral preparation is used. Broaching is performed in 10° to 15° of anteversion, as dictated by the patient's anatomy. The trial neck and head are assembled on the final broach according to the preoperative plan. The LTC distance is measured and compared with the templated and intraoperatively measured values (**Fig. 8**). The distance between the vascular foramen along the intertrochanteric ridge and the head center can also be measured. This distance should be slightly increased from the previous measurement if the acetabular center of rotation has been medialized. Adjustments are made as necessary to recreate the surgical plan.

Trial reduction is performed. Standard manual assessments of combined anteversion, stability, rectus femoris and iliotibial band tension, and impingement-free range of motion can be performed. Leg length change can be estimated using the Steinman pin or other manual techniques.[35] As always, navigation is a helpful augment to clinical judgment and manual techniques, but is not a replacement.

To navigate leg length and offset, the limb is placed back in the standardized position and the probe is used to identify the femoral checkpoint and the ECG lead. The quality of the information gleaned from this assessment relies on the pelvic array remaining fixed during acetabular and femoral preparation and impaction. It also relies on reproduction of the original limb position and accurate palpation of the ECG lead through the drapes.

If navigation measurements conflict with the clinical assessment, the pelvic checkpoint can be verified to confirm that the pelvic array has not moved. If discordance remains, an informed compromise between assessments prevents large errors from occurring. When combined with precise robotic restoration of the planned acetabular center of rotation and 3D CT-based planning of femoral length and offset, the author has found the LTC to be an invaluable double check against both navigation and manual leg length assessments.

If the goal LTC was restored, adjustments are rarely appropriate. The trials are removed and the stem is impacted. The trial head is replaced and the appropriate final LTC distance is confirmed. The femoral trunnion is cleaned and dried, the final femoral head is impacted, and the hip is reduced.

The checkpoints are removed, as are the pins anchoring the pelvic array.

The superior capsule is repaired to the posterior capsule with absorbable suture. The short external rotators and posterior capsule are repaired to the inner aspect of the greater trochanter using transosseous sutures. The quadratus femoris is repaired to its femoral insertion, along with the gluteal sling (if released). Periarticular soft tissue injection with a pain control cocktail is performed. Layered closure is performed. Radiographs confirm that component position matches the preoperative plan (**Fig. 9**).

Enhanced workflow

With the enhanced workflow, a modular array is placed on the proximal femur in the area of the greater trochanter, along with a femoral checkpoint (**Fig. 10**A). Femoral registration is performed after dislocation. The planned neck cut is identified with the navigation probe and marked. Manual femoral preparation is performed before acetabular exposure. A femoral broach array is used to measure the anteversion achieved and the position of the broach relative to the templated plan, along with the anticipated effect on limb length and offset. Once the femoral preparation has been performed, the modular array is disassembled, leaving the anchor point fixed within the femur (see **Fig. 10**B). Acetabular preparation is performed as described earlier. The femoral stem is impacted and trial reduction is performed. The modular femoral array is reassembled and change in limb length and offset is determined with the navigation. This requires moving the hip to define the center of rotation, and relies on the position of the femoral and pelvic arrays for accuracy. Combined anteversion is also reported. Following the reconstruction, both arrays and checkpoints are removed. Depending on bone quality, the current modular femoral array can create a noticeable defect in the greater trochanter. Although this is unlikely to be clinically significant, bone grafting can be performed with acetabular reamings if desired.

Author's cup-only workflow

With the cup-only workflow, the planned acetabular center of rotation is precisely achieved with robotic assistance. Leg length and offset are restored by 3D templating of the femoral plan and surgical restoration of the planned LTC distance. No femoral registration is performed and no femoral checkpoint or array is needed. After acetabular exposure, the pelvic array is secured with in-wound pins placed immediately superior to the acetabulum, eliminating the need for percutaneous fixation in the iliac crest. Acetabular registration, cup insertion, and verification of cup position are performed as described earlier. The pelvic array and checkpoint are removed after cup insertion. Manual femoral preparation is performed. The LTC measurement guides restoration of the leg length and offset, complimented by other standard manual assessments. The secondary measurement from the vascular foramen at the intertrochanteric crest to head center is a helpful adjunct in cases in which the top of the lesser trochanter is ill defined, and allows triangulation for precise placement of the head center. This workflow maximizes surgical efficiency. Given the accuracy and precision of robotic cup placement and 3D CT templating, navigation of the femur may be redundant for routine cases in which bone landmarks can easily be identified.

Immediate Postoperative Care

Use of a robot does not influence postoperative care, because the fundamentals of THR are not changed. In the author's experience, the robot does not meaningfully affect surgical duration or blood loss. Multimodal regimens are used for control

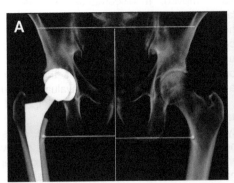
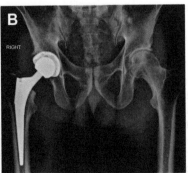

Fig. 9. Comparison of the preoperative plan (*A*) to the postoperative radiograph (*B*) demonstrates excellent correspondence.

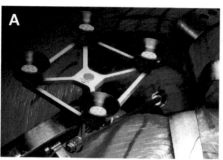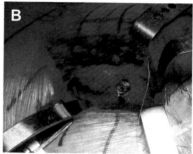

Fig. 10. In the enhanced workflow, a modular femoral array is used (*A*) that can be disassembled (*B*) to facilitate acetabular work, and later reassembled to give navigation feedback about leg length, offset, and combined anteversion. The express workflow gives feedback about leg length and offset without need for a femoral array or formal registration.

of pain and prophylaxis against venous thromboembolism. Rapid mobilization is encouraged.

TECHNIQUE MODIFICATIONS FOR THE DIRECT ANTERIOR APPROACH
Preoperative Planning

Ideal acetabular anteversion is closer to 15° for the anterior approach, but varies with anatomy. Excessive anteversion can create anterior instability, but inadequate anteversion can cause tendon irritation at the psoas recess. A smaller implant and deeper socket position can resolve this conflict of priorities. The LTC distance is not used from the anterior approach, but anticipating the ideal femoral stem size and offset is helpful.

Preparation and Patient Positioning

The patient is positioned supine. The author uses a standard radiolucent table with a table-mounted retractor. Custom tables designed for direct anterior THR can also be used. An ECG lead is placed at the superior aspect of the ipsilateral patella before skin preparation, so it is palpable through the drapes. The iliac crest and the proximal half of the femur on the operative side are included in the sterile field, as is the contralateral iliac crest, which is used for attachment of the pelvic array.

Surgical Approach and Procedure

Direct anterior exposure is performed as described by Lovell.[36] Because the LTC cannot be reproducibly measured from the anterior approach, the author routinely navigates femoral preparation. The enhanced workflow could theoretically aide in optimal placement of the femoral neck cut, but the express workflow is adequate to facilitate leg length and offset restoration, particularly with the ability to directly assess leg

length from the anterior approach on a standard table.

A single checkpoint is placed on the greater trochanter. The pelvic array is attached to the contralateral hemipelvis using 3 half pins placed percutaneously in the iliac crest. Registration of limb length and offset is performed before the femoral neck cut by identifying the femoral checkpoint and ECG lead with the navigation probe. The pelvic array is used for reference. Limb position must be reproducible.

The femoral neck is cut and the femoral head is removed from the wound. Labrum and foveal soft tissues are removed. A pelvic checkpoint is placed and acetabular registration is performed. Placing the reamer and reamer shaft into the acetabulum before connecting the shaft to the robot facilitates effortless insertion without trauma to the tensor muscle. The reamer shaft can be detached from the robot before removal. A similar set of maneuvers can be useful for before and after cup impaction, which is performed using haptic robotic guidance. The author digitally palpates the cup to confirm that it is not prominent at the psoas recess before placing screws or the acetabular liner.

Once the acetabular liner is placed, a table-mounted retractor is used to elevate the femur and additional retractors are placed to optimize exposure. Capsular releases are completed, followed by standard femoral preparation. A trial neck and head are assembled on the final broach and trial reduction is performed.

Stability is assessed by extension and external rotation of the hip. If instability is detected, length may be inadequate or there may be posterior impingement. With robotic acetabular placement, impingement should be uncommon. Leg length equality is assessed by gross palpation and by using navigation. The limb is brought to the neutral position and the navigation probe is used to locate the femoral checkpoint and the ECG probe at the knee. The navigation reports leg length and offset compared with the preoperative state and the contralateral side. Adjustments are made as necessary to achieve desired length and stability. Trials are removed and the definitive femoral stem is implanted. A final trial reduction confirms the ideal modular head. Robotic guidance may render intraoperative fluoroscopy redundant, but the author continues to evaluate the reconstruction fluoroscopically before selecting the final head.

REHABILITATION AND RECOVERY

Weight bearing is determined by quality of fixation. Most primary and revision cases can bear full weight. Hip precautions are influenced by surgical approach, and perhaps parameters such as bearing diameter, combined anteversion, soft tissue repair, surgeon experience, and hospital protocol. No precautions are typically used with the anterior approach. For the posterior approach, the author uses posterior hip precautions until the first postoperative visit at 2 to 3 weeks after surgery. Patients considered to be at increased risk of dislocation (such as patients with hip fractures and female patients with good preoperative range of motion) are asked to observe precautions for 6 weeks, whereas patients at low risk of dislocation who present with stiffness at the first visit are told to relax precautions. The combination of a meticulous soft tissue repair, accurate acetabular position, and precise information about combined anteversion gives the author confidence in relaxing precautions. Functional motions such as abduction and external rotation are emphasized early for all patients.

RESULTS IN THE LITERATURE

Prior research has found improved precision with computer navigation, but failed to show meaningful improvements in clinical outcomes at short-term follow-up. Possible explanations include lack of a clinical difference, lack of statistical power, and lack of adequately sensitive instruments for assessment. Improved precision has the potential to reduce both short-term complications (like dislocation, leg length inequality, and psoas tendinitis from soft tissue impingement) and long-term failures related to increased wear from edge loading and/or implant impingement. A recent retrospective review of 180 ceramic-on-ceramic THRs observed a significantly higher frequency of placement within the safe zone for 60 navigated cups (100% within the Lewinnek safe zone) versus 120 manual cups (74% within the Lewinnek safe zone).[37] There was a significant

difference in dislocation rate between the 2 groups (8% in manual hips and 0% with navigations; $P = .03$). The 13-year survival was 100% in navigated hips and 95.6% in manual hips, but this did not reach statistical significance.[37]

ROBODOC achieved improvements in implant fit and fill as well as reduction in the incidence of periprosthetic fracture compared with manual techniques, but surgical times averaged 240 minutes in the early experience with an associated increase in blood loss.[22] Surgeon experience and improvements in the robotic workflow allowed a decrease in surgical times,[22] but technical complications related to the use of the robot have been reported to occur in 9.3% of cases.[24] Some investigators found no decrease in the incidence of femoral fracture,[24] and other users experienced increase in dislocation, which was attributed to soft tissue damage.[23] These results may have been technique related, but enthusiasm for the ROBODOC system waned among some users. The system has undergone changes and more recent studies have shown the use of ROBODOC to result in more reliable limb length restoration and reduced stress shielding of the proximal femur compared with manual techniques,[25] without an increase in dislocations. The system received 510(k) clearance from the FDA in 2008, but updated outcomes studies on the United States experience are not yet available.

Although there is limited information available about clinical outcomes, the accuracy and precision of robotic acetabular placement using the Mako RIO robot has been documented. Cadaveric studies show markedly greater precision for both inclination and anteversion with the robot compared with a manual bone preparation.[38,39] A clinical study of 100 hips showed significant decrease in outliers with Mako robotic posterior THR compared with manual posterior THR.[40] As assessed using the Lewinnek safe zone, there were no outliers among the 50 patients who underwent robotic surgery, whereas there were 10 outliers among the 50 patients in the manual group.[40] Using the Callanan safe zone, there were 4 outliers with robotic assistance and 19 outliers with manual techniques.[40] A single-surgeon series investigating clinical and radiographic outcomes with the Mako surgical robot revealed a marked reduction in the rate of radiographic outliers in 100 robotic THRs compared with 200 manual THRs.[41] An interesting finding of this study was that 10 years of surgeon experience resulted in a 45% increase in precision with manual THR, whereas subsequent addition of Mako robotic assistance resulted in a 139% increase in precision compared with the same baseline.[41] A multicenter study comparing intraoperative assessment of cup position with the Mako robot with postoperative cup position measured on plain radiographs confirmed that the cup was placed within the Lewinnek safe zone 88% of the time.[42]

Published data regarding limb length discrepancy after Mako robot–assisted THR are limited. Radiographic discrepancy was 5 mm or less in 89.6% of robot-assisted posterior THRs, with no discrepancies greater than 1 cm.[43] These data showed no improvement from manual techniques,[43] but Mako software used at the time did not measure contralateral limb length. New software improves planning of limb length equalization, but does not eliminate the need for assessment of clinical leg length difference. The same investigators found greater than 5-mm discrepancy between radiographic and robot-measured leg length change in 30.6% of cases.[44] Radiographic measurement is not a perfect surrogate for clinical length. Nevertheless, navigation of limb length should be viewed as a complement to manual techniques rather than a replacement.

A retrospective review of the first year of experience using the Mako robot for THR is underway (Hepinstall MS, unpublished data, 2014). Results are consistent with the published literature, with a significant decrease in radiographic outliers, a slight increase in surgical time, and no increase in surgical complications. No obvious robotic malfunction occurred during surgery, the robot caused no damage to bone or soft tissue, and no atypical complications were experienced. Whether objective improvements in precision will deliver expected improvements in clinical outcome remains an important question.

SUMMARY

With improvements in implant design and materials, most well-positioned THRs have avoided mechanical failure for decades. In the absence of trauma, mechanical failures are primarily caused by technical factors that could potentially be avoided with more accurate and precise surgical planning and execution, including bone preparation and prosthesis implantation. The coupling of 3D image–based planning with robotic surgical precision offers the opportunity to improve markedly in both areas. Robotic surgery now allows markedly improved precision without significantly increasing surgical complexity.

Twenty-degree ranges of abduction and anteversion seem broad, but without computer assistance the surgeons have been unable to consistently place implants within the Lewinnek safe zone. Robotic precision may help clinicians to move past staying within safe zones, to defining and consistently achieving patient-specific target positions. As society increasingly demands objective measures of the quality of care, the accuracy of component positioning is an important metric that arthroplasty surgeons should actively seek to control.

ACKNOWLEDGMENTS

The author acknowledges the valuable feedback provided by José A. Rodriguez, MD during the preparation of this article.

REFERENCES

1. Learmonth ID, Young C, Rorabeck C. The operation of the century: total hip replacement. Lancet 2007; 370:1508–19.
2. Anand R, Graves SE, de Steiger RN, et al. What is the benefit of introducing new hip and knee prostheses? J Bone Joint Surg Am 2011;93(Suppl 3):51–4.
3. Bozic KJ. Femoral and acetabular component utilization in the United States. In: Proceedings of the Thirty-Ninth Open Meeting of the Hip Society. San Diego (CA); 2011. p. 15.
4. Austin MA, Higuera CA, Rothman RH. Total hip arthroplasty at the Rothman Institute. HSS J 2012; 8:146–50.
5. Gonzalez MH, Mihalko WM. Total joint arthroplasty: is perfection attainable. AAOS Now 2014;8(5).
6. Barrack RL, Schmalzried TP. Impingement and rim wear associated with early osteolysis after a total hip replacement: a case report. J Bone Joint Surg Am 2002;84:1218–20.
7. Walter WL, Insley GM, Walter GK, et al. Edge loading in third generation alumina ceramic-on-ceramic bearings: stripe wear. J Arthroplasty 2004;19:402–13.
8. Malik A, Maheshwari A, Dorr LD. Impingement with total hip replacement. J Bone Joint Surg Am 2007; 89:1832–42.
9. Wan Z, Boutary M, Dorr LD. The influence of acetabular component position on wear in total hip arthroplasty. J Arthroplasty 2008;23:51–6.
10. Katz JN, Wright EA, Wright J, et al. Twelve-year risk of revision after primary total hip replacement in the U.S. Medicare population. J Bone Joint Surg Am 2012;94:1825–32.
11. Overgaard S, Peterson A, Havelin L, et al. The prognosis of total hip arthroplasty (THA) in patients younger than 50 years of age, results of 14,610 primary THA. J Bone Joint Surg Br 2011;96(Suppl II):87.
12. Lewinnek GE, Lewis JL, Tarr R, et al. Dislocation after total hip-replacement arthroplasties. J Bone Joint Surg Am 1978;60:217–20.
13. Biederman R, Tonin A, Kriskmer M, et al. Reducing the risk of dislocation after total hip arthroplasty: the

effect of orientation of the acetabular component. J Bone Joint Surg Br 2005;87:762–9.

14. Walter WL, O'Toole GC, Walter WK, et al. Squeaking in ceramic-on-ceramic hips: the importance of acetabular component orientation. J Arthroplasty 2007;22: 496–503.

15. Langton DJ, Jameson SS, Joyce TJ, et al. The effect of component size and orientation on the concentrations of metal ions after resurfacing arthroplasty of the hip. J Bone Joint Surg Br 2008;90:1143–51.

16. Morlock MM, Bishop N, Zustin J, et al. Modes of implant failure after hip resurfacing: morphological and wear analysis of 267 retrieval specimens. J Bone Joint Surg Am 2008;90(Suppl 3):89–95.

17. Pearle AD, Kendoff D, Musahl V. Perspectives on computer-assisted orthopaedic surgery: movement toward quantitative orthopaedic surgery. J Bone Joint Surg Am 2009;91(Suppl 1):7–12.

18. Widmer KH, Zurfluh B. Compliant positioning of total hip components for optimal range of motion. J Orthop Res 2004;22:815–21.

19. Callanan MC, Jarrett B, Bragdon CR, et al. The John Charnley award: risk factors for cup malpositioning; quality improvement through a joint registry at a tertiary hospital. Clin Orthop Relat Res 2011;469:319–29.

20. Murphy WS, Werner SD, Kowal JH, et al. The safe zone for acetabular component orientation. Bone Joint J 2013;95(Suppl 28):44.

21. McGrory BJ, Morrey BF, Cahalan TD, et al. Effect of femoral offset on range of motion and abductor muscle strength after total hip arthroplasty. J Bone Joint Surg Br 1995;77:865–9.

22. Bargar WL, Bauer A, Borner M. Primary and revision total hip replacement using the Robodoc system. Clin Orthop Relat Res 1998;354:82–91.

23. Honl M, Dierk O, Gauck C, et al. Comparison of robotic-assisted and manual implantation of a primary total hip replacement: a prospective study. J Bone Joint Surg Am 2003;85:1470–8.

24. Schulz A, Seide K, Queitsch C, et al. Results of total hip replacement using the Robodoc surgical assistant system: clinical outcome and evaluation of complications for 97 procedures. Int J Med Robot 2007; 3:301–6.

25. Nakamura N, Sugano N, Nishii T, et al. A comparison between robotic-assisted and manual implantation of cementless total hip arthroplasty. Clin Orthop Relat Res 2010;468:1072–81.

26. Lonner JH, John TK, Conditt MA. Robotic arm-assisted UJA improves tibial component alignment: a pilot study. Clin Orthop Relat Res 2010;468:141–6.

27. Dunbar NJ, Roche MW, Park BH, et al. Accuracy of dynamic tactile-guided unicompartmental knee arthroplasty. J Arthroplasty 2012;37:803–8.

28. Citak M, Suero EM, Citak M, et al. Unicompartmental knee arthroplasty: is robotic technology more accurate than conventional technique. Knee 2013;20:268–71.

29. Mofidi A, Plate AF, Lu B, et al. Assessment of accuracy of robotically assisted unicompartmental arthroplasty. Knee Surg Sports Traumatol Arthrosc 2014. [Epub ahead of print].

30. Dorr LD, Jones RE, Padgett DE. Robotic guidance in total hip arthroplasty: the shape of things to come. Orthopedics 2011;34:652–5.

31. Parratte S, Pagnano MW, Coleman-Wood K, Kaufman KR, Berry DJ. The 2008 Frank Stinchfield award: variation in postoperative pelvic tilt may confound the accuracy of hip navigation systems. Clin Orthop Relat Res 2009;467:43–9.

32. Charnley J. Low friction arthroplasty of the hip: theory and practice. Berlin: Springer-Verlag; 1979.

33. Dorr LD, Malik A, Dastan M, et al. Combined anteversion technique for total hip arthroplasty. Clin Orthop Relat Res 2009;467:119–27.

34. Schmalzried TP. The importance of proper acetabular component positioning and the challenges to achieving it. Oper Tech Orthop 2009;19:132–6.

35. Ranawat CS, Rao RR, Rodriguez JA, et al. Correction of limb length inequality during total hip arthroplasty. J Arthroplasty 2001;16:715–20.

36. Lovell TP. Single-incision direct anterior approach for total hip arthroplasty using a standard operating table. J Arthroplasty 2008;23(Suppl 7):64–8.

37. Sugano N, Takao M, Sakai T, et al. Does CT-based navigation improve the long-term survival in ceramic-on-ceramic THA? Clin Orthop Relat Res 2012;470:3054–9.

38. Dorr L, Pagnano M, Trousdale R, et al. Accuracy of robotically assisted acetabular cup implantation. J Bone Joint Surg Br 2012;94(Suppl XXV):104.

39. Nawabi DH, Conditt MA, Ranawat AS, et al. Haptically guided robotic technology in total hip arthroplasty - a cadaveric investigation. Proc Inst Mech Eng H 2013;227:302–9.

40. Domb BG, El Bitar YF, Sadik AY, et al. Comparison of robotic-assisted and conventional acetabular cup placement in THA: a matched-pair controlled study. Clin Orthop Relat Res 2014;472:329–36.

41. Conditt M, Illgen R. Robotic assisted THA improves accuracy compared with manual THA technique. Bone Joint J 2013;95(Suppl 34):35.

42. Dounchis J, Elson L, Bragdon CR. A multi-centre evaluation of acetabular cup positioning in robotic-assisted total hip arthroplasty. Bone Joint J 2013; 95(Suppl 28):1.

43. Domb B, El Bitar Y, Stone JC, et al. Leg length discrepancy following total hip arthroplasty: comparing anterior, posterior and MAKO-assisted posterior approaches. Bone Joint J 2013;95(Suppl 34):49.

44. Domb B, El Bitar Y, Jackson T, et al. Radiographic results of total hip arthroplasty using the MAKO robotic guidance system. Bone Joint J 2013; 95(Suppl 34):289.

Trauma

Preface
Trauma

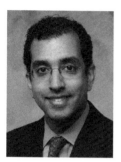

Saqib Rehman, MD
Editor

We have three trauma articles in the current issue of the *Orthopedic Clinics of North America,* which I think you will enjoy reading. Periprosthetic fractures of the lower extremity will continue to challenge orthopedic surgeons as more baby boomers with total joint replacements sustain fragility fractures. Drs Kancherla and Nwachuku discuss the treatment principles of periprosthetic fractures of the femur after total knee arthroplasty.

In another article, Drs Amorosa, Kloen, and Helfet share their clinical experience and review the evaluation and management of high-energy pediatric pelvic and acetabular fractures. Although these are injuries that often present to pediatric hospitals, the surgeons who usually manage these types of injuries typically treat adults. I think that both pediatric orthopedic surgeons at trauma centers and orthopedic trauma surgeons who treat mostly adult patients can learn quite a bit from this article.

The management of traumatic bone loss in the lower extremities continues to be a topic of interest to orthopedic surgeons who manage open fractures. I frequently get asked, "which bone graft should I use for this?", or "how should we address the bone loss in this patient?" from my colleagues. Dr Pipitone and I have attempted to address the basic principles and strategies for the management of bone loss in our article in this issue.

Saqib Rehman, MD
Department of Orthopaedic Surgery
Temple University Hospital
3401 North Broad Street
Philadelphia, PA 19140, USA

E-mail address:
Saqib.rehman@tuhs.temple.edu

Orthop Clin N Am 45 (2014) xv
http://dx.doi.org/10.1016/j.ocl.2014.07.002
0030-5898/14/$ – see front matter © 2014 Elsevier Inc. All rights reserved.

orthopedic.theclinics.com

The Treatment of Periprosthetic Femur Fractures After Total Knee Arthroplasty

Vamsi K. Kancherla, MD*, Chinenye O. Nwachuku, MD

KEYWORDS

- Periprosthetic • Femur fracture • Knee arthroplasty

KEY POINTS

- The incidence of periprosthetic femur fractures after total knee arthroplasty is 2.5%.
- Fracture displacement, implant stability, and the presence of osteoporotic bone are a few factors that help determine management.
- Open reduction internal fixation with locking plates and retrograde intramedullary nail fixation, each with their own advantages and disadvantages, are excellent treatment options that can yield favorable results.
- The primary complications from operative intervention include nonunion, malunion, hardware failure, infection, and refracture.

BACKGROUND

Total knee arthroplasty (TKA) outcomes have historically been largely positive; however, the increased activity of an aging baby boomer population has led to a notable presence of periprosthetic fractures, with an incidence as high as 5.5%.[1] Periprosthetic fractures after TKA are defined as fractures occurring in the femur, tibia, and/or patella and within 15 cm of the joint line or 5 cm of the intramedullary stem.[2,3] With the number of primary TKAs annually being greater than 300,000 a year in the United States,[4] the incidence of postoperative periprosthetic femur, tibia, and patella fractures have ranged from 0.3% to 2.5%, 0.4%, and 0.68%, respectively.[1,4,5] Risk factors have included osteoporosis, osteolysis, rheumatoid arthritis, anterior notching of the femoral cortex, poor knee flexion, neuromuscular disorders, corticosteroid therapy, cemented prostheses, and revision procedures.[5–9] After appropriate diagnostic workup and classification of these peri-implant failures, management often requires critical assessment of patient health, fracture location, bone quality, implant stability, presence of proximal femoral implants (arthroplasty, nail, plate), surgeon experience and training, operative costs, and reoperation rates.

Treatment options for periprosthetic supracondylar femur fractures, each with their own advantages and disadvantages, range from nonoperative to operative fixation (**Box 1**) in the form of skeletal traction, external fixation, plate fixation (nonlocked vs locked), flexible (Rush rods, Enders nails) or rigid intramedullary nails (IMNs), revision arthroplasty, and distal femoral replacement (DFR).[10–14] Each of

Funding Sources: None.
Conflict of Interest: None.
Department of Orthopaedic Surgery, St. Luke's University Health Network, 801 Ostrum Street, PPHP2, Bethlehem, PA 18015, USA
* Corresponding author.
E-mail address: KancheV@slhn.org

orthopedic.theclinics.com

Box 1
Operative options

Skeletal traction

External fixation

Open reduction internal fixation

Anterograde intramedullary nail fixation

Retrograde intramedullary nail fixation

Revision arthroplasty

Distal femoral replacement

---

these modalities can be augmented with cerclage wires, cement, and/or allograft. Alternative, less popular methods have included thin-wire external fixation, the so-called "nailed cementoplasty," fibular allograft supplementation of plate fixation, and upside down use of a proximal femoral nail.[7] In a 2008 systematic review by Herrera and colleagues[15] of 29 case series totaling 415 cases, analysis of various treatment methods (nonoperative, nonlocked and locked plating, retrograde IMN [RIMN], and external fixation) yielded an overall nonunion rate of 9%, fixation failure rate of 4%, infection rate of 3%, and revision surgery rate of 13%.

More recent literature has come to support operative intervention in the form of locked plating (LP) and RIMN fixation; however, much controversy remains on which is superior biomechanically and clinically.[4,7,16–28] A 2013 systematic review by Ristevski and colleagues[24] analyzed 44 studies (719 fractures) and found both LP and RIMN to offer significant advantages over nonoperative treatment and conventional (nonlocked) plating techniques. They also noted that LP trended toward increased nonunion rates compared with RIMN, whereas RIMN had a significantly higher malunion rate. No difference was seen with regard to need for secondary surgical procedures. Meneghini and colleagues[22] in 2014 compared modern RIMN with periarticular LP and found no significant difference in nonunion (9% in RIMN vs 19% in LP; $P = .34$) despite a significantly different mean number of screws in the distal fracture fragment (3.8 in RIMN vs 5.0 in LP; $P \leq .001$).

Nevertheless, regardless of treatment option, this era of personalized care requires that each patient be scrutinized not only from a fracture standpoint but also based on overall health goals. Because of patient age and baseline health status, complication rates and mortality can be expected to be high[29]; mortality rates are as high as 17% at 6 months and 30% at 1 year. A systematic,

individualized approach to the management of periprosthetic femur fractures after a TKA can result in favorable outcomes.

CLASSIFICATION

Historically, classification systems for periprosthetic femur fracture after a TKA have focused exclusively on fracture displacement without assessing for implant involvement,[14] including those by Neer and colleagues[30] in 1967, DiGioia and Rubash[31] in 1991, and Chen and colleagues in 1994.[32] Since 1997, two systems (**Figs. 1** and **2**) have accounted for implant stability and the relationship of the fracture to the implant. Rorabeck and Taylor[33] described 3 types of periprosthetic distal femur fractures. Type I are nondisplaced fractures with a stable prosthesis, type II are 5 mm displaced or 5° angulated with a stable prosthesis, and type III are those with an unstable prosthesis.[32] As per the system by Su and colleagues,[14] the 3 types of fractures are type 1, which are proximal to the femoral component; type II, which start at the proximal end of the component and extend proximally; and type III, which extend distal to the proximal border of the femoral component. Additionally, the presence of an interprosthetic fracture, one that occurs between a hip and knee arthroplasty implant, can be classified by either the Vancouver or Rorabeck systems.[31,32] Implant stability and fracture location will guide utility of either classification system and subsequent treatment options.

DIAGNOSIS AND IMAGING

A thorough history and physical examination can help identify the cause and mechanism of a periprosthetic femur fracture. Each patient should be evaluated for cause of fracture (low vs high energy) and preexisting knee pain that may suggest loosening. Additionally, obtaining a detailed medical and surgical history is critical in identifying potential for poor healing and previous implant sizes. All fractures should be evaluated to document a neurovascular examination and rule out an open fracture. Occasionally, when a patient has clinical signs of infection, septic loosening cannot be excluded. Therefore, a microscopic (microbiological) analysis of the intra-articular fluid for white blood cells and bacteria may be recommended.[7,25]

From an imaging stand point, standard anteroposterior and lateral radiographic views can help classify the fracture and assess the stability of the prosthesis. Because implant stability may not be obvious on plain radiographs, a computed tomography scan may help find signs of loosening,

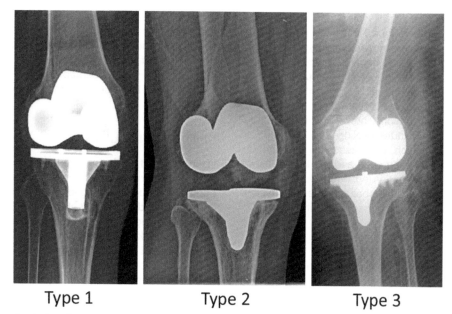

Fig. 1. Rorabeck classification.

particularly around the femoral component. Even such advanced imaging may not detect a loose implant if it is merely partial. Therefore, the surgeon should be prepared to eventually change to a revision prosthesis when an osteosynthesis is initially planned.[7,23,25]

MANAGEMENT

In general, treatment options should allow for immediate stabilization of the fracture and rapid mobilization of the patient, with the ultimate goal of safely returning the patient to preinjury level of function. Ultimately, the goals of treatment are to maintain at least a 90° knee range of motion, with less than 2 cm of shortening and less than 5° of varus or valgus malalignment.[16]

NONOPERATIVE

Although most displaced periprosthetic distal femur fractures are treated operatively, the utility of

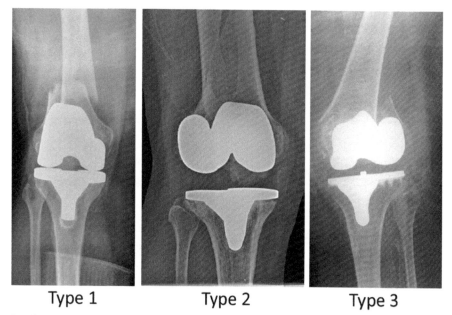

Fig. 2. Su classification.

nonoperative treatment (splint, cast, immobilizer, or cutaneous traction) cannot be ignored in non-displaced fractures, nonambulatory patients, or patients who have too many comorbid conditions to survive surgical intervention (**Fig. 3**). The extremity should be immobilized in extension for 4 to 6 weeks and the patient kept non–weight-bearing. These options, however, require extensive time for fracture healing and can lead to malunion, nonunion, decreased range of motion, difficulty with nursing care, and morbidity associated with immobilization (eg, deep vein thrombosis formation, pulmonary emboli, muscle atrophy, respiratory deconditioning, bed sores, infection).[14]

OPERATIVE

Among the several operative options available, open reduction internal fixation (ORIF), rigid RIMN, and distal femoral replacement have risen to the forefront of modern orthopedics. The advantages and disadvantages of each stem from factors such as patient health, patients goals, fracture location, bone quality, component type and stability, presence of other hardware, and miscellaneous variables, such as surgeon preference and operative costs. For patients who may not tolerate a more aggressive intervention, less invasive operative options, such as skeletal traction and external fixation, can be placed without incurring significant blood loss, operative time, and anesthesia-related complications. Although

they are safe, easy to place, and cost-effective, they share the same potential outcome profile as the aforementioned nonoperative modalities, with the addition of pin site infection. Because of this, for a patient with acceptable risks, ORIF and RIMN fixation have become more popular (**Figs. 4–7**).

ORIF: LOCKING PLATES

In the setting of stable implants with adequate bone stock, plate and IMN fixation are ideal operative options. Although plating choices are vast (locking, buttress, condylar screw, blade plate), locking plate technology has largely supplanted conventional (nonlocked) plating because of its stiffer biomechanical strength, improved outcomes in osteoporotic bone, lower rates of nonunion, and decreased need for secondary surgical procedure.[24,25,34] Locking plate fixation also allows for fixation using a less invasive stabilization system (Synthes, Paoli, PA, USA) or a minimally invasive plate osteosynthesis technique, which can reduce the incidence of soft tissue injury and periosteal stripping. When compared with RIMN, Horneff and colleagues[20] found that LP fixation led to significantly greater radiographic union, no difference in time to full weight-bearing, and an overall lower reoperation rate.

Despite these attractive outcomes, other clinical outcomes studies have shown potential for increased operative time, blood loss, and need for

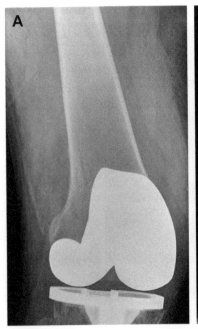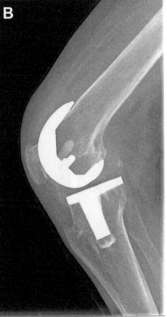

Fig. 3. Nonoperative treatment, (*A*) anteroposterior and (*B*) lateral views.

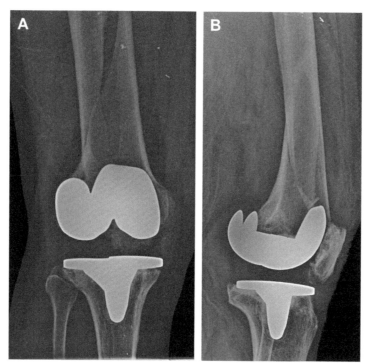

Fig. 4. Locking plate fixation, preoperative (A) anteroposterior and (B) lateral views.

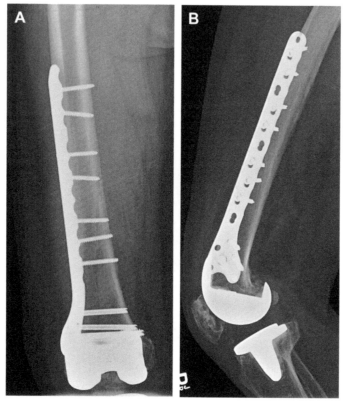

Fig. 5. Locking plate fixation, postoperative (A) anteroposterior and (B) lateral views.

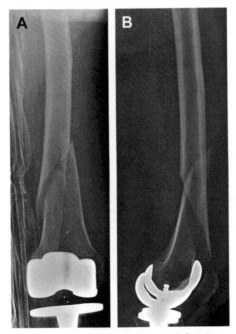

Fig. 6. Retrograde intramedullary nail fixation, preoperative (*A*) anteroposterior and (*B*) lateral views.

transfusion.[20] Furthermore, biomechanical studies have suggested that LP technology can be too stiff, leading to decreased micromotion at the fracture site and an increased risk for nonunion, with rates as high as 20%.[34,35] To address this concern, however, far cortical locking screws were introduced in 2005. Far cortical locking screws obtain fixation only in the far cortex and have been shown in an ovine model to result in 36% greater callus volume, 44% higher bone mineral content, and 54% more strength in torsion.[34,35]

IMN FIXATION

When compared with LP constructs, the use of IMN fixation for a fracture with a stable implant has been controversial. The RIMN can be advantageous because of its potential for load-sharing stabilization of the fracture, reduced estimated blood loss and operative time, and conservative soft tissue dissection.[3,7,10,20,36] In a polytrauma patient, avoiding periosteal stripping while effectively introducing growth factors to the fracture site via

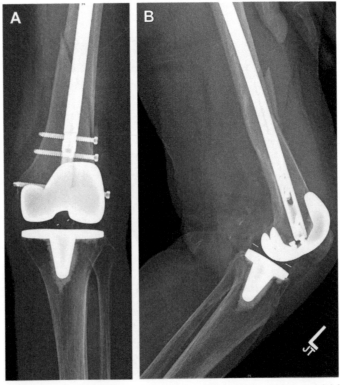

Fig. 7. Retrograde intramedullary nail fixation, postoperative (*A*) anteroposterior and (*B*) lateral views.

reaming may be critical.[14] From a logistics standpoint, IMN fixation allows for supine positioning of the patient and can be a useful incision for a floating knee.[37] Additionally, in the setting of a TKA, avoiding a lateral-based incision for plate fixation can reduce the chance of developing skin bridge problems.[14] Although conventional treatment has focused primarily on rigid retrograde nailing, the use of anterograde intramedullary fixation has also been reported. Although evidence is weak, a few reports of this technique have demonstrated acceptable results for Brooker-Wills distal locking IMNs, Rush rods, Enders nails, and fibular graft.[8,14] An anterograde rigid IMN (**Figs. 8** and **9**) can be used if no proximal implant is already present, enough length to the distal fracture fragment is available to allow for multiple interlocking screws, or in the presence of a femoral component that will not allow for retrograde nail insertion (closed box, stemmed component).

The most commonly discussed disadvantages of a retrograde IMN have included its limited use in cruciate-sacrificing (posterior stabilized) TKAs with a closed or narrow intercondylar box and difficulty in achieving 2 interlocking screws in the distal fracture fragment.[7,20,36,38] In the setting of a cruciate-retaining femoral prosthesis, the diameter of the intercondylar box is variable because of vendor design. Most notch diameters range from 11 to 20 mm, allowing for a nail that is at least 1 mm smaller in size.[14] Therefore, preoperative planning is crucial to identify the total knee prosthesis and

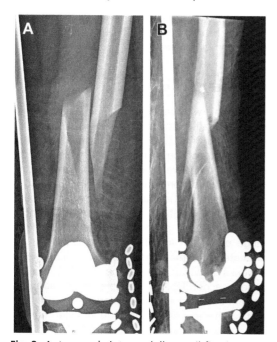

Fig. 8. Anterograde intramedullary nail fixation, preoperative (*A*) anteroposterior and (*B*) lateral views.

determine the femoral canal width so that an appropriately sized nail can be used.[14,39] From a reduction standpoint, because of the poor supracondylar fit of an IMN and lack of solid fixation in osteoporotic bone, varus malalignment can occur.[8] Nonunion, loosening of locking screws with migration of the nail into the knee joint, and decreased range of motion have also been reported.[8] Finally, other concerns have been pulmonary fat microemboli from nail insertion,[20] metallosis and accelerated polyethylene wear from interaction at the rod-prosthesis interface,[8] and metal debris created secondary to the use of a diamond-tip metal cutting burr for opening a narrow or closed box.[40]

REVISION TKA AND MEGAPROSTHESIS RECONSTRUCTION

Other options in the surgeon's armamentarium for the treatment of periprosthetic femur fractures include revision arthroplasty with a stemmed femoral component (**Figs. 10** and **11**) and modular DFR (**Figs. 12** and **13**). In the setting of significant comminution, a fracture too distal that prevents multiple screw insertion, and/or implant instability, LP and RIMN fixation may not be feasible. Therefore, the use of a stemmed femoral component or DFR can allow for rapid mobilization and weight-bearing.[4,11,41] Furthermore, Chen and colleagues[41] found that primary reconstruction via ORIF is beneficial for preserving bone stock, but primary distal femoral arthroplasty may be preferred in patients with osteopenia or those at high risk for nonunion.

Indications for long-stemmed femoral revision include fractures with associated implant loosening and/or wear[42] without metaphyseal bone loss.[12] Srinivasan and colleagues[42] noted that with this type of prosthesis, appropriate diaphyseal fixation and alignment can be obtained and allows for early mobilization. Few studies, however, have concentrated on DFR for periprosthetic femur fractures after TKA. Pour and colleagues[43] found that DFR was best used as a salvage device for the elderly, sedentary patient with complex knee abnormalities.[44] Indications for using DFR include fractures that have a significant amount of bone stock deficiency from fracture pattern and bone loss, loose femoral prosthesis, ligamentous compromise, coronal plane instability, and fractures not amendable to other types of internal fixation.[44,45] Jassim and colleagues[45] noted that this method of treatment was able to compensate for bone loss, relieve knee pain, and provide immediate stability to the knee. Despite these potential advantages, the complication rate is high and encompasses infection, loosening, femoral

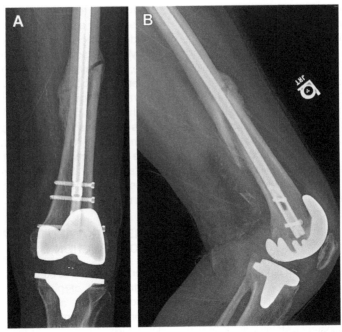

Fig. 9. Anterograde intramedullary nail fixation, postoperative (*A*) anteroposterior and (*B*) lateral views.

fractures,[46] and intraoperative blood loss requiring transfusions.

AUGMENTATION

Although modern implants can be low profile and have the ability for multiple polyaxial screw fixation,[47,48] complications still occur, which suggests

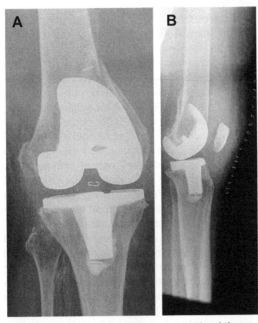

Fig. 10. Revision arthroplasty, preoperative (*A*) anteroposterior and (*B*) lateral views.

that biologically friendly augmentation may have a role in achieving favorable outcomes. Regardless of the fixation used, each construct can be supplemented with cerclage wires, bone graft (autograft, allograft, cortical strut), and/or polymethylmethacrylate.[10,14] Kassab and colleagues[49] noted that revision with a distal femoral allograft can be a viable salvage procedure for reinforcing cortical defects; however, there remains an 8% to 12% infection risk and potential for nonunion, fracture, resorption, and instability.

POSTOPERATIVE MANAGEMENT

For patients who undergo less aggressive fixation or nonoperative treatment, therapy can work on strength and mobilization. However, this is often limited and can be painful for the patient. In the setting of operative treatment, all patients should receive some form of deep vein thrombosis prophylaxis (mechanical and/or chemical), postoperative antibiotics, and early rehabilitation concentrated on patient mobilization and knee range of motion (ROM). Weight-bearing can be protected to some degree for approximately 6 to 8 weeks; however, this can be adjusted for each patient according to variable bone strength, implant use, and surgeon preference.[7,25] Postoperative therapy should include transfer training and the use of an assistive device. Additionally, the utility of a continuous passive motion device for periprosthetic supracondylar femur fracture

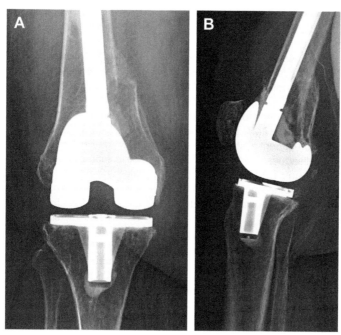

Fig. 11. Revision arthroplasty, postoperative (*A*) anteroposterior and (*B*) lateral views.

fixation is unknown but can be useful to obtain early functional ROM. Because weight-bearing, knee ROM, and pain improve over a period of 6 to 8 weeks, weight-bearing can be advanced and the patient can begin formal strengthening and gait training therapy.[7,25]

COMPLICATIONS

Periprosthetic-treated femur fractures in patients who have undergone TKA have an overall complication rate up to 41% and revision rate of 29%.[25] Nonoperatively treated fractures have an overall

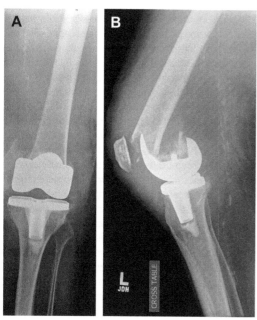

Fig. 12. Distal femoral replacement, preoperative (*A*) anteroposterior and (*B*) lateral views.

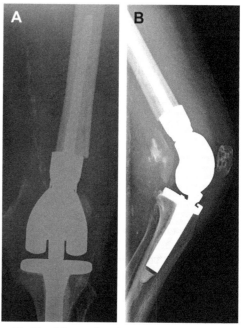

Fig. 13. Distal femoral replacement, postoperative (*A*) anteroposterior and (*B*) lateral views.

complication rate of 31%, nonunion rate of 14%, and malunion rate of 18%.[14] Additionally, operatively treated fractures have rates of 19% for complications, 7% for nonunion, 4% for malunion, 3% for infection, and 3% for hardware failure.[14] A systematic review by Herrera and colleagues[15] in 2008 found that RIMN had a nonunion rate of 1.5% compared with 5.3% for LP; the need for a secondary procedure was 4.6% in the RIMN group and 8.8% in the LP group. A more recent systematic review by Meneghini and colleagues[22] in 2014 found the nonunion rate to be 9% and 19% for RIMN and LP, respectively. Despite this difference, the RIMN group showed a significantly higher malunion rate (11% vs 9% for LP).[36]

SUMMARY

The rise of TKA in an aging and active population will be met with the challenge of managing periprosthetic fractures. In addressing the femoral side, a thorough evaluation of the patient and their goals will help diagnose and effectively treat a complex problem. Despite the occasional value of a nonoperative route, the use of locking plates, IMNs, or arthroplasty have often yielded better clinical and radiographic results. The patient, injury pattern, and surgeon are all important factors in obtaining a favorable outcome.

REFERENCES

1. Chimutengwende-Gordon M, Khan W, Johnstone D. Recent advances and developments in knee surgery: principles of periprosthetic knee fracture management. Open Orthop J 2012;6:301–4.
2. Dennis DA. Periprosthetic fractures following total knee arthroplasty. Instr Course Lect 2001;50:379–89.
3. Han HS, Oh KW, Kang SB. Retrograde intramedullary nailing for periprosthetic supracondylar fractures of the femur after total knee arthroplasty. Clin Orthop Surg 2009;1(4):201–6.
4. Saidi K, Ben-Lulu O, Tsuji M, et al. Supracondylar periprosthetic fractures of the knee in the elderly patients: a comparison of treatment using allograft-implant composites, standard revision components, distal femoral replacement prosthesis. J Arthroplasty 2014;29(1):110–4.
5. Meyer C, Alt V, Schroeder L, et al. Treatment of periprosthetic femoral fractures by effective lengthening of the prosthesis. Clin Orthop Relat Res 2007;463:120–7.
6. Masri BA, Meek RM, Duncan CP. Periprosthetic fractures evaluation and treatment. Clin Orthop Relat Res 2004;(420):80–95.
7. Ricci W. Classification and treatment of periprosthetic supracondylar femur fractures. J Knee Surg 2013;26(1):9–14.
8. Tharani R, Nakasone C, Vince KG. Periprosthetic fractures after total knee arthroplasty. J Arthroplasty 2005;20(4 Suppl 2):27–32.
9. Zuurmond RG, Pilot P, Verburg AD. Retrograde bridging nailing of periprosthetic femoral fractures. Injury 2007;38(8):958–64.
10. Bezwada HP, Neubauer P, Baker J, et al. Periprosthetic supracondylar femur fractures following total knee arthroplasty. J Arthroplasty 2004;19(4):453–8.
11. Lundh F, Sayed-Noor AS, Brosjo O, et al. Megaprosthetic reconstruction for periprosthetic or highly comminuted fractures of the hip and knee. Eur J Orthop Surg Traumatol 2014;24(4):553–7.
12. McGraw P, Kumar A. Periprosthetic fractures of the femur after total knee arthroplasty. J Orthop Traumatol 2010;11(3):135–41.
13. Sarmah SS, Patel S, Reading G, et al. Periprosthetic fractures around total knee arthroplasty. Ann R Coll Surg Engl 2012;94(5):302–7.
14. Su ET, DeWal H, Di Cesare PE. Periprosthetic femoral fractures above total knee replacements. J Am Acad Orthop Surg 2004;12(1):12–20.
15. Herrera DA, Kregor PJ, Cole PA, et al. Treatment of acute distal femur fractures above a total knee arthroplasty: systematic review of 415 cases (1981-2006). Acta Orthop 2008;79(1):22–7.
16. Bong MR, Egol KA, Koval KJ, et al. Comparison of the LISS and a retrograde-inserted supracondylar intramedullary nail for fixation of a periprosthetic distal femur fracture proximal to a total knee arthroplasty. J Arthroplasty 2002;17(7):876–81.
17. Chen SH, Chiang MC, Hung CH, et al. Finite element comparison of retrograde intramedullary nailing and locking plate fixation with/without an intramedullary allograft for distal femur fracture following total knee arthroplasty. Knee 2014;21(1):224–31.
18. Gavaskar AS, Tummala NC, Subramanian M. The outcome and complications of the locked plating management for the periprosthetic distal femur fractures after a total knee arthroplasty. Clin Orthop Surg 2013;5(2):124–8.
19. Ha CW, Shon OJ, Lim SW, et al. Minimally invasive plate osteosynthesis for periprosthetic distal femoral fractures after total knee arthroplasty. Knee Surg Relat Res 2014;26(1):27–32.
20. Horneff JG 3rd, Scolaro JA, Jafari SM, et al. Intramedullary nailing versus locked plate for treating supracondylar periprosthetic femur fractures. Orthopedics 2013;36(5):e561–6.
21. Kilucoglu OI, Akgul T, Saglam Y, et al. Comparison of locked plating and intramedullary nailing for periprosthetic supracondylar femur fractures after knee arthroplasty. Acta Orthop Belg 2013;79(4):417–21.

22. Meneghini RM, Keyes BJ, Reddy KK, et al. Modern retrograde intramedullary nails versus periarticular locked plates for supracondylar femur fractures after total knee arthroplasty. J Arthroplasty 2014;29(7): 1478–81.

23. Platzer P, Schuster R, Aldrian S, et al. Management and outcome of periprosthetic fractures after total knee arthroplasty. J Trauma 2010;68(6):1464–70.

24. Ristevski B, Nauth A, Williams D, et al. Systematic review of the treatment of periprosthetic distal femur fractures. J Orthop Trauma 2014;28(5):307–12.

25. Ruchholtz S, Tomas J, Gebhard F, et al. Periprosthetic fractures around the knee-the best way of treatment. Eur Orthop Traumatol 2013;4(2):93–102.

26. Salas C, Mercer D, DeCoster TA, et al. Experimental and probabilistic analysis of distal femoral periprosthetic fracture: a comparison of locking plate and intramedullary nail fixation. Part B: probabilistic investigation. Comput Meth Biomech Biomed Eng 2011;14(2):175–82.

27. Salas C, Mercer D, DeCoster TA, et al. Experimental and probabilistic analysis of distal femoral periprosthetic fracture: a comparison of locking plate and intramedullary nail fixation. Part A: experimental investigation. Comput Meth Biomech Biomed Eng 2011;14(2):157–64.

28. Singh SP, Bhalodiya HP. Outcome and incidence of periprosthetic supracondylar femoral fractures in TKA. Indian J Orthop 2013;47(6):591–7.

29. Streubel PN, Ricci WM, Wong A, et al. Mortality after distal femur fractures in elderly patients. Clin Orthop Relat Res 2011;469(4):1188–96.

30. Neer CS 2nd, Grantham SA, Shelton ML. Supracondylar fracture of the adult femur. A study of one hundred and ten cases. J Bone Joint Surg Am 1967; 49(4):591–613.

31. DiGioia AM 3rd, Rubash HE. Periprosthetic fractures of the femur after total knee arthroplasty. A literature review and treatment algorithm. Clin Orthop Relat Res 1991;(271):135–42.

32. Chen F, Mont MA, Bachner RS. Management of ipsilateral supracondylar femur fractures following total knee arthroplasty. J Arthroplasty 1994;9(5): 521–6.

33. Rorabeck CH, Taylor JW. Classification of periprosthetic fractures complicating total knee arthroplasty. Orthop Clin N Am 1999;30(2):209–14.

34. Ries Z, Hansen K, Bottlang M, et al. Healing results of periprosthetic distal femur fractures treated with far cortical locking technology: a preliminary retrospective study. The Iowa orthopaedic journal 2013; 33:7–11.

35. Ries ZG, Marsh JL. Far cortical locking technology for fixation of periprosthetic distal femur fractures:

a surgical technique. The journal of knee surgery 2013;26(1):15–8.

36. Hou Z, Bowen TR, Irgit K, et al. Locked plating of periprosthetic femur fractures above total knee arthroplasty. J Orthop Trauma 2012;26(7):427–32.

37. Funovics PT, Vecsei V, Wozasek GE. Mid- to long-term clinical findings in nailing of distal femoral fractures. Journal of surgical orthopaedic advances 2003;12(4):218–24.

38. Large TM, Kellam JF, Bosse MJ, et al. Locked plating of supracondylar periprosthetic femur fractures. The Journal of arthroplasty 2008;23(6 Suppl 1):115–20.

39. Heckler MW, Tennant GS, Williams DP, et al. Retrograde nailing of supracondylar periprosthetic femur fractures: a surgeon's guide to femoral component sizing. Orthopedics 2007;30(5):345–8.

40. Maniar RN, Umlas ME, Rodriguez JA, et al. Supracondylar femoral fracture above a PFC posterior cruciate-substituting total knee arthroplasty treated with supracondylar nailing. A unique technical problem. The Journal of arthroplasty 1996;11(5):637–9.

41. Chen AF, Choi LE, Colman MW, et al. Primary versus secondary distal femoral arthroplasty for treatment of total knee arthroplasty periprosthetic femur fractures. J Arthroplasty 2013;28(9):1580–4.

42. Srinivasan K, Macdonald DA, Tzioupis CC, et al. Role of long stem revision knee prosthesis in periprosthetic and complex distal femoral fractures: a review of eight patients. Injury 2005;36(9):1094–102.

43. Pour AE, Parvizi J, Slenker N, et al. Rotating hinged total knee replacement: use with caution. J Bone Joint Surg Am 2007;89(8):1735–41.

44. Mortazavi SM, Kurd MF, Bender B, et al. Distal femoral arthroplasty for the treatment of periprosthetic fractures after total knee arthroplasty. J Arthroplasty 2010;25(5):775–80.

45. Jassim SS, McNamara I, Hopgood P. Distal femoral replacement in periprosthetic fracture around total knee arthroplasty. Injury 2014;45(3):550–3.

46. Merkel KD, Johnson EW Jr. Supracondylar fracture of the femur after total knee arthroplasty. J Bone Joint Surg Am 1986;68(1):29–43.

47. Hanschen M, Aschenbrenner IM, Fehske K, et al. Mono- versus polyaxial locking plates in distal femur fractures: a prospective randomized multicentre clinical trial. Int Orthop 2014;38(4):857–63.

48. Ruchholtz S, El-Zayat B, Kreslo D, et al. Less invasive polyaxial locking plate fixation in periprosthetic and peri-implant fractures of the femur—a prospective study of 41 patients. Injury 2013;44(2):239–48.

49. Kassab M, Zalzal P, Azores GM, et al. Management of periprosthetic femoral fractures after total knee arthroplasty using a distal femoral allograft. J Arthroplasty 2004;19(3):361–8.

Management of Traumatic Bone Loss in the Lower Extremity

Paul S. Pipitone, DO*, Saqib Rehman, MD

KEYWORDS

- Lower extremity trauma • Segmental bone loss • Critical sized defects • Limb reconstruction

KEY POINTS

- Critically sized defects are defined as smallest sized defects, in a specific bone and species of animal, which do not heal or undergo 10% regeneration. This condition generally occurs when the size of the defect is 2 to 3 times the diameter of the involved bone.
- The initial assessment of the patient with an injured extremity with bone loss should begin with Advanced Trauma Life Support (ATLS) protocol, focusing initially on resuscitation measures and determining whether the injured limb is salvageable.
- Initial fracture care should focus on thorough irrigation and debridement and fracture stabilization with either temporary external or definitive internal fixation.
- Defects less than 4 cm may be treated with autogenous iliac crest bone grafting. Defects between 3 and 7 cm may be treated with a bone shortening/relengthening procedure. Defects between 2 and 10 cm may be treated with autogenous bone graft obtained via the Reamer-Irrigator-Aspirator (RIA), or with distraction osteogenesis. Defects greater than 10 cm may be treated with vascularized fibular grafting.
- The RIA system allows for the procurement of greater than 50 cm^3 of bone graft rich in several growth factors.
- The Masquelet technique, although a 2-stage procedure, offers advantages such as local antibiotic delivery, mechanical stability, and production of a biomembrane that protects autograft resorption.
- Bone morphogenetic proteins (BMPs) may be used as treatment adjuncts and demonstrate equivalent efficacy and safety as autogenous bone graft. However, nonvascularized autogenous bone graft remains the gold standard for bone grafting.

INTRODUCTION

Significant bone loss may occur as a result of high-energy trauma, infection, tumor resection, revision surgery, and developmental deformities.[1] This entity has a dramatic effect on both the surrounding soft tissue and the healing potential of the injured bone. Fracture nonunions occur for various reasons, and this well-established complication is quoted in the literature as having a 2.5% prevalence after long-bone fractures.[1] However, in the setting of segmental bone loss, this rate approaches 100% secondary to the limited ability of the skeletal system to repair and fill defects.[2] Based on several animal studies, critically sized defects are defined as the smallest sized defect,

Conflict of interest statement: The authors certify that they have no commercial associations (eg, consultancies, stock ownership, equity interest, patent/licensing arrangements, and so forth) that might pose a conflict of interest in connection with the submitted article.
Location statement: Research for this article was conducted at Temple University Hospital and its affiliates.
Department of Orthopaedic Surgery and Sports Medicine, Temple University School of Medicine, 3401 North Broad Street, Philadelphia, PA 19140, USA
* Corresponding author.
E-mail address: pspipitone@gmail.com

Orthop Clin N Am 45 (2014) 469–482
http://dx.doi.org/10.1016/j.ocl.2014.06.008
0030-5898/14/$ – see front matter © 2014 Elsevier Inc. All rights reserved.

in a specific bone and species of animal, which does not heal or undergoes 10% regeneration; this is considered to be the case when the length of the deficiency is 2 to 3 times the diameter.[3]

Treatment of large segmental bone defects presents a challenge for the treating orthopedic surgeon. Historically, management of these injuries consisted of amputation, which provided a short recovery period but resulted in a significant loss of limb function. At present, the focus of treatment has shifted toward limb salvage procedures and includes the following treatment options: bone shortening; distraction osteogenesis, the use of vascularized and nonvascularized bone grafts; and bone substitutes. This article reviews the various treatment strategies available for the management of critically sized defects in lower extremity trauma.

INITIAL MANAGEMENT

The initial approach to the traumatized limb with associated bone loss should follow the ATLS protocol. Once the primary survey is completed and resuscitation measures have been initiated, the secondary survey in then commenced. During this phase of the protocol, an assessment of whether or not the injured limb is salvageable is made.

Once limb salvage has been decided, the injured extremity should undergo thorough irrigation and debridement and initial fracture stabilization. The initial debridement may result in further loss of soft tissue and/or bone when grossly contaminated and devitalized tissue is removed. A plastic surgeon should be consulted in the initial phases of care to assist in definitive soft-tissue coverage. In cases in which a plastic surgeon is unavailable, negative pressure wound therapy may be used to initially manage wounds with significant soft-tissue injury (**Fig. 1**). In addition, antibiotic-impregnated polymethylmethacrylate (PMMA) cement beads may be used at this stage to manage dead space created after removal of all dead or nonviable tissue (**Fig. 2**). The use of antibiotic beads also allows for local antibiotic delivery at the site of injury. In most cases with significant soft-tissue and bone loss, a temporary external fixator provides initial fracture stabilization (see **Fig. 2**). However, in those cases in which bone loss is limited and the condition of the soft tissue is favorable, definitive internal fixation may be a primary option.

IMMEDIATE BONE SHORTENING

Immediate limb shortening and lengthening has been described for the management of longitudinal bone defects with or without soft-tissue loss

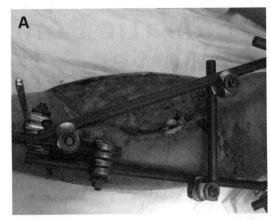

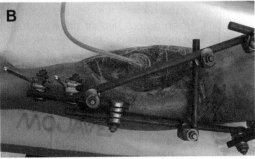

Fig. 1. Negative pressure wound therapy (NPWT) use in a grade IIIB open tibia-fibula fracture with associated degloving injury from all-terrain vehicle crash. (*A*) Clinical photograph demonstrating significant soft-tissue injury. (*B*) Clinical photograph demonstrating the use of NPWT as initial strategy for temporary wound coverage.

due to different causes.[4] This method not only allows for the management of bony defects but also assists in soft-tissue coverage by reducing the defect size or soft-tissue tension.[1] Therefore, immediate shortening with subsequent progressive lengthening of the bone is an accepted treatment alternative for those who have absolute or relative contraindications for free or local flaps.[5] In addition, this method results in an inherently stable facture pattern that allows the patient to walk and bear weight soon after surgery. Furthermore, this active and functional management can shorten the treatment time and reduce costs and absence from work.[4] The degree of shortening that can be tolerated is multifactorial and depends on the following: the bone involved, the location within the bone itself, and whether it is a 1-bone segment (eg, humerus or femur) in which shortening is better tolerated or a 2-bone segment (eg, radius and ulna, tibia and fibula). With respect to the bone involved, immediate shortening of the upper extremity is tolerated well, as limb length discrepancy does not significantly alter function.[6]

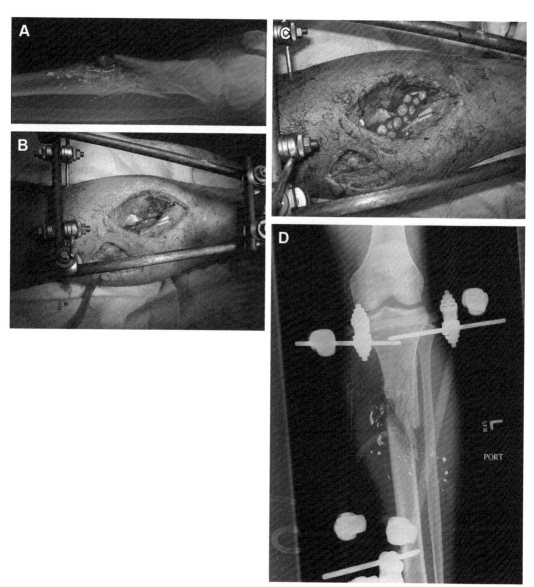

Fig. 2. Dead space management of an open fracture with antibiotic cement beads. (*A*) Significant comminution as a result of a gunshot injury to the tibia. (*B*) Significant bone loss and soft-tissue injury. (*C*) Use of antibiotic beads in the area of bone loss. (*D*) The injury was initially stabilized with an external fixator.

In the tibia and humerus, immediate shortening can be performed for defects of 3 to 4 cm and in the femur for defects of 5 to 7 cm.[1] Femoral shortening may also be managed with compensatory shortening of the contralateral extremity, especially in patients with more than average height.[6]

Bone defects less than 3 cm can usually be acutely shortened.[7,8] Acute shortening of greater than 3 cm may be safe if the result of the vascular physical examination does not change. However, acute shortening of greater than 4 cm may result in venous congestion, edema, tissue necrosis, and infection. In situations in which the defect is too large to close immediately, gradual shortening

(5 mm/day) may be undertaken to avoid any untoward complications.[1]

DISTRACTION OSTEOGENESIS

The first successful bone lengthening was reported by Codivilla in 1905, who described the osteotomy of a cortex and the application of an immediate traction force via a calcaneal pin. In 1913, Obredanne was the first to use an external fixator for limb lengthening. However, it was Ilizarov, in the 1950s, who developed the modern-day technique of distraction osteogenesis.[9] This technique refers to the production of new bone between vascular bone surfaces created by an osteotomy and separated by gradual distraction.[10]

The basic components of distraction osteogenesis include the following:

1. Use of an external fixator that affords stability and applies corrective forces that produce lengthening, angular correction, or transportation of bone.
2. A corticotomy, defined by Ilizarov as a low-energy osteotomy of the cortex, with preservation of the blood supply to the both periosteum and medullary canal.
3. A postoperative period
   - This period may be divided into 3 consecutive periods: latency, distraction, and consolidation.[10]
     - The latency period is the time from corticotomy until distraction begins and ranges between 3 and 10 days. This period is generally thought to enhance bone formation.[9]
     - During the distraction period, the apparatus is adjusted by 1 mm per day at a sequence of 0.25 mm 4 times per day.
       - Clinical studies have confirmed that this technique promoted osteogenesis in humans, but it was noted that the rate and frequency of distraction may have to be adjusted depending on factors such as the quality of bone formation and the response of the soft tissues.[11]
     - The final and longest phase is the consolidation period.
       - During this period, the newly formed bone in the distraction gap is allowed to bridge and corticalize. The external fixation index denotes the number of days the external fixator is attached to the bone per centimeter of length gained. This index is typically 30 days per centimeter of length gained. The bone healing index is the time to union in months divided by amount of lengthening in centimeters.[12]

This technique offers many advantages when used to treat bone defects in the lower extremity. It has the ability to correct deformity and lengthen an extremity; it eliminates donor site morbidity seen with autologous grafting or free tissue transfer.[13] It allows the patient to remain ambulatory, as it enables early weight bearing and active range of motion. In addition, it may be used to treat massive bone loss ranging from 2 to 10 cm in size (**Fig. 3**).

Despite these advantages, this technique requires long-term placement of external fixators

and may be associated with complications.[14] Neurovascular damage is a potential immediate complication but may be avoided with a thorough knowledge of anatomy.[15] Frame-related complications are the most common and include pin tract infections, broken wires, and joint contractures.[13] Patient intolerance of the frame is also another important factor to consider. Distraction osteogenesis using the Ilizarov technique requires almost 2 months in fixation for every centimeter of defect reconstructed in a single level transport.[13,16,17] Therefore, there should be extensive preoperative education of the patient and the family to increase compliance, as the treatment is lengthy and painful.[9]

After frame-related complications, the second most common complication is nonunion at the docking site.[18] Several options exist to augment and enhance union at the docking site, including autologous bone graft, shingling or reshaping of the bone edges,[19] bifocal transport over an intramedullary IM nail,[14] secondary IM nailing,[20] and application of low-intensity pulsed ultrasound.[21]

In general, good results have been achieved with the use of the Ilizarov fixator. Studies have shown it to be a reliable method to treat segmental bone loss, with researchers reporting between 75% to 100% success.[22–29] Despite these results, the Ilizarov system uses hinge and translation mechanisms that are specifically oriented for a given case and requires sequential correction of multiaxial deformities.[30] Because of this, there is a steep learning curve in using the Ilizarov system.

The Taylor Spatial Frame (TSF) (Smith & Nephew, Memphis, TN, USA) is a multiplanar external hexapod frame that consists of 2 rings or partial rings connected by 6 telescopic struts at special universal joints. The TSF offers many advantages including reliability and the versatility to simultaneously correct rotation, angulation, and translation deformities by adjusting the strut lengths.[31] Several clinical studies have reported favorable outcomes with the TSF in terms of healing traumatic bone defects and deformity correction.[32–36]

NONVASCULARIZED BONE GRAFT OPTIONS

Nonvascularized bone grafts remain the gold standard for autologous bone grafts, as they contain the 3 components necessary to promote or enhance bone regeneration.[37] These components include osteoconductivity, osteoinduction, and osteogenicity. Possible donor sites include the iliac crest, distal femur, proximal tibia, fibula, distal radius, and olecranon.[1] The iliac crest is the most common donor site and is facile to harvest. It

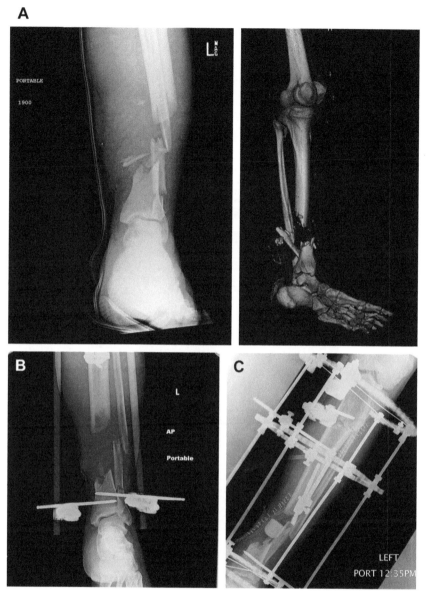

Fig. 3. Ilizarov bone transport as a method for reconstruction of a massive skeletal defect in a grade IIIB open tibia-fibula fracture after motorcycle crash. (*A*) Initial radiograph and three-dimensional reconstruction computed tomographic scan demonstrating a comminuted distal tibia-fibula fracture with significant tibial bone loss. The injury was initially managed with irrigation and debridement and placement of an external fixator. The wound was managed with delayed primary closure during the initial hospitalization. No soft-tissue flap was required in this particular case. (*B*) The area of traumatic bone loss was subsequently managed 10 weeks after initial injury with a bone transport procedure. (*C*) Postoperative radiograph 10 weeks after initial injury demonstrating conversion of the external fixator to a bone transport ring fixator (Smith & Nephew, Memphis, TN, USA). A proximal tibial corticotomy is noted, as well as a distal antibiotic cement spacer block, which was removed 6 weeks later. After 4 months, autogenous iliac crest bone grafting of the docking site was performed. (*D*) Postoperative radiograph demonstrating bone regeneration proximally and a clinical photograph after autogenous iliac crest bone grafting of the docking site. (*E*) Postoperative radiograph after frame removal 11 months later demonstrating bone consolidation proximally at the corticotomy site and union at the docking site distally.

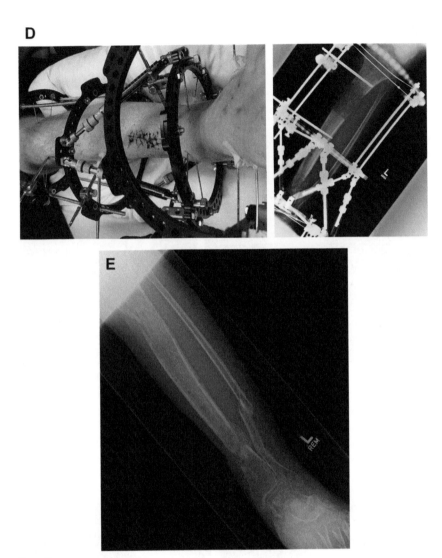

Fig. 3. (*continued*)

offers advantages such as good-quality bone with a high concentration of progenitor cells and growth factors.[38] However, its use may be limited to smaller defects ranging from 0.5 to 3 cm,[1] and there may be significant morbidity with harvesting large quantities of bone. Several studies have shown high incidences of complications related to iliac crest harvest, including donor site pain and injury to cutaneous nerves resulting in painful neuromas.[39–43] In addition, bridging large bone defects by avascular grafts involves creeping substitution, with cells migrating from the well-perfused resection and junction area into an almost acellular matrix.[44] Therefore, the use of avascular grafts not only requires time but also bears a high risk for complications, including bone atrophy, transplant fracture, and nonunion.[44–46]

REAMER-IRRIGATOR-ASPIRATOR

The RIA device (Synthes, West Chester, PA, USA) was originally designed as a simultaneous reaming, irrigation, and aspiration system to reduce the IM pressure, cortical heat generation, and systemic effects during IM nailing.[47–51] The RIA device now offers an additional source of bone to treat traumatic bone defects (**Fig. 4**).

This method of obtaining bone graft is quite practical, as the IM canals of the femur and tibia are easy to access and contain large amounts of cancellous bone graft.[39] In addition, the biological content of the RIA graft has been shown to be superior to iliac crest bone graft (ICBG), and the volume available is regularly 50 cm^3 or more.[2] Research comparing the quantitative levels of growth factors from RIA aspirate, ICGB, and

A

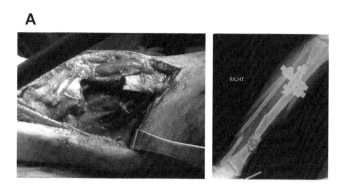

B

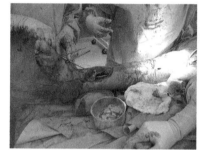
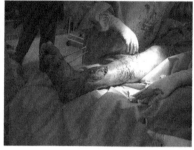
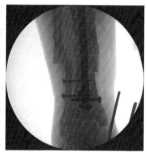

Fig. 4. Reconstruction of a skeletal defect with the use of the Reamer-Irrigator-Aspirator (RIA) in a grade IIIB open tibia-fibula fracture in a pedestrian stuck by an automobile. The injury was managed initially with irrigation and debridement and external fixation. (*A*) Clinical photograph and radiograph demonstrating temporary stabilization with an external fixator. Note both the degree of soft-tissue injury and bone loss. Three days after initial presentation, repeat irrigation and debridement was performed and the area of bone loss was managed with antibiotic beads. (*B*) Repeat irrigation and debridement procedures were performed during a 1-week period, and the injury was stabilized definitively with an intramedullary nail and syndesmotic screws. An antibiotic cement spacer block was also used. (*C*) After 7 weeks, the cement spacer was removed and autogenous femoral canal bone graft was harvested with the RIA system. (*D*) Postoperative radiograph after autogenous femoral canal bone grafting. (*E*) Postoperative radiograph 18 months after autogenous femoral canal bone grafting demonstrating union at the area of bone loss.

platelet preparations found higher levels of 5 of 7 growth factors obtained from IM reamings compared with iliac crest graft.[52] These growth factors included fibroblast growth factor, platelet-derived growth factor, insulinlike growth factor, BMP, and transforming growth factor (TGF).

Studies have shown the utility of RIA bone graft in treating bone defects. McCall and colleagues[39] reported on large segmental bone defects treated with RIA bone graft. The average defect size in their study population of 21 patients was 6.6 cm, and 85% of the defects were healed at 11 months. However, 7 of the 17 healed defects required additional surgery. Stafford and Norris[2] treated 25 patients with 27 segmental defect nonunions with RIA graft. The overall average segmental defect measured 5.8 cm in length, and at 6 months and 1 year postoperatively, 70% and 90% of the nonunions were healed both clinically and radiographically.

Although there are many reports on the potential benefit of the RIA graft, there are concerns about the mechanical changes that occur in the donor femur after graft harvesting. For example, its use in the elderly is one that should be exercised with caution because of reduced cortical thickness and potential for postoperative fracture.[53] Lowe and colleagues[54] reported a case series of postoperative fractures that occurred after RIA graft harvesting and suggested the following:

1. Preoperative assessment of cortical diameters at long-bone harvest sites
2. Careful monitoring during intraoperative reaming
3. Avoidance of RIA bone graft harvesting in patients with a history of osteoporosis or osteopenia unless postharvest IM stabilization is considered

Others have demonstrated that attention must be paid to technique as eccentric femoral reaming

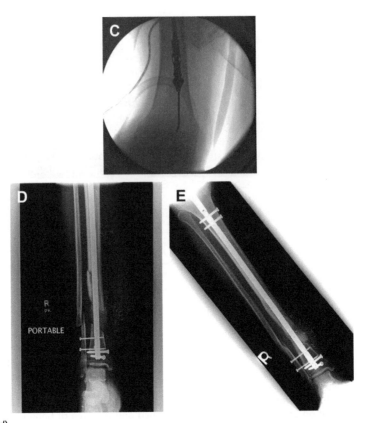

Fig. 4. (*continued*)

either proximally or distally may result in catastrophic failure.[55]

MASQUELET TECHNIQUE

The notion of creating a membrane to protect and enhance the local environment was introduced in the early 1960s. The initial materials tested were nonabsorbable substances such as Teflon and polyurethane sponges.[56–58] Masquelet and colleagues[59,60] developed the use of induced membrane-assisted massive autograft for segmental bony defects and successfully managed defects 25 cm or less with associated severe soft-tissue injury by use of this technique. This is a 2-stage procedure. The first stage involves complete removal of all devitalized bone and soft tissue. This step is followed by implantation of a PMMA cement spacer. The injury is then stabilized by either internal or external fixation methods. The second stage is usually undertaken 6 to 8 weeks later and involves careful removal of the cement spacer with preservation of the resultant induced membrane and substitution with autologous cancellous bone graft (**Fig. 5**).[61]

The induced membrane offers the advantages of preventing autograft resorption, maintaining graft position, and preventing soft-tissue interposition.[62] The induced membrane is a unique and potent tissue made of type I collagen–heavy matrix, and fibroblastic cells are the dominant cell type.[62,63] The tissue is highly vascularized, and the cement spacer causes a mild foreign body inflammatory response that decreases 2 weeks after implantation, with resolution 6 months after bone grafting.[64,65] Immunochemical assessment has shown that the induced membrane secretes growth and osteoconductive factors, such as vascular endothelial growth factor, TGF-β1, and BMP-2. BMP-2 production peaks at 4 weeks postimplantation. This finding indicates that an optimal time for definitive bone grafting exists.[64]

There are several clinical case series that have demonstrated satisfactory outcomes with the use of this technique. In 2000, Masquelet and colleagues[60] reported a union rate of 100% in a series of patients with upper and lower extremity segmental defects that measured 4 to 25 cm in length. McCall and colleagues[39] reported on a series of 20 patients with upper and lower extremity segmental bone defects treated with the induced membrane technique and fixation with either IM nails or plate and screw constructs. They reported a union rate of 85% at final follow-up. However, 7

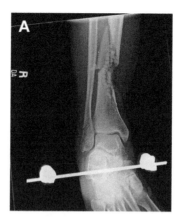

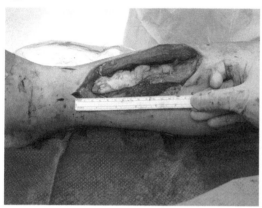

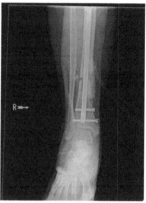

Fig. 5. Use of the Masquelet technique in the management of a skeletal defect in a grade IIIB open tibia fracture treatment. The injury was initially stabilized at an outside facility with an external fixator and subsequently underwent irrigation and debridement and definitive fixation with an intramedullary nail. The area of bone loss was managed with the induced membrane technique. (*A*) Intraoperative photograph demonstrating the antibiotic cement spacer in the area of bone loss. (*B*) Postoperative radiograph demonstrating fracture stabilization with an intramedullary nail and antibiotic cement spacer. (*C*) After 8 weeks, the cement spacer was removed and autogenous iliac crest bone graft was harvested. (*D*) Intraoperative photograph demonstrating the induced membrane held within the forceps and iliac crest bone packed into the defect. (*E*) Postoperative radiograph 12 months after antibiotic cement spacer removal and autogenous iliac crest bone grafting demonstrating union at the area of bone loss.

patients required additional surgery after the second stage. Apard and colleagues[66] reported a union rate of 92% in 12 patients with segmental bone loss of the tibia treated with the induced membrane technique and IM nailing.

VASCULARIZED BONE GRAFTS

The history of free vascularized bone grafts dates back to 1905, when Huntington successfully used a pedicled fibular graft to fill a large tibial defect.[67] Fredrickson published his experimental work in the successful transfer of living ribs for mandible reconstruction in dogs in conjunction with McCullogh[68] in 1972 and later with Ostrup[69] in 1975. Also in 1975, Taylor[70] became the first to report the successful microsurgical transfer of

a free living fibular graft to manage large tibial defects in 2 clinical cases. In 1979, Pho[71] reported on the transfer of a vascularized proximal fibula as a hemivascularized joint transplant to replace the distal end of the radius after resection of a giant cell tumor.

When approaching limb reconstruction in the setting of trauma, one must consider the viability of the vascular supply of the surrounding environment. Avascularity of the remaining environment is now recognized as a central component of the pathogenesis following large defects induced by high-energy trauma and other causes.[72] In cases such as these, the choice of a vascularized bone graft seems inevitable, as bone grafts with intrinsic blood supply lead to higher success rates and to acceleration of the repair process in the

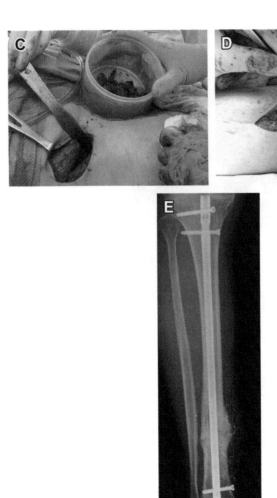

Fig. 5. *(continued)*

reconstruction of defects and necrotic lesions of the skeleton.[44,45,73]

The fibula remains one of the most frequent donor sites for free vascularized bone transfers. Its vascular anatomy is well understood, with the peroneal artery and veins providing an adequate vascular pedicle. Transfer is straightforward, and approximately 25 cm of fibula graft can be harvested. The graft should be 4 cm longer than the defect, which enables a 2-cm overlap proximally and distally.[74] At the donor site, 5 cm should be left distally to avoid ankle problems and 7 cm proximally to avoid knee problems as well as damage to the peroneal nerve.[1] The use of the vascularized fibular graft offers several advantages with respect to the biology of bone healing. First, the vascularity and viability of the graft is maintained. Second, the process of creeping substitution, as seen with non-vascularized grafts, is bypassed, and the stronger mechanical properties of the graft allows for faster

incorporation and graft hypertrophy.[44] These factors contribute to the fact that vascularized autografts are more likely to achieve union in a short time frame. On average, the time to union is between 3 and 6 months.[75] Furthermore, the graft is less likely to undergo cortical resorption and less likely to sustain stress fractures as compared with an avascular graft.[44] In addition, the use of a vascularized fibula graft may be considered for managing bone defects larger than 10 cm, smaller defects that have failed to heal with nonvascularized bone grafting, and previously infected bone nonunion with or without a defect associated with osteonecrosis.[74,76] However, this technique does have disadvantages, including donor site morbidity, limited graft availability, a demanding surgical technique with prolonged anesthesia time, extended non–weight bearing, and the risk of inadequate graft hypertrophy and stress fracture.[1] Rates of stress fracture associated with this technique have been quoted between 7.7% and 22.2 % in the literature.[77] In addition, vessels are sacrificed and the progress of bony healing and vascular viability are both difficult to monitor.[44]

Alternative donor sites available for vascularized bone transfer include the iliac crest, which can be harvested with a vascular pedicle, based on the deep circumflex iliac artery; the lateral border of the scapula, based on the thoracodorsal vessels; and the ribs, based on the intercostal vessels.[37] These sites are reasonable alternative donor sites to the vascularized fibular graft. However, they are also associated with their own inherent disadvantages. The vascularized iliac crest is associated with donor site complications including bowel herniation, contour defects, and injury to the lateral femoral cutaneous nerve. The lateral border of the scapula may be taken as a composite free flap together with the latissimus dorsi muscle. Although this allows the simultaneous coverage of large soft-tissue defects together with bone reconstruction, the strength of the bone graft does not equal that provided by the fibular graft. Finally, the vascularized rib graft does not have significant strength and requires time to hypertrophy before significant loads can be applied.[37]

BONE MORPHOGENETIC PROTEINS AND REGIONAL GENE THERAPY

In 1965, Marshall R. Urist discovered the so-called bone induction principle. The theory postulated that bone matrix contained inducing agents that could help generate new bone formation when implanted into an extraskeletal site.[78] Urist[79] identified this factor as a protein and named it bone morphogenetic protein. Since their discovery, BMPs have been studied extensively and may be considered to be the most important growth factors for bone healing owing to their potent osteoinductive properties.[80,81] Currently, nearly 20 structurally related BMPs have been discovered, and these proteins are known to be members of the TGF-β superfamily. Recombinant DNA technology has allowed for their production, and 2 BMPs are commercially available in the recombinant form: rhBMP-2 and rhBMP-7.

The clinical utility of these proteins in the management of critical sized defects in humans has been in shown the literature. Using a clinical model, Geesink and colleagues[82] were the first to demonstrate that recombinant BMPs can induce healing in cortical bone defects in humans. RhBMP-7 bound to collagen particles was shown to be effective in 5 of 6 patients with a critically sized fibular defect. Only 3 of 6 patients treated with a type I collagen carrier alone had bone

formation. Jones and colleagues[83] compared the use of rhBMP-2 combined with allograft versus autogenous bone graft in the delayed reconstruction of posttraumatic tibial diaphyseal defects with mean lengths of 4 cm. The defects treated with rhBMP-2/allograft showed no difference with respect to union or complication rates. The investigators concluded that rhBMP-2/allograft is as safe and as effective as traditional autogenous bone grafting for the treatment of tibial fractures associated with extensive traumatic diaphyseal bone loss. These results demonstrate that there might be an indication for BMP use in the treatment of critical sized defects in combination or as an alternative to established therapies. However, there is need for further studies to clearly define the indications and treatment strategies. It has been shown that large doses of BMPs have been required to induce adequate bone formation in humans.[84] The side effects of such large protein doses are unknown. Furthermore, there are concerns that a single dose of recombinant protein may not be sufficient to yield an adequate response, particularly in the case in which there is compromised bone stock and vascularity.[85,86] Regional gene therapy is another approach to deliver proteins to a specific anatomic site.

Regional gene therapy can be used via an in vivo or an ex vivo approach. In an in vivo technique, the vector is delivered directly to the anatomic site. In an ex vivo approach, specific cells are harvested from the patient and then transduced outside the body; the transduced cells are then reimplanted into a specific anatomic site.[87] However, getting gene therapy protocols into human clinical trials is a lengthy, expensive, and frustrating process, especially for a condition that is not lethal.[88] Before gaining US Food and Drug Administration approval, the safety and efficacy of any potential gene therapy for bone regeneration would need to be confirmed in large animals, and at the present state, human clinical trials will not be underway for several years.[89]

SUMMARY

Bone defects represent a challenging clinical problem for the treating orthopedic surgeon. Various treatment options exist with differing advantages and disadvantages. There is no one strategy that can be recommended for all conditions. Therefore, the treating surgeon must be aware of all options available and make decisions on an individual basis. This decision-making process must be a flexible one and take into account several factors, including the amount of bone loss, the degree of soft-tissue injury, and the patient's overall health status and willingness to comply with prolonged treatment strategies. Therefore, careful preoperative planning and counseling with patients and family members are necessary when dealing with these injuries. The patient must understand that the course of treatment is long, complications may be encountered, and eventual amputation may be required.

REFERENCES

1. Ashman O, Phillps AM. Treatment of non-unions with bone defects: which options and why? Injury 2013;44(Suppl 1):S43–5.
2. Stafford RP, Norris LN. Reamer-irrigator-aspirator bone graft and bi Masquelet technique for segmental bone defect nonunions: a review of 25 cases. Injury 2010;41(Suppl 2):S72–7.
3. Pneumaticos S, Triantafyllopoulos G, Basdra E, et al. Segmental bone defects: from cellular and molecular pathways to the development of novel biological treatments. J Cell Mol Med 2010; 14(11):2561–9.
4. El-Rosasy MA. Acute shortening and re-lengthening in the management of bone and soft tissue loss in complicated fractures of the tibia. J Bone Joint Surg Br 2007;89(1):80–8.
5. Bundgaard GK, Christensen SK. Tibial bone loss and soft tissue defect treated simultaneously with Ilizarov technique - a case report. Acta Orthop Scand 2000;71(5):534–6.
6. DeCoster TA, Gehlert RJ, Mikola EA. Management of posttraumatic segmental bone defects. J Am Acad Orthop Surg 2004;12:28–38.
7. Nho SJ, Helfet DL, Rozbruch SR. Temporary intentional leg shortening and deformation to facilitate wound closure using the Ilizarov/Taylor spatial frame. J Orthop Trauma 2006;20(6):419–24.
8. Sen C, Kocaoglu M, Eralp L, et al. Bifocal compression-distraction in the acute treatment of grade III open tibia fractures with bone and soft-tissue loss: a report of 24 cases. J Orthop Trauma 2004;18(3):150–7.
9. Aronson J. Limb-lengthening, skeletal reconstruction and bone transport with the Ilizarov method. J Bone Joint Surg Am 1997;79(8):1243–58.
10. Fischgrund J, Paley D, Sutter C. Variables affecting time to bone healing during limb lengthening. Clin Orthop Relat Res 1994;301:31–7.
11. Ilizarov GA. Clinical application of tension-stress effect for limb lengthening. Clin Orthop Relat Res 1990;250:8–26.
12. Sabharwal S. Enhancement of bone formation during distraction osteogenesis: pediatric applications. J Am Acad Orthop Surg 2011;19:101–11.
13. Girard PJ, Kuhn KM, Bailey JR, et al. Bone transport combined with locking bridge plate for the treatment of tibial segmental defects: a report of 2 cases. J Orthop Trauma 2013;27(8):220–6.
14. Oh CW, Song HR, Roh JY, et al. Bone transport over an intramedullary nail for reconstruction of long bone defects in tibia. Arch Orthop Trauma Surg 2008;128:801–8.
15. Speilberg B, Parrat T, Dheerendra KS, et al. Ilizarov principles of deformity correction. Ann R Coll Surg Engl 2010;92(2):101–5.
16. Green SA. Skeletal defects. A comparison of bone grafting and bone transport for segmental skeletal defects. Clin Orthop Relat Res 1990;301:111–7.
17. Paley D. Problems, obstacles and complications of limb lengthening by the Ilizarov technique. Clin Orthop Relat Res 1990;250:81–104.
18. Watson JT. Distraction osteogenesis. J Am Acad Orthop Surg 2006;14:S168–74.
19. Dhar SA, Mir MR, Ahmed MS, et al. Acute peg in hole docking in the management of infected nonunion of long bones. Int Orthop 2008;32(4):559–66.
20. Wantanabe K, Tsuchiya H, Sakurakichi K, et al. Tibial lengthening over an intramedullary nail. J Orthop Sci 2005;10(5):480–5.
21. Gold SM, Wassereman R. Preliminary results of tibial bone transports with pulsed low intensity ultrasound (Exogen). J Orthop Trauma 2005;19(1):10–6.
22. Cattaneo R, Catagni M, Johnson EE. The treatment of infected nonunions and segmental defects of the tibia by methods of Ilizarov. Clin Orthop 1992;280:143–52.
23. Cierny G 3rd, Zorn KE. Segmental tibial defects. Comparing convential and Ilizarov methodologies. Clin Orthop 1994;301:118–23.
24. Green SA, Jackson JM, Wall DM, et al. Management of segmental defects by the Ilizarov intercalary bone transport method. Clin Orthop 1992;280:136–42.
25. Marsh JL, Prokuski L, Biermann JS. Chronic infected tibial nonunions with bone loss. Conventional techniques versus bone transport. Clin Orthop 1994;301:139–46.
26. Paley D, Maar DC. Ilizarov bone transport treatment for tibial defects. J Orthop Trauma 2000;14:76–85.
27. Polyzois D, Papachristou G, Kotsiopoulos K, et al. Treatment of tibial and femoral bone loss by distraction osteogenesis. Experience in 28 infected and 14 clean cases. Acta Orthop Scand Suppl 1997;275:84–8.
28. Saleh M, Rees A. Bifocal surgery for deformity and bone loss after lower-limb fractures. Comparison of bone-transport and compression-distraction methods. J Bone Joint Surg Br 1995;77:429–34.
29. Song HR, Cho SH, Koo KH, et al. Tibial bone defects treated by internal bone transport using the Ilizarov method. Int Orthop 1998;22:293–7.

30. Feldman DS, Shin SS, Madan S, et al. Correction of tibial malunion and nonunion with six-axis analysis deformity correction using the Taylor spatial frame. J Orthop Trauma 2000;17(8):549–54.

31. Rozbruch SR, Weitzman AM, Watson JT, et al. Simultaneous treatment of tibial and soft tissue defects with the Ilizarov method. J Orthop Trauma 2006;20:197–205.

32. Sala F, Elabatrawy Y, Thabet AM, et al. Taylor spatial frame fixation in patients with multiple traumatic injuries: study of 57 long-bone fractures. J Orthop Trauma 2013;27(8):442–50.

33. Sala F, Albisetti W, Capitani D. Versatility of Taylor Spatial Frame in Gustilo-Anderson III C femoral fractures: report of three cases. Musculoskelet Surg 2010;94:103–8.

34. Granger R, Radler C, Speigner B, et al. Correction of post-traumatic lower limb deformities using the Taylor Spatial Frame. Int Orthop 2010;34:723–30.

35. Nakase T, Kitano M, Kawai H, et al. Distraction osteogenesis for the correction of three-dimensional deformities with shortening of lower limbs by Taylor spatial frame. Arch Orthop Trauma Surg 2009;129: 1197–201.

36. Dammerer D, Kirchbichler K, Donnan L, et al. Clinical value of the Taylor Spatial Frame: a comparison with the Ilizarov and Orthofix fixators. J Child Orthop 2011;5:343–9.

37. Gan A, Puhaindran ME, Pho R. The reconstruction of large bone defects in the upper limb. Injury 2013;44:313–7.

38. Sen M, Miclau T. Autologous iliac crest bone graft: should it still be the gold standard for treating nonunions? Injury 2007;38:S75–80.

39. McCall TA, Brokow DS, Jelen BA, et al. Treatment of large segmental bone defects with reamer-irrigator-aspirator bone graft: technique and case series. Orthop Clin North Am 2010;41:63–73.

40. Ahlmann E, Patzakis M, Roidis N, et al. Comparison of anterior and posterior iliac crest bone grafts in terms of harvest site morbidity and functional outcomes. J Bone Joint Surg Am 2002;84(5): 716–20.

41. Seiler JG 3rd, Johnson J. Iliac crest autogenous bone grafting: donor site complications. J South Orthop Assoc 2000;9(2):91–7.

42. Arrington ED, Smith WJ, Chambers HG, et al. Complications of iliac crest bone graft harvesting. Clin Orthop Relat Res 1996;329:300–9.

43. Silber JS, Anderson DG, Daffner SD, et al. Donor site morbidity after anterior iliac crest bone harvest for single level anterior cervical discectomy and fusion. Spine 2003;28(2):134–9.

44. Soucacos PN, Kokkalis ZT, Piagkou M, et al. Vascularized bone grafts for the management of skeletal defects in orthopedic trauma and reconstructive surgery. Injury 2013;44(Suppl.1):S70–5.

45. Soucacos PN, Johnson EO, Babis G. An update on recent advances in bone regeneration. Injury 2008; 39:S1–4.

46. Soucacos PN, Dailana Z, Beris AE, et al. Vascularized bone grafts for the management of non-union. Injury 2006;37:S41–50.

47. Masquelet AC, Benko PE, Mathevon H, et al. Harvest of cortico-cancellous intramedullary femoral bone graft using the Reamer-Irrigator-Aspirator (RIA). Orthop Traumatol Surg Res 2012;98:227–32.

48. Huseby EE, Lyberg T, Opdahl H, et al. Cardiopulmonary response to reamed intramedullary nailing of the femur comparing traditional reaming with one step Reamer-Irrigator-Aspirator reaming system: an experimental study in pigs. J Trauma 2010;69:E6–14.

49. Huseby EE, Lyberg T, Madsen JE, et al. The influence of one step Reamer-Irrigator-Aspirator technique on the intramedullary pressure in the pig femur. Injury 2006;37:935–40.

50. Higgins TF, Casey V, Bachus K. Cortical heat generation using an irrigating/aspirating single pass reaming vs. conventional stepwise reaming. J Orthop Trauma 2007;21:192–7.

51. Green J. History and development of suction-irrigation-reaming. Injury 2010;41(Suppl 2):S24–31.

52. Schmidmaier G, Herrmann S, Green J, et al. Quantitative assessment of growth factors in reaming aspirate, iliac crest, and platelet preparation. Bone 2006;39(5):1156–63.

53. Pape H, Tarkin IS. Reamer Irrigator Aspirator: a new technique for bone graft harvesting from the intramedullary canal. Oper Tech Orthop 2008;18: 108–13.

54. Lowe J, Della Rocca GJ, Murtha Y, et al. Complications associated with negative pressure reaming for harvesting autologous bone graft: a case series. J Orthop Trauma 2010;24(1):46–52.

55. Silva JA, McCormick JJ, Reed MA, et al. Biomechanical effects of harvesting bone graft with the Reamer/Irrigator/Aspirator on the adult femur: a cadaver study. Injury 2010;41(Suppl 2):S85–9.

56. Gilmer WS Jr, Tooms RE, Salvatore JE. An experimental study of the influence of implanted polyurethane sponges upon subsequent bone formation. Surg Gynecol Obstet 1961;113:143–8.

57. Eickholz P, Pretzl B, Holle R, et al. Long-term results of guided tissue regeneration therapy with non-resorbable and bioabsorbable barriers: III. Class II furcations after 10 years. J Periodontol 2006;77(1):88–94.

58. Meinig RP, Rahn B, Perren SM, et al. Bone regeneration with resorbable polymeric membranes: treatment of diaphyseal bone defects in the rabbit radius with poly(L-lactide) membrane. A pilot study. J Orthop Trauma 1996;10(3):178–90.

59. Masquelet AC. Muscle reconstruction in reconstructive surgery: soft tissue repair and long bone reconstruction. Langenbecks Arch Surg 2003; 338(5):344–6.

60. Masquelet AC, Fitoussi F, Begue T, et al. Reconstruction of the long bones by the induced membrane and spongy autograft. Ann Chir Plast Esthet 2000;45(3):346–53 [French].

61. Giannoudis PV, Omar F, Goff T, et al. Masquelet technique for the treatment of bone defects: tips-tricks and future directions. Injury 2011;42:591–8.

62. Viateau V, Bensidhoum M, Guillemin G, et al. Use of the induced membrane technique for bone tissue engineering purposes: animal studies. Orthop Clin North Am 2010;41(1):49–56.

63. Pelissier P, Masquelet AC, Bareille R, et al. Induced membranes secrete growth factors including vascular and osteoinductive factors and could stimulate bone regeneration. J Orthop Res 2004; 22(1):73–9.

64. Viateau V, Guillemin G, Bousson V, et al. Long-bone critical-size defects treated with tissue-engineered grafts: a study on sheep. J Orthop Res 2007;25(6): 741–9.

65. Viateau V, Guillemin G, Calando Y, et al. Induction of a barrier membrane to facilitate reconstruction of massive segmental diaphyseal bone defects: an ovine model. Vet Surg 2006;35(5):445–52.

66. Apard T, Bigorre N, Cronier P, et al. Two-stage reconstruction of post-traumatic segmental tibia bone loss with nailing. Orthop Traumatol Surg Res 2010;96(5):549–53.

67. Huntington TW VI. Case of bone transference: use of a segment of fibula to supply a defect in tibia. Ann Surg 1905;41:249–51.

68. McCullough DW, Frederickson JM. Composite neovascularized rib grafts for mandibular reconstruction. Surg Forum 1972;23:492–4.

69. Ostrup LT, Frederickson JM. Distant transfer of a free, living bone graft by microvascular anastomoses. An experimental study. Plast Reconstr Surg 1974;54:274–85.

70. Taylor GI, Miller GD, Ham FJ. The free vascularized bone graft - a clinical extension of microvascular techniques. Plast Reconstr Surg 1975;55:533–44.

71. Pho RW. Free vascularized fibular transplant for replacement of the lower radius. J Bone Joint Surg Br 1979;61:362–5.

72. Stevenson S. Enhancement of fracture healing with autogenous and allogenic bone grafts. Clin Orthop Relat Res 1998;355:S239–46.

73. Beris AE, Payatakes AJ, Kostopoulos VK, et al. Nonunion of femoral neck fractures with osteonecrosis of the femoral head: treatment with combined free vascularized fibular grafting and subtrochanteric valgus osteotomy. Orthop Clin North Am 2004;35: 335–43, ix.

74. Wood MB. Free vascularized fibular grafting - 25 years of experience: tips, techniques and pearls. Orthop Clin North Am 2007;38:1–12, v.

75. Weiland AJ. Current concepts review: vascularized free bone transplants. J Bone Joint Surg Am 1981; 63:166–9.

76. Pederson WC, Pearson DW. Long bone reconstruction with vascularized bone grafts. Orthop Clin North Am 2007;38:23–5, v.

77. Beris A, Lykissas M, Korompilias A. Vascularized fibula transfer for lower limb reconstruction. Microsurgery 2011;31:205–11.

78. Argintar E, Edwards S, Delahay J. Bone morphogenetic proteins in orthopaedic trauma surgery. Injury 2011;42:730–4.

79. Urist MR. A morphogenetic matrix for differentiation of bone tissue. Calcif Tissue Res 1970;(Suppl):98–101.

80. Dimitriou R, Jones E, McGonagle D, et al. Bone regeneration: current concepts and future directions. BMC Med 2011;9:66.

81. De Biase P, Capanna R. Clinical applications of BMPs. Injury 2005;36(Suppl):S43–6.

82. Geesink R, Hoefnagels H, Bulstra S. Osteogenic activity of OP-1 bone morphogenetic protein (BMP-7) in a human fibular defect. J Bone Joint Surg Br 1999;81:710–8.

83. Jones AL, Bucholz RW, BMP-2 Evaluation in Surgery for Tibial Trauma-Allograft (BESTT-ALL) Study Group, et al. Recombinant human BMP-2 and allograft compared with autogenous bone graft for reconstruction of diaphyseal tibial fractures with cortical defects. A randomized, controlled trial. J Bone Joint Surg Am 2006;88(7):1431–41.

84. Govender S, Csimma C, Genant HK, et al. Recombinant human bone morphogenetic protein-2 for treatment of open tibial fractures: a prospective, controlled, randomized study of four hundred and fifty patients. J Bone Joint Surg Am 2002;84: 2123–34.

85. Lieberman JR, Ghivizzani SC, Evans CH. Gene transfer approaches to the healing of bone and cartilage. Mol Ther 2002;6:141–7.

86. Oakes DA, Lieberman JR. Osteoinductive applications of regional gene therapy: ex vivo gene transfer. Clin Orthop 2000;379(Suppl):S101–12.

87. Baltzer AW, Lieberman JR. Regional gene therapy to enhance bone repair. Gene Ther 2004; 11:344–50.

88. Evans CH, Ghivizzani SC, Robins PD. Getting arthritis gene therapy into the clinic. Nat Rev Rheumatol 2011;7(4):244–9.

89. Evans C. Gene therapy for the regeneration of bone. Injury 2011;42:599–604.

High-energy Pediatric Pelvic and Acetabular Fractures

Louis F. Amorosa, MD[a],*, Peter Kloen, MD, PhD[b],
David L. Helfet, MD[c]

KEYWORDS

- High-energy fracture • Pelvis • Acetabulum • Pediatric

KEY POINTS

- Pediatric pelvic fractures are markers of high-energy injuries and are unlikely to be the cause of death, but are a sign of other associated life-threatening injuries such as head or thoracoabdominal trauma.
- Pelvic hemorrhage may go unrecognized in pediatric patients because of a more effective vasoconstriction mechanism and the ability of the immature periosteum to tamponade bleeding.
- Operative indications for pediatric pelvic fractures are based on amount of displacement and degree of instability and are indicated to prevent deformity and long-term disability and pain.
- Pediatric posterior wall acetabular fractures may be misinterpreted as small fragments when magnetic resonance imaging (MRI) reveals a large osteocartilaginous wall fragment requiring operative fixation. Most pediatric acetabular fractures involving the posterior wall require MRI to better judge the size of the fracture fragment(s).
- There is little evidence for the optimal treatment of triradiate acetabular fractures, and outcomes are poor for the most severe crush injuries.

INTRODUCTION

Pediatric pelvic and acetabular fractures are rare, with a reported incidence of 1 per 100,000 children per year.[1,2] Pediatric pelvic fractures caused by high-energy injury mechanisms are a marker of impending death because of associated head and other injuries.[3] Long-term outcome studies of pediatric pelvic fractures are lacking because of their rarity. Treatment can differ significantly between skeletally immature and skeletally mature pelvic fractures. Depending on the injury, the potential exists for long-term disability from residual deformity, growth disturbance, compensatory scoliosis, and pain. Literature specifically on pediatric acetabular fractures is even more scarce than literature on pediatric pelvic fractures. This article presents the anatomy, general considerations, classification systems, and treatment strategies for high-energy pelvic and acetabular fractures in skeletally immature patients based on the best available evidence and our own experience in treating these patients. Pediatric pelvic avulsion fractures, which are usually caused by low-energy mechanisms such as athletic events, are not addressed in this article.

The authors have nothing to disclose.
[a] Department of Orthopaedic Surgery, New York Medical College, Westchester Medical Center, Valhalla, NY, USA; [b] Department of Orthopaedic Surgery, Academic Medical Center, Amsterdam, The Netherlands; [c] Orthopaedic Trauma Service, Hospital for Special Surgery, New York, NY, USA
* Corresponding author.
E-mail address: amorosal@wcmc.com

ANATOMY
Pelvis

The pelvis begins to form during the first 2 months of embryologic development. The acetabulum, formed by the convergence of the ilium, ischium, and pubis, begins to cavitate and by the eighth week a fully developed hip joint exists. By 9 weeks, endochondral ossification of the ilium begins, with the ischium beginning to ossify at about 16 weeks, and the pubis a few weeks following this. The epiphyseal centers of the pelvis, including the triradiate cartilage, are visible at this time.[4]

The pubic symphysis, composed of thick cartilaginous endplates, has a variable rate of ossification until about age 10 years. The iliac crest and spines remain cartilaginous until adolescence, at which time secondary ossification centers develop along the anterolateral iliac crest at 13 to 15 years of age. As ossification of the wing advances posteriorly toward the posterior superior iliac spine, fusion to the rest of the ilium occurs from 15 to 17 years, with complete fusion often not occurring until age 25 years. The ilium is thought to develop normally based partly on the pull of the gluteal muscles on its outer wing.[4,5]

Acetabulum

The first ossification center of the acetabulum begins in infancy as woven bone at the level of the acetabular fossa. The triradiate cartilage is composed of 3 secondary ossification centers at the periphery of the acetabulum, with the pubis, the ilium, and ischium each contributing to an arm of growth (**Fig. 1**). These 3 secondary ossification centers begin to develop within the acetabular cartilage in the prepubescent period. The os acetabuli, part of the pubis, appears at 8 years of

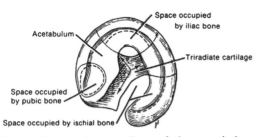

Fig. 1. The triradiate cartilage of the acetabulum, lateral view. Growth occurs outward from the triradiate cartilage until fusion occurs with the secondary ossification centers of the pubis, ilium, and ischium at skeletal maturity, and the acetabulum is fully ossified. (*From* Ponseti IV. Growth and development of the acetabulum in the normal child. Anatomical, histological, and roentgenographic studies. J Bone Joint Surg Am 1978;60(5):575–85; with permission.)

age, and develops into the anterior acetabular wall, with fusion normally by age 15 years. The acetabular epiphysis, the secondary ossification center of the ilium, appears between 8 and 9 years, and contributes to most of the roof of the acetabulum, and fully fuses by 18 years. The ischial epiphysis appears between 9 and 10 years with the secondary ossification center in the ischium continuing to develop through adolescence.[5] Before the visualization of secondary ossification centers during adolescence, injuries to this region can be missed with radiographs.

The triradiate cartilage and other ossification centers contribute to the widening of both the pelvic ring and the acetabulum. Interstitial growth in the triradiate cartilage contributes to the height and width of the acetabulum, but much of the growth as well as its depth are stimulated by mechanical stimuli. The acetabulum cavitates as a result of the pressure of the femoral head and also symbiotically contributes to the normal development of the femoral head. As the triradiate cartilage grows and develops into the acetabulum it also grows outward, contributing to the length of the pelvic bones.[4,5]

PATTERN OF TRAUMATIC ACETABULAR DYSPLASIA

Dysplasia caused by injury is distinct from developmental dysplasia of the hip (DDH). In DDH, the femoral neck is typically anteverted and the femoral head subluxes laterally and anteriorly while the pelvic ring remains symmetric and relatively unaffected. The acetabulum has a decreased lateral and anterior center edge angle. In posttraumatic hip dysplasia, proximal femoral anatomy is normal, but the true pelvis deforms and appears lengthened on the side of the injured acetabulum. The teardrop and inner wall of the acetabulum appear increased in size and the femoral head lateralizes. Patients usually have symmetric leg lengths but the leg can appear shortened because of the upward migration of the femoral head into the growth-arrested acetabulum. A positive Trendelenburg sign toward the uninjured side may be present because of an increased lever arm of the abductor muscle tendon-tendon unit on the injured side.[6]

CAUSE OF TRAUMATIC ACETABULAR DYSPLASIA

The exact cause of premature closure of the triradiate cartilage has yet to be elucidated. Rodrigues[7] suggested that the hematoma that forms after injury ossifies creating a bony bridge that halts growth of the physis. Trousdale and Ganz[6] suggested a combination of direct injury to the growth plate chondroblasts during the trauma and subsequent scarring as likely contributing to growth arrest. Bucholz and colleagues[8] suggested that the hypoxia caused by traumatic disruption of precarious microcirculation to the chondroblasts causes growth arrest.

Animal studies have contributed to the knowledge on traumatic acetabular dysplasia. Delgado and colleagues[9] found in a rat model that selective injuries to different flanges of the triradiate cartilage resulted in different patterns of growth arrest and deformity of the acetabulum. Gepstein and colleagues[10] showed in a study of selective fusion of rabbit triradiate cartilage that injury to the ilioischial flange has the greatest negative effect on growth and development with 100% of rabbit acetabuli having dysplasia and 66% of hips dislocated by 9 weeks after iatrogenic injury.

GENERAL CONSIDERATIONS
The Unique Characteristics of the Skeletally Immature Pelvis

Elasticity
The distinction between adult and pediatric pelvic fractures is not only related to anatomy and development but also to injury mechanism, associated injuries, and mortality. Depending on the age of the child, much of the pelvis is composed of cartilage, and the bone has thicker periosteum. These factors make the pediatric pelvis more elastic than the adult pelvis. Pediatric sacroiliac and pubic symphyseal joints are wider and thicker in children than in adults, and they are capable of absorbing a greater amount of force without frank rupture. These anatomic considerations may account for the lower incidence of pelvic fractures in children than in adults.[11] Because the immature pelvis is more resistant to sustaining a fracture, when a fracture does occur, unless it is an avulsion fracture, it should be assumed that it is caused by a high-energy mechanism. When a pelvic fracture occurs in a child, there should be a high suspicion for associated head injury, thoracic injuries, and abdominal injuries.[12]

Lower mortality
Even though pelvic fractures in children are harbingers of other associated life-threatening bodily injuries, children who sustain pelvic fractures have an overall lower mortality from pelvic fractures than adults.[13] Over a 6 year period at a level I trauma center, of 57 children diagnosed with a pelvic fracture, only 1 patient had significant hemorrhage directly related to a pelvic fracture, and the

3 mortalities were caused by other injuries.[14] Another retrospective study found similarly low mortalities in pediatric pelvic fractures.[15]

Better hemorrhagic control
Skeletally immature pelvic fractures are associated with less blood loss than in adults.[14] Because the thicker periosteum is more resistant to fracture, incomplete greenstick pelvic fractures can occur. The unruptured periosteum contains and tamponades bleeding fracture hematoma. Furthermore, children have vasculature that is more vasoreactive and bleeding vessels in the pelvis are more likely to effectively constrict, limiting hemorrhage. Although this is protective for the child, it also can mask earlier stages of hemorrhagic shock. When a child with a high-energy pelvic fracture is hemodynamically unstable and is bleeding into the pelvis, the trauma team should immediately stabilize the pelvis provisionally and aggressively resuscitate the child with blood and blood products, because the child is likely in late stages of hemorrhagic shock. However, mortality in a child with a pelvic fracture is usually not from the pelvic fracture but approximately 75% of time from an associated head injury.[16]

Injury mechanism
The mechanism of injury is another distinction between adult and pediatric pelvic fractures, and may also be a factor in why mortalities in children are lower. Pediatric pelvic fractures are more likely to be the result of a pedestrian being struck by a motor vehicle than from a head-on motor vehicle accident, which is a common injury mechanism in adult pelvic fractures.[2,15,16] Pedestrians are most likely to be struck on the side of the body, which is likely to cause a lateral compression injury. Lateral compression injuries are also associated with head and thoracic injuries, whereas head-on motor vehicle collisions are more likely to cause an anterior-posterior compression or open-book pelvic fracture, more commonly associated with life-threatening hemorrhage and death than lateral compression fractures.[17]

Status of the triradiate cartilage
Deciding when to treat a child as skeletally immature or as an adult should largely be based on the status of the triradiate cartilage. Silber and Flynn[2] performed a retrospective review of 166 pediatric pelvic fractures and evaluated several different radiographic parameters for gauging skeletal maturity, including the Risser stage, closure of the triradiate cartilage, closure of the ischial physis, closure of the proximal femur physis, and closure of the greater trochanter apophysis. They concluded that, in the context of pelvic fractures,

the most reliable method of deciding on skeletal maturity was the status of the triradiate cartilage. Before triradiate closure, the pelvis is considered skeletally immature and can show injury patterns unique to this age group. Silber and Flynn[2] found single, isolated pelvic ring injuries such as iliac wing fractures or isolated rami fractures 29% of the time in skeletally immature patients, which is an extremely rare pattern in adult patients. These isolated injury patterns are likely caused by the greater elasticity of the immature cartilaginous pelvis and thicker periosteum. After triradiate closure, injury patterns are identical to those of adults and can be treated as such (**Fig. 2**). Therefore, one of the guiding principles of treating pediatric pelvic and acetabular fractures is the status of the triradiate cartilage. On average, the triradiate cartilage closes at 14 years in boys and at 12 years in girls.

EVALUATION AND INITIAL TREATMENT

The trauma evaluation begins following advanced pediatric life support (APLS) protocol, beginning with airway, breathing, circulation, and exposure followed by a full musculoskeletal examination evaluating the spine, pelvis, and extremities.[18] The hips should be tested for range of motion to help determine whether there is a hip dislocation or acetabular fracture. A Morel-Lavallée lesion (internal deglovement) is uncommon in children but can be seen in overweight adolescents.[19]

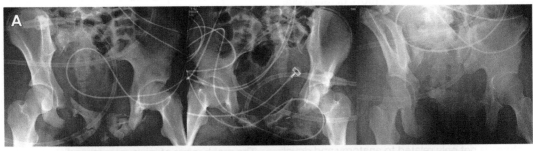

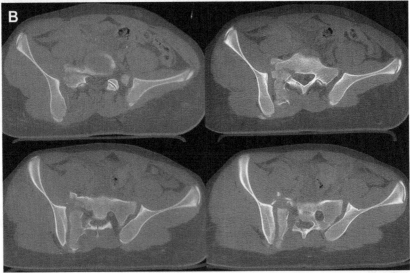

Fig. 2. (*A*) A 13-year-old girl was struck by a car moving 40 km/h (25 miles per hour) while walking. Initial anteroposterior (AP), inlet, and outlet radiographs show a complex pelvic ring open-book injury with widening of the pubic symphysis and a vertical shear fracture of the right sacrum involving the sacral foramen and bilateral superior and inferior pubic rami fractures. (*B*) Computed tomography (CT) images further delineate the fracture/dislocation and fracture pattern. (*C*) Initial resuscitation included 8 units of blood, and anterior pelvic external fixation. Definitive fixation of the pelvic ring injury was performed when the patient was hemodynamically stable with spinopelvic fixation posteriorly and external fixation anteriorly. (*D*) AP, inlet, and outlet radiographs and CT image showing healed sacral and pelvic fractures with maintenance of adequate pelvic symmetry at 19 months after surgery. (*E*) Removal of spinopelvic hardware was performed at 19 months. Radiographs at last follow-up, 5 years after surgery. By then the patient was asymptomatic and had long since returned to all prior athletic activities, including soccer.

C

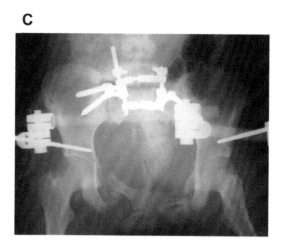

D

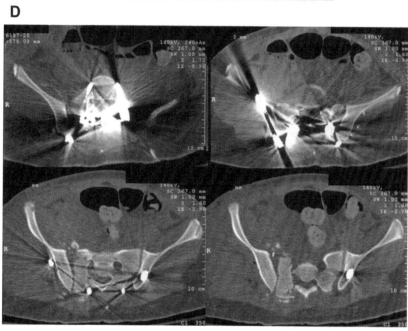

E

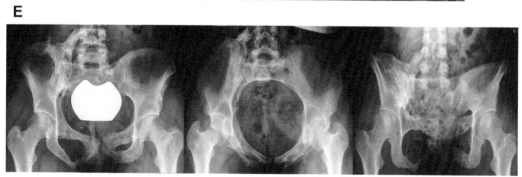

Fig. 2. (*continued*).

The pelvis should be palpated for tenderness and crepitus over the pubic rami, laterally over the iliac wings, and posteriorly over the sacrum. Pelvic stability should be evaluated with antero-posterior (AP) and lateral compression forces to the iliac wings. In an unstable pelvic fracture, this should only be performed once in order not to disrupt any clot that may have previously formed.

When a displaced pelvic fracture is diagnosed in a hemodynamically unstable patient, a pelvic binder or sheet should be placed during the trauma evaluation to decrease intrapelvic volume and potentially tamponade off any bleeding from vessels and bone. Vertically unstable pelvic fractures and hip dislocations after reduction should be treated with skeletal traction. If the patient does not respond to initial resuscitative measures and pelvic binder application, bleeding secondary to fracture is most often caused by bleeding veins or bone and is not arterial. Computed tomography (CT) scan with contrast shows a characteristic extravasating contrast blush, which is sensitive for arterial bleeding 80% to 84% of the time.[20–22] More studies are needed to definitively determine the best treatment protocol; however, angiography is still the next step in the treatment algorithm at most trauma centers.[23]

Open pelvic fractures can easily be missed and therefore suspicion should always be high in the setting of high-energy trauma. A thorough examination for blood around the urethral meatus, the vagina, the scrotum, and the rectum should be performed. A retrograde urethrogram should be performed by a urologic specialist to evaluate the urogenital pathway before placement of a Foley catheter if any suspicion exists for a urologic injury. If a bladder injury has occurred and a suprapubic catheter is placed, and if anterior fixation of the associated pelvic fracture is planned, the orthopedic surgery team should be present when the catheter is placed to ensure that it does not compromise future incisions.[24] During the digital rectal examination, bony fragments in the rectal vault indicate an open pelvic fracture and high-riding prostate signifies urologic injury. Open pelvic fractures communicating with the colon or rectum usually require a temporary diverting colostomy to help prevent infection and osteomyelitis.[24] The site of colostomy should be planned in conjunction with the orthopedic team in order to prevent interference with and contamination of future surgical approaches to the pelvis. An open pelvic fracture requires intravenous antibiotics and urgent irrigation and debridement and external fixation.

PELVIC FRACTURES
Classification

Several classification systems exist for pediatric pelvic fractures. Quinby[25] classified pediatric pelvic fractures into 3 groups based on a series of 20 patients less than 14 years of age. The classification was most useful for general trauma surgeons and was based on the severity of injury to multiple organ systems and who required laparotomy: Group I were mild or stable fractures not requiring laparotomy; group II were fractures with internal organ injury that require surgical exploration; group III were fractures associated with massive hemorrhage and multiple fractures. Watts[3] later classified pelvic fractures in children as follows: simple avulsion fracture; fracture of the pelvic ring, either stable or unstable; acetabular fracture.

The Torode and Zieg[15] classification is most widely used today (**Fig. 3**). Type I fractures are avulsion fractures of bony insertions of muscles attaching to the pelvis, commonly occurring during a sporting event. Type II injuries are iliac wing fractures, usually caused by a direct force on the lateral side, such as in a pedestrian who is struck. Type III fractures are simple ring fractures involving the pubic rami or a pubic symphysis disruption. Type IV pelvic injuries are ring fractures or joint disruptions, resulting in instability of at least part of the pelvic ring. Type IV fractures include straddle injuries in which the bilateral superior and inferior pubic rami are fractured, combined fractures, or dislocations of both the anterior and posterior ring, as well as combined pelvic ring injury and acetabular fractures. Type IV fractures are more serious injuries associated with life-threatening internal injuries, and are more often associated with progressive growth disturbance and deformity.[15] More recently, this classification was modified by using CT findings in addition to plain radiographs.[26] The original classification was changed into type I, II, III-A, III-B, and IV. The difference between type III-A and III-B is that, in addition to an anterior ring injury, there is also a posterior ring fracture in type III-B.

Pediatric patients with closed triradiate cartilage are considered to be skeletally mature and therefore pelvic fractures in this group should be classified using the same system used in adult injuries, the Tile and Pennal classification system, later adopted by the Arbeitsgemeinschaft für Osteosynthesefragen/Orthopaedic Trauma Association (AO/OTA) classification system for pelvic fractures.[27] Young and Burgess later modified this classification system to add subclassifications based on increasing amounts of force with

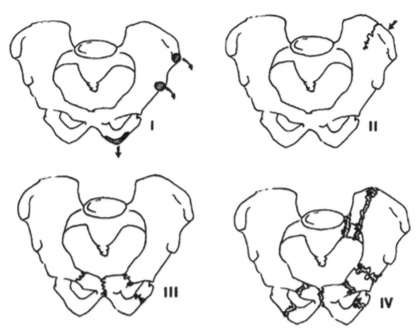

Fig. 3. The Torode and Zieg[15] classification is commonly used for pediatric pelvic fractures. Type I fractures are avulsions of bony insertions of muscles attaching to the pelvis. Type II are iliac wing fractures. Type III fractures involve the pubic rami or a pubic symphysis disruption, which may not disrupt the posterior pelvic ring. Type IV fractures are combined fractures or disruptions of the anterior and posterior pelvic ring or acetabulum and result in pelvic instability. (*From* Torode I, Zieg D. Pelvic fractures in children. J Pediatr Orthop 1985;5(1):76–84; with permission.)

resultant increased disruption of the pelvic ring.[28] They also added a combined injury mechanism as a fourth class of pelvic ring disruption. This classification is important because the subgroups have different associated injury patterns, blood transfusion requirements, and mortalities. Furthermore, it helps guides treatment. Although this classification system does not specifically differentiate adults from children, it is applicable to skeletally mature adolescents, and in a skeletally mature adolescent the Tile and Pennal/AO/OTA system or the Young and Burgess system is more commonly used.

Diagnostic Imaging

Standard trauma films include an AP radiograph of the pelvis in addition to the lateral cervical spine and chest radiographs. Some trauma centers have stopped obtaining initial radiographs and use standard full-body screening CT scan instead.[29,30] The normal pubic symphysis in very young children is 10-mm to 12-mm wide, whereas in adult patients the width of the symphysis is 2 to 4 mm.[31]

Some clinicians have questioned the utility of regularly obtaining a CT scan in pediatric pelvic fractures, given the risks of radiation in pediatric patients and the question of whether or not CT

scans result in a change of management. The addition of CT scans to standard AP pelvis radiographs in 62 patients who sustained pelvic fractures at a level I pediatric trauma center changed the classification in 9 patients (15%) and definitive management in 2 patients (3%).[32] Given that most patients with trauma require CT scans to rule out associated head, thoracic, abdominal and pelvic visceral, and spinal injuries, CT scans should be obtained for any pediatric patient with suspected instability or significant anterior disruption, or when posterior ring disruption is suspected based on plain films. Acetabular fractures merit a CT scan to fully evaluate the articular surface. In addition, standard inlet and outlet views or Judet radiographic views are performed in pelvic and acetabular fractures respectively. CT scans are typically not necessary for apophyseal avulsion fractures that occur from low-energy mechanisms.

In young children, in whom much of the pelvis is not ossified, and if there is a high index of suspicion but no fracture is clearly seen on radiographs, the more advanced imaging of choice is magnetic resonance imaging (MRI), which is most sensitive at showing the degree of soft tissue disruption and displacement, including nonossified portions of the acetabulum (**Fig. 4**).[33,34]

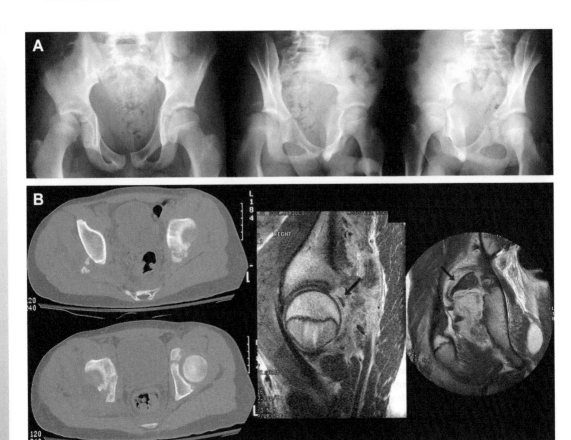

Fig. 4. (*A*) AP, obturator oblique, and iliac oblique pelvic radiographs of an 11-year-old boy who fell while walking on stairs; radiographs show a right posterior hip fracture-dislocation. The small lucent area proximal to the femoral head corresponds with the affected posterior wall. Neither the size of the fragment nor the need for its internal fixation can be determined using plain radiographs because of the significant unossified bone present in the skeletally immature acetabulum. (*B*) Axial CT images (*left*) showing the affected right hip and contralateral hip. The ossification nuclei of the left acetabulum posterior wall are seen. On the right acetabulum, only small ossified fragments are evident. Sagittal MRI cartilage-specific pulse sequence (*right images*) show a 75% posterior wall involvement compared with the contralateral noninjured side. The black arrows point to a large posterior wall fragment, displaced vertically. (*C*) Through a Kocher-Langenbeck approach, the right hip joint was exposed. The posterior wall fragment measured 4 cm × 3 cm, and comprised the whole posterior coverage of the femoral head (*black arrow*). A postoperative AP radiograph shows a concentric and stable reduction of the right hip. The posterior wall of the acetabulum was reconstructed using a 3.5 pelvic reconstruction plate and a one-third tubular spring plate. (*D*) AP and Judet radiographs at 3.5 years show a healed posterior wall fracture with excellent maintenance of joint space and fixation and Brooker grade II heterotopic ossification. (*E*) AP and lateral radiographs at 5.5 years with maintenance of joint space. The patient resumed all preinjury activities, and reported complete resolution of pain, participating in regular wilderness camps and hiking. (*From* Rubel IF, Kloen P, Potter HG, et al. MRI assessment of the posterior acetabular wall fracture in traumatic dislocation of the hip in children. Pediatr Radiol 2002;32(6):435–9; with permission.)

Pelvic Fractures: Treatment

In the past, nonoperative treatment was recommended for the same reasons it is often the treatment of choice in skeletally immature extremity fractures: immature bone and cartilage have the ability to remodel. It was also thought that iatrogenic injury to the triradiate cartilage and other ossification centers during the operative procedure would result in growth arrest.[3,35]

Pelvic fractures: nonoperative indications and management

Nonoperative treatment of skeletally immature pelvic fractures or ring disruptions is indicated for minimally displaced Torode and Zieg[15] type I avulsion fractures, type II iliac wing fractures that do not extend into the dome of the acetabulum, and most type III fractures without significant displacement or signs of instability. Straddle fractures, characterized by bilateral superior and inferior

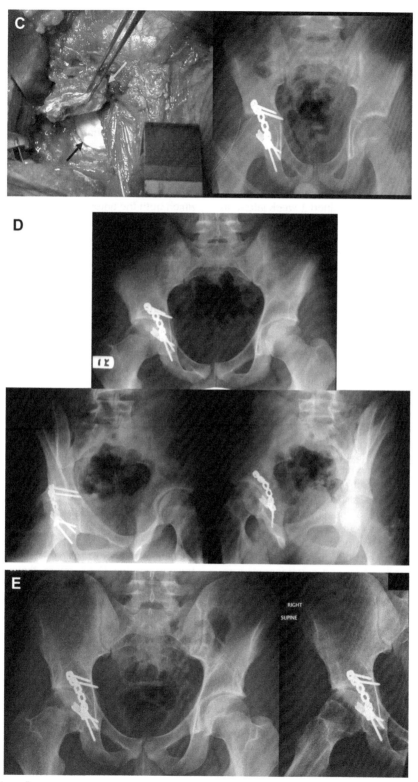

Fig. 4. (*continued*).

pubic rami fractures, considered type IV injuries, are generally treated nonoperatively because only the anterior ring is disrupted. Although past methods of nonoperative treatment have included bed rest, skeletal traction, pelvic sling, and spica cast immobilization, these methods have fallen out of favor because they tend to interfere with early rehabilitation and mobilization, especially in patients with polytrauma with multiorgan system injuries, and risks of prolonged bed rest outweigh the benefit to fracture immobilization and stability. Therefore the patient is kept non–weight bearing on the affected side(s) initially. Repeat radiographs of the pelvis should be obtained 1 week later and followed on a weekly basis for signs of displacement until callus has begun to form, at which point the patient can be progressed to partial weight bearing and rehabilitation, and isometric muscle strengthening begun. The period of non–weight bearing is usually short, because by 2 weeks after injury most skeletally immature pelvic fractures show radiographic evidence of callus formation. Fracture healing can be expected by 4 to 6 weeks, at which time the patient can be advanced to weight bearing as tolerated. Radiographs should be obtained every few months in the year following injury to monitor for any signs of growth arrest.

Pelvic fractures: operative indications

Available evidence suggests that unstable and displaced pelvic fractures in pediatric patients have poor functional and clinical outcomes if treated nonoperatively.[36–38] Schwarz and colleagues[36] reported on 17 patients, all less than 12 years old at the time of injury, who sustained unstable pelvic fractures that were treated nonoperatively, and by 2 years all showed poor clinical results, with various degrees of growth arrest and pain. Smith and colleagues,[37] performed a retrospective review of 20 patients with open triradiate cartilage who were treated for an unstable pelvic fracture. Pelvic asymmetry did not remodel in these children, and pelvic asymmetry greater than 1 cm was associated with compensatory scoliosis, low back pain, sacroiliac pain, and a Trendelenburg sign. The investigators recommended operative treatment of all unstable pelvic fractures with greater than 1 cm of asymmetry to reduce long-term morbidity. Blasier and colleagues[39] proposed the following indications for operative fixation in pediatric pelvic fractures: to allow better wound care in open fractures, to control hemorrhage during resuscitation, to allow earlier mobilization and ease nursing care, to prevent deformity, and to improve overall patient care in patients with polytrauma. The best available evidence leads to the following conclusions: pelvic fractures that are unstable or displaced significantly merit operative reduction and fixation, regardless of the patient's age or skeletal maturity.

In skeletally immature patients with pelvic fractures, the injuries that are treated with surgery are mostly Torode and Zieg[15] type IV injuries, in which part of the pelvic ring is disrupted and unstable. Pelvic instability is defined by displacement of the pelvic ring that occurs with normal weight bearing.[24] Displacement that results in pelvic asymmetry of greater than 1 cm is considered significant and should be corrected.[37] Specific indications include the equivalent of Tile C injuries in which both the anterior and posterior ring are disrupted, displaced vertical sacral fractures or sacroiliac dislocations in which the posterior ring is disrupted and unstable, and displaced iliac wing fractures that extend into the sacroiliac joint or the acetabulum. In these cases, the specific type of operative treatment depends on the injury pattern and the overall medical stability of the patient. The goals of surgery are anatomic reduction and stable fixation that attempts to avoid violation of growth centers as far as possible.

Operative treatment of the pelvic ring: open reduction and internal fixation versus external fixation

Whether to primarily use closed reduction and external fixation versus open reduction and internal fixation (ORIF) of the pelvis in skeletally immature patients as a definitive treatment is a matter of debate. ORIF of the pubic symphysis is a straightforward procedure and has been described for children as young as 3 years of age.[40] However, in children, the pubic symphysis has physes bilaterally, and a plate placed over the symphysis necessitates removal to allow increasing growth of the anterior ring. Furthermore, the surgeon should leave as small a footprint as possible in order to not violate the growing physes at the symphysis. Often in children, pubic symphysis disruption occurs not though the fibrocartilage of the symphysis but through the physis itself on one or both sides at the symphysis, just as in a Salter-Harris type of injury of long bones.[41] Because of the concern for iatrogenic physeal injury at the symphysis and the necessity for later implant removal, we reserve internal fixation of the pubic symphysis in skeletally immature patients in cases when the anterior ring cannot be reduced acceptably under closed means with external fixation. Suturing of the symphysis can alternatively be performed instead of plate and screws and may obviate implant removal at a later date. External fixation is indicated for patients with open pelvic fractures and in polytrauma situations.[42]

Technical Considerations in Pelvic Ring Surgery

Anterior pelvic ring

External fixation The location of the physes and apophyses are identified on standard radiographs. The size, type, number, location, and configuration of pins can vary with the age of the child and injury pattern. Only 1 pin on each side of the pelvis is usually necessary in children if using iliac wing or supra-acetabular pins. Supra-acetabular (anteroinferior) pins have been shown to be biomechanically stronger than iliac crest (anterosuperior) pins in adult pelvic bones.[43] With image intensification orientation in the proper plane, supra-acetabular pins should not risk violation of the triradiate cartilage, which lies caudal to the path of the supra-acetabular pin.[31] They do violate the apophysis of the anterior inferior iliac spine; however, this has no known clinical significance (**Fig. 5**). Iliac crest pins alternatively can be used but this requires violation of the iliac wing apophysis and risks growth arrest of the iliac wing, which may have an effect on the abdominal muscles that insert on the iliac wing. In children younger than 8 years old, smaller-sized 4-mm smooth pins can be used.[44] In children more than 8 years old, smooth 5-mm Steinmann pins can be used. If placed into the iliac crests, a combination of palpation and fluoroscopic imaging is used. Smooth pins are used instead of standard threaded Steinmann pins in order to decrease the risk of iatrogenic growth arrest of the apophysis.[42] For supra-acetabular pin placement, the pins are placed using obturator oblique views for the starting point and trajectory, and the iliac oblique view to judge depth, keeping in mind the importance of staying in bone, cephalad to the hip joint and triradiate cartilage.[45] Once pins have been placed on both sides of the pelvis, the reduction and frame are applied in standard fashion. Weekly radiographs should be checked to ensure that there is no displacement and the external fixator can be removed when there is abundant callus formation on radiographs, which is usually by 4 weeks in this population.[31]

Posterior pelvic ring

Posterior fixation of the pelvic ring is indicated in the presence of a displaced sacral fracture, sacroiliac joint dislocation, or a displaced posterior iliac wing fracture with concomitant anterior ring disruption.[24] Previous studies have shown a high incidence of pelvic asymmetry, pain, and disability if displaced posterior pelvic ring injuries in children are treated nonoperatively or not addressed with direct posterior fixation.[46] When reduction of the anterior ring either via closed or open means does not indirectly reduce an unstable posterior ring disruption adequately, the Ganz pelvic C-clamp can be used to reduce sacroiliac joint disruption.[47] If this is not possible, then open reduction may be necessary. Operative approach to reduction and fixation depends on the location of the posterior ring fracture, amount of displacement, as well as other injury factors, such as amount of soft tissue injury posteriorly. These are the same considerations as in adults with similar injury patterns.

For posterior ring injuries that can be adequately reduced through closed methods, percutaneous sacroiliac screw fixation is preferred. Preoperative CT scan should be analyzed for templating and to fully delineate the safe corridor of screw passage at S1 and S2. Some investigators have advocated placing sacroiliac screws percutaneously in the CT scanner under local anesthesia and sedation.[48] Others have considered this an ideal method for pediatric patients given that CT-guided screw placement allows passage of screws safely through a smaller corridor.[24] With the introduction of intraoperative CT scans such as the O-arm (Medtronic Corporation), computer navigation may be more commonly used to perform screw

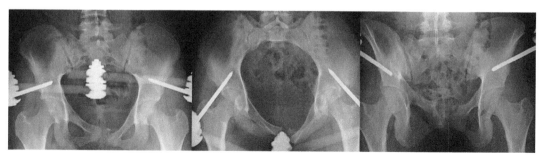

Fig. 5. Supra-acetabular pins used for external fixation of an anterior-posterior pelvic ring injury in a skeletally mature adolescent. The triradiate cartilage is closed but the iliac apophyses remain open so supra-acetabular pins were preferred for fixation.

placement while in the operating room. Sacroiliac screw size should be based on the diameter and length of the safe corridor on preoperative CT scan (**Fig. 6**). Percutaneous placement of sacroiliac screws has been described in a child as young as 20 months old.[49] The screw(s) should be removed at 6 months after surgery to prevent bony overgrowth, growth arrest, and deformity.

ACETABULAR FRACTURES
Epidemiology

Acetabular fractures account for between 4% and 20% of all pediatric pelvic fractures.[8,50–52] Most pediatric acetabular fractures are in adolescents, with few reported at less than 10 years of age.[53]

Classification

The Watts[3] classification is based on radiographs and is centered on hip joint stability. Type I are small fragments associated with a hip dislocation. Type II are linear fractures associated with pelvic fractures and are usually stable injuries. Type III are linear fractures with associated hip joint instability. Type IV fractures occur with central fracture-dislocations of the hip. In skeletally mature patients in whom the triradiate cartilage has closed, the standard classification system of Letournel and Judet[54] is used.

Diagnostic Imaging

Standard radiographs are obtained including Judet views, followed by CT scan to delineate the full extent and pattern of injury. Radiographs of the acetabulum tend to underestimate the size of posterior wall fractures because of the cartilaginous portion of the acetabulum that is not yet ossified.[34] MRI is especially useful to evaluate nonosseous injury to the acetabulum, including the joint surface, nonossified cartilage and labrum, and triradiate cartilage.

Treatment

After standard trauma evaluation, the most urgent situation specific to an acetabular fracture is a concomitant hip dislocation, which should be reduced urgently to try to preserve the blood supply to the femoral head. This reduction can be performed in the emergency department under conscious sedation with strong muscle relaxation. Postreduction radiographs should be obtained afterward and, if any residual incongruency of the hip joint is seen, CT scan followed possibly by MRI to look for bony fragments in the joint or soft tissue labrum serving as mechanical blocks to reduction. In fracture-dislocations, skeletal traction can be applied to hold the joint reduced until definitive operative fixation and to take pressure off cartilage in the presence of displaced fragments. In skeletally mature adolescents who have closed triradiate cartilages, acetabular fractures are treated using the same algorithm and methods as in adult patients. However, acetabular fracture healing is faster than in adults. In skeletally immature patients, there is extensive callus within 2 weeks that can complicate reduction and fixation. Also in skeletally immature patients, implants are typically removed 6 to 18 months after surgery to prevent growth disturbance.

Nonoperative treatment

If nonoperative treatment is indicated, patients should be kept non–weight bearing on the affected leg until 6 to 8 weeks after injury and radiographic evidence of healing. They should be followed with radiographs in the first year and until skeletal maturity if there is any concern for growth arrest.[51,55] Heeg and colleagues[53] reported on 29 pediatric patients ranging in age from 2 to 16 years who sustained acetabular fractures not involving the triradiate cartilage. Patients who had minimal displacement of the fracture, a concentric hip after reduction of a fracture-dislocation, or a fracture

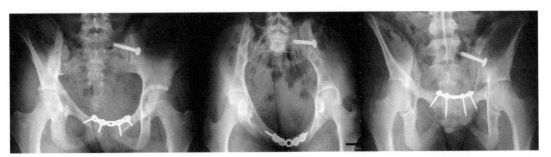

Fig. 6. Skeletally mature adolescent with pubic symphysis and left sacroiliac joint disruption treated with pubic symphysis ORIF and left posterior sacroiliac percutaneous screw placement. The screw is short because the dysmorphic first sacral segment does not allow safe passage for a longer screw.

with severe comminution but little displacement were treated nonoperatively. Better functional outcome scores were associated with minimal displacement and small fragments.

Operative treatment

There are few outcome data on ORIF of acetabular fractures in skeletally immature patients because of the rarity of the injury, but multiple case reports and series have shown that skeletally immature patients have good outcomes with ORIF of appropriately indicated fractures.[33,34,56] Indications for operative treatment of acetabular fractures not involving the triradiate cartilage are displacement of greater than 2 mm of the articular surface as seen on MRI, which is the most sensitive imaging test; an incongruous hip joint after a fracture-dislocation and subsequent reduction; incarcerated fragments of bone or soft tissue in the hip joint; an open acetabular fracture; and an acetabular fracture associated with a displaced pelvic fracture.

The operative approach to an acetabular fracture in pediatric patients is essentially the same as in that of adults, dictated by the fracture pattern. For primarily posteriorly based fracture patterns, a Kocher-Langenbeck approach is used. The blood supply to the femoral head should be protected and preserved. Depending on the size of the patient, fixation can be used with 2.0-mm, 2.4-mm, 2.7-mm, or 3.5-mm screws and reconstruction plates. The posterior wall fragment is often larger than expected (**Fig. 7**).[34] In children, the periosteum of the pelvis is thicker than in adults and often the fracture is an incomplete greenstick type that can be reduced without completion. Pure soft tissue and cartilaginous unossified injuries can be repaired with suture anchors to intact acetabulum in an anatomic fashion. If fragments are too small to be fixated, they can be excised in order to allow a concentric reduction but only if the hip has been taken through a stable range of motion once the fragments and tissue have been removed from the joint. For anterior-based fracture patterns the classic ilioinguinal or Stoppa approach can be used.[57]

After surgery, patients are kept toe-touch weight bearing with posterior precautions when the Kocher-Langenbeck is used. Implants usually require removal 6 to 12 months after surgery in children with significant growth remaining to prevent growth disturbance and difficulty with removal once they become enveloped within new bone.

Triradiate injuries

Triradiate injuries are less common than nonphyseal acetabular fractures, and few have been reported in the literature.[53]

Triradiate injuries: classification

Bucholz and colleagues[8] introduced a classification system specifically for triradiate injuries in skeletally immature patients based on the Salter-Harris type of injury patterns in a small series of patients. Type I triradiate injuries are simple fractures through the physis. Type II go through the physis and then extend into a noncartilaginous region of a ramus, pelvic brim, or iliac wing causing a Thurston Holland fragment similar to that seen in distal tibia physeal fractures. Type V injuries are crush injuries to the triradiate cartilage, can easily be missed on standard radiographs, and are thought to have the highest risk of growth arrest and subsequent deformity. Type I and II fractures are thought to be caused by shearing mechanisms, whereas type V injuries are caused by an impaction or crush injury.

Triradiate injuries: treatment and outcomes

Evidence for treatment of triradiate injuries in skeletally immature patients is lacking because of the rarity of these injuries.[58] In the past, nonoperative treatment of triradiate injuries was recommended.[59] Bucholz and colleagues'[8] original description of the triradiate physeal classification concerned 9 patients who sustained triradiate injuries. In the 4 patients with type V crush injuries, all experienced growth arrest of the triradiate cartilage, whereas 3 of 4 patients with a type I injury did not, and the 1 patient with a type II injury did not.[8] Trousdale and Ganz[6] reported on 5 patients who sustained acetabular fractures before skeletal maturity and developed severe posttraumatic acetabular dysplasia, 4 of whom required corrective osteotomies as adults.[6] Heeg and colleagues[59] reported on 2 patients with Bucholz type I injuries, 1 patient with a type II injury, and 3 patients with type V crush injury. All type I and type II injuries were treated nonoperatively and had satisfactory radiographic and functional outcomes. However, the 3 type V crush injuries resulted in growth arrest and posttraumatic dysplasia requiring reconstructive osteotomies. The same group had reported on 4 patients with triradiate injuries, all of whom experienced concomitant sacroiliac joint disruption.[51] One patient with a type I injury and associated sacroiliac disruption went on to develop a normal hip joint but pelvic obliquity and leg length discrepancy caused by the pelvic ring injury. All 3 of the patients who sustained type V injuries had triradiate growth arrest, and 2 of the 3 developed posttraumatic acetabular dysplasia. A case report of a 13-year-old boy who sustained a type I triradiate fracture with minimal displacement treated nonoperatively had no growth arrest and no residual deformity.[60]

496

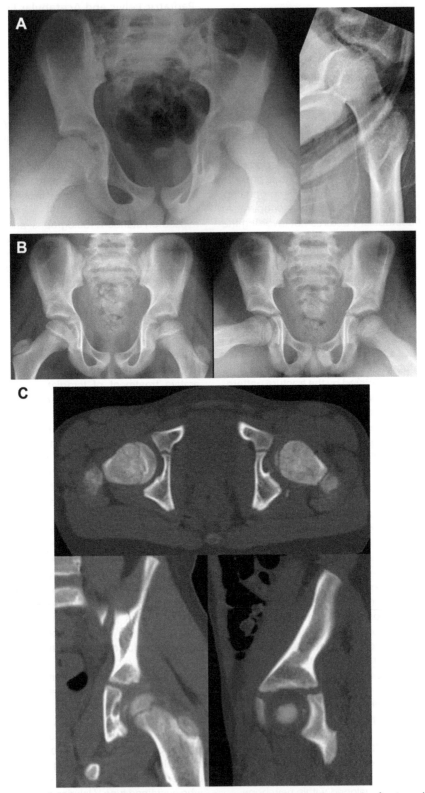

Fig. 7. (A) An 8-year-old boy was tackled while playing football and sustained a posterior fracture-dislocation of his left hip. He was taken to a local hospital where AP and lateral radiographs were obtained. A closed reduction was attempted unsuccessful. He was emergently taken to the operating room for an open reduction of his hip dislocation. (B) Two weeks following injury he presented for a second opinion. AP and lateral radiographs were obtained suggesting slight lateral subluxation of the hip and the possibility of an interarticular fragment within the hip joint. (C) CT imaging was performed, confirming presence of an intraarticular fragment.

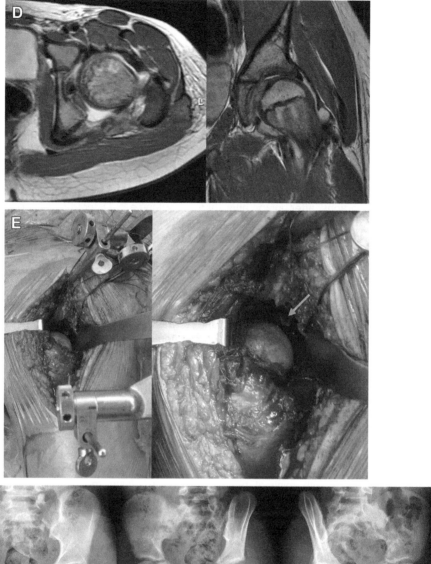

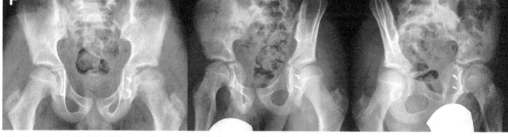

Fig. 7. (*continued*). (*D*) MRI was also used to fully assess the injuries associated with his posterior hip dislocation including the unossified part, the posterior wall fragment, and the cartilage of the femoral head and acetabulum. The MRI imaging showed a posterior wall acetabular fracture with a significant fragment of acetabular cartilage, 1.3 cm in size, interposed in the hip joint along with the attached transverse ligament, all contributing to the observed subluxation of the left hip. A focal, small, high-grade partial-thickness chondral defect to the parafoveal margin of the femoral head was also observed near the intraarticular fragment. (*E*) ORIF was performed expeditiously, on the same day as presentation, to prevent further damage to the hip joint associated with a retained intraarticular fragment (*white arrow*). Through a Kocher-Langenbeck approach, and using a femoral distractor to achieve adequate joint access, the intraarticular fragment was carefully identified and repaired along with the labral and capsular attachment using 2 suture anchors with additional suture repairs of the labrum and hip capsule. (*F*) The patient returned for regular follow-up and healed uneventfully. He last followed up at 2 years following surgery with excellent radiographic results as shown, including maintenance of fixation and joint space.

Sener and colleagues[61] reported on a case of an 8-year-old girl who sustained a sacroiliac joint disruption and concomitant disruption of the triradiate cartilage. The triradiate injury was indirectly reduced once the sacroiliac joint was reduced. However, at 20 months' follow-up, she had developed osseous bridging of the triradiate cartilage and mild coxa valga.

Some investigators have proposed initial nonoperative treatment of all triradiate injuries because of the technical difficulty of initial operative treatment, and recommend instead corrective salvage osteotomy if growth arrest and deformity occurs.[59] Others have advocated observing closely with radiographs after injury and then intervening early to remove osseous bridges if they arise, similar to the technique used in premature long bone physeal closures described by Langenskiold.[62] Dias described resecting a physeal bar in a 3-year-old girl with premature partial closure of the triradiate cartilage from a septic hip in the neonatal period. The iliofemoral approach was used, the bar was drilled out, and an autogenous fat graft was placed into the defect. However, infection recurred, as did the physeal bar.[63] Peterson and Robertson had more success in their case report, describing a 7-year-old boy who 2 years previously had incurred several injuries, including a triradiate injury that had been treated nonoperatively, and went on to develop an osseous bridge and increasing deformity. The investigators used the lateral window of the ilioinguinal approach to remove the physeal bar with minimal periosteal stripping and placed bone wax over the defect. The acetabulum went on to grow and develop normally until it closed slightly prematurely near the end of adolescence.[64]

Some conclusions can be drawn from these small case reports and series on triradiate injuries: type I and type II injuries have a better prognosis than type V injuries; younger patients have a higher likelihood of a poor outcome[8,51,55]; and many of the most severe triradiate injuries are associated with a pelvic ring injury, most often a sacroiliac disruption.[46,51] When the sacroiliac joint is concurrently dislocated, it should be reduced by either open or closed means, at which time the triradiate cartilage may be reduced indirectly. If there is a displaced triradiate injury of greater than 2 mm that is not reducible by closed means, operative intervention through the lateral 1 or 2 windows of the ilioinguinal approach can be used to reduce the pelvic brim, taking care not to disrupt the overlying periosteum and perichondrium.[8,55] Minifragment or small fragment reconstruction plates are used to buttress the

reduction and bridge the triradiate without any screws through it in order not to iatrogenically injure the physes.

COMPLICATIONS

Given the healing potential of the immature skeleton, nonunions after pelvic and acetabular fractures are rare. Malunions do occur and recent evidence suggests that the remodeling potential of the pelvis and acetabulum might not be as good as has been described in the past. Smith and colleagues[37] showed that pelvic asymmetry of more than 1 cm correlates with poor functional outcome.[65] Osteotomy of a posttraumatic pelvic deformity is a possible salvage operation but is technically demanding and there is little evidence for long-term results.[51] Premature closure of the triradiate cartilage or bar formation across the physis, especially in children younger than 10 years, may lead to acetabular dysplasia with the potential for hip subluxation and early posttraumatic arthrosis.[7] Other complications are heterotopic ossification, injuries to the lumbosacral plexus, and urologic injuries.

SUMMARY

Pediatric pelvic and acetabular fractures are rare injuries. The skeletally immature pelvic fracture is a distinct entity from the skeletally mature pelvic fracture. With the exception of avulsion injuries, they are almost always the result of a high-energy injury mechanism. A full trauma protocol should be instituted, having a high index of suspicion for associated life-threatening injuries, including head, thoracic, and abdominal injuries. Most pediatric patients with a pelvic fracture are more likely to die of these associated injuries than of the pelvic fracture.

Treatment of pediatric pelvic and acetabular fractures has largely been based on small case series and case reports. In the past, it was recommended that almost all of these injuries be treated nonoperatively. However, pelvic and acetabular fractures do not all remodel well. Prospective studies are needed to establish optimal treatment guidelines. Until then, in the presence of instability or significant displacement, operative fixation by a pelvic and acetabular fracture specialist should be considered to allow the best possible outcome.

REFERENCES

1. Karunakar MA, Goulet JA, et al. Operative treatment of unstable pediatric pelvis and acetabular fractures. J Pediatr Orthop 2005;25(1):34–8.

2. Silber JS, Flynn JM. Changing patterns of pediatric pelvic fractures with skeletal maturation: implications for classification and management. J Pediatr Orthop 2002;22(1):22–6.

3. Watts HG. Fractures of the pelvis in children. Orthop Clin North Am 1976;7(3):615–24.

4. Delaere O, Dhem A. Prenatal development of the human pelvis and acetabulum. Acta Orthop Belg 1999;65(3):255–60.

5. Ponseti IV. Growth and development of the acetabulum in the normal child. Anatomical, histological, and roentgenographic studies. J Bone Joint Surg Am 1978;60(5):575–85.

6. Trousdale RT, Ganz R. Posttraumatic acetabular dysplasia. Clin Orthop Relat Res 1994;(305):124–32.

7. Rodrigues KF. Injury of the acetabular epiphysis. Injury 1973;4(3):258–60.

8. Bucholz RW, Ezaki M, et al. Injury to the acetabular triradiate physeal cartilage. J Bone Joint Surg Am 1982;64(4):600–9.

9. Delgado-Baeza E, Sanz-Laguna A, et al. Experimental trauma of the triradiate epiphysis of the acetabulum and hip dysplasia. Int Orthop 1991;15(4):335–9.

10. Gepstein R, Weiss RE, et al. Acetabular dysplasia and hip dislocation after selective premature fusion of the triradiate cartilage. An experimental study in rabbits. J Bone Joint Surg Br 1984;66(3):334–6.

11. Demetriades D, Karaiskakis M, et al. Pelvic fractures in pediatric and adult trauma patients: are they different injuries? J Trauma 2003;54(6):1146–51 [discussion: 1151].

12. Spiguel L, Glynn L, et al. Pediatric pelvic fractures: a marker for injury severity. Am Surg 2006;72(6):481–4.

13. Ismail N, Bellemare JF, et al. Death from pelvic fracture: children are different. J Pediatr Surg 1996;31(1):82–5.

14. Grisoni N, Connor S, et al. Pelvic fractures in a pediatric level I trauma center. J Orthop Trauma 2002;16(7):458–63.

15. Torode I, Zieg D. Pelvic fractures in children. J Pediatr Orthop 1985;5(1):76–84.

16. Bond SJ, Gotschall CS, et al. Predictors of abdominal injury in children with pelvic fracture. J Trauma 1991;31(8):1169–73.

17. Dalal SA, Burgess AR, et al. Pelvic fracture in multiple trauma: classification by mechanism is key to pattern of organ injury, resuscitative requirements, and outcome. J Trauma 1989;29(7):981–1000 [discussion: 1000–2].

18. ATLS. Advanced trauma life support. American College of Surgeons. 2008.

19. Holden CP, Holman J, Herman MJ. Pediatric pelvic fractures. J Am Acad Orthop Surg Mar 2007;15(3):172–7.

20. Cerva DS Jr, Mirvis SE, et al. Detection of bleeding in patients with major pelvic fractures: value of contrast-enhanced CT. AJR Am J Roentgenol 1996;166(1):131–5.

21. Pereira SJ, O'Brien DP, et al. Dynamic helical computed tomography scan accurately detects hemorrhage in patients with pelvic fracture. Surgery 2000;128(4):678–85.

22. Stephen DJ, Kreder HJ, et al. Early detection of arterial bleeding in acute pelvic trauma. J Trauma 1999;47(4):638–42.

23. Osborn PM, Smith WR, et al. Direct retroperitoneal pelvic packing versus pelvic angiography: a comparison of two management protocols for haemodynamically unstable pelvic fractures. Injury 2009;40(1):54–60.

24. Smith WR, Oakley M, et al. Pediatric pelvic fractures. J Pediatr Orthop 2004;24(1):130–5.

25. Quinby WC Jr. Fractures of the pelvis and associated injuries in children. J Pediatr Surg 1966;1(4):353–64.

26. Shore BJ, Palmer CS, et al. Pediatric pelvic fracture: a modification of a preexisting classification. J Pediatr Orthop 2012;32(2):162–8.

27. Pennal GF, Tile M, et al. Pelvic disruption: assessment and classification. Clin Orthop Relat Res 1980;(151):12–21.

28. Burgess AR, Eastridge BJ, et al. Pelvic ring disruptions: effective classification system and treatment protocols. J Trauma 1990;30(7):848–56.

29. Guillamondegui OD, Mahboubi S, et al. The utility of the pelvic radiograph in the assessment of pediatric pelvic fractures. J Trauma 2003;55(2):236–9 [discussion: 239–240].

30. Kessel B, Sevi R, et al. Is routine portable pelvic X-ray in stable multiple trauma patients always justified in a high technology era? Injury 2007;38(5):559–63.

31. Schlickewei W, Keck T. Pelvic and acetabular fractures in childhood. Injury 2005;36(Suppl 1):A57–63.

32. Silber JS, Flynn JM, et al. Role of computed tomography in the classification and management of pediatric pelvic fractures. J Pediatr Orthop 2001;21(2):148–51.

33. Hearty T, Swaroop VT, et al. Standard radiographs and computed tomographic scan underestimating pediatric acetabular fracture after traumatic hip dislocation: report of 2 cases. J Orthop Trauma 2011;25(7):e68–73.

34. Rubel IF, Kloen P, et al. MRI assessment of the posterior acetabular wall fracture in traumatic dislocation of the hip in children. Pediatr Radiol 2002;32(6):435–9.

35. Musemeche CA, Fischer RP, et al. Selective management of pediatric pelvic fractures: a conservative approach. J Pediatr Surg 1987;22(6):538–40.

36. Schwarz N, Posch E, et al. Long-term results of unstable pelvic ring fractures in children. Injury 1998; 29(6):431–3.

37. Smith W, Shurnas P, et al. Clinical outcomes of unstable pelvic fractures in skeletally immature patients. J Bone Joint Surg Am 2005;87(11): 2423–31.

38. Upperman JS, Gardner M, et al. Early functional outcome in children with pelvic fractures. J Pediatr Surg 2000;35(6):1002–5.

39. Blasier RD, McAtee J, et al. Disruption of the pelvic ring in pediatric patients. Clin Orthop Relat Res 2000;(376):87–95.

40. Gansslen A, Pohlemann T, et al. Internal osteosynthesis after unstable pelvic ring fracture in a 3-year-old child. Unfallchirurg 1998;101(7):570–3 [in German].

41. Ogden J. Injury to the pelvis and acetabulum in the pediatric patient (the immature skeleton). In: Helfet D, Tile M, Kellam JF, editors. Fractures of the pelvis and acetabulum. Philadelphia: Lippincott Williams & Wilkins; 2007. p. 351–75.

42. Reff RB. The use of external fixation devices in the management of severe lower-extremity trauma and pelvic injuries in children. Clin Orthop Relat Res 1984;(188):21–33.

43. Kim WY, Hearn TC, et al. Effect of pin location on stability of pelvic external fixation. Clin Orthop Relat Res 1999;(361):237–44.

44. Podeszwa D, Wilson P. Pelvic and acetabular fractures. In: Herring J, editor. Tachdjian's pediatric orthopaedics. Philadelphia: Saunders; 2007. p. 3.

45. Haidukewych GJ, Kumar S, et al. Placement of half-pins for supra-acetabular external fixation: an anatomic study. Clin Orthop Relat Res 2003;(411): 269–73.

46. Heeg M, Klasen HJ. Long-term outcome of sacroiliac disruptions in children. J Pediatr Orthop 1997;17(3):337–41.

47. Holt GE, Mencio GA. Pelvic C-clamp in a pediatric patient. J Orthop Trauma 2003;17(7):525–7.

48. Ziran BH, Smith WR, et al. Iliosacral screw fixation of the posterior pelvic ring using local anaesthesia and computerised tomography. J Bone Joint Surg Br 2003;85(3):411–8.

49. Starr AJ, Ortega G, et al. Management of an unstable pelvic ring disruption in a 20-month-old patient. J Orthop Trauma 2009;23(2):159–62.

50. Bryan WJ, Tullos HS. Pediatric pelvic fractures: review of 52 patients. J Trauma 1979;19(11):799–805.

51. Heeg M, Visser JD, et al. Injuries of the acetabular triradiate cartilage and sacroiliac joint. J Bone Joint Surg Br 1988;70(1):34–7.

52. Reed MH. Pelvic fractures in children. J Can Assoc Radiol 1976;27(4):255–61.

53. Heeg M, de Ridder VA, et al. Acetabular fractures in children and adolescents. Clin Orthop Relat Res 2000;(376):80–6.

54. Letournel E, Judet R. Fractures of the acetabulum. New York: Springer-Verlag; 1993.

55. Scuderi G, Bronson MJ. Triradiate cartilage injury. Report of two cases and review of the literature. Clin Orthop Relat Res 1987;(217):179–89.

56. Brooks E, Rosman M. Central fracture-dislocation of the hip in a child. J Trauma 1988;28(11):1590–2.

57. Elmadag M, Acar MA. A modified Stoppa (technique) approach for treatment of pediatric acetabular fractures. Case Rep Orthop 2013;2013:478131.

58. Liporace FA, Ong B, et al. Development and injury of the triradiate cartilage with its effects on acetabular development: review of the literature. J Trauma 2003;54(6):1245–9.

59. Heeg M, Klasen HJ, et al. Acetabular fractures in children and adolescents. J Bone Joint Surg Br 1989;71(3):418–21.

60. McDonnell M, Schachter AK, et al. Acetabular fracture through the triradiate cartilage after low-energy trauma. J Orthop Trauma 2007;21(7): 495–8.

61. Sener M, Karapinar H, et al. Fracture dislocation of sacroiliac joint associated with triradiate cartilage injury in a child: a case report. J Pediatr Orthop B 2008;17(2):65–8.

62. Langenskiold A. An operation for partial closure of an epiphysial plate in children, and its experimental basis. J Bone Joint Surg Br 1975;57(3): 325–30.

63. Dias L, Tachdjian MO, et al. Premature closure of the triradiate cartilage. Report of a case. J Bone Joint Surg Br 1980;62B(1):46–8.

64. Peterson HA, Robertson RC. Premature partial closure of the triradiate cartilage treated with excision of a physical osseous bar. Case report with a fourteen-year follow-up. J Bone Joint Surg Am 1997;79(5):767–70.

65. Keshishyan RA, Rozinov VM, et al. Pelvic polyfractures in children. Radiographic diagnosis and treatment. Clin Orthop Relat Res 1995;(320): 28–33.

Pediatric Orthopaedics

Preface
Pediatric Orthopaedics

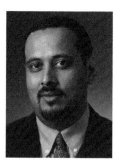

Shital N. Parikh, MD
Editor

Early-onset scoliosis is defined as scoliosis of any cause in children younger than five years of age. Such deformities at an early age can have a deleterious effect on the development of the immature skeleton and cardiopulmonary system. The goal of treatment is to control or correct these deformities. Adultlike fusion of multiple spinal segments has been used in the past but is considered undesirable in this age group due to the permanent restrictions in growth that accompany it. Several recent developments have led to progressive improvement in the management of this condition. Like Ponseti clubfoot casting, serial casting for early-onset scoliosis, as popularized by Mehta, has shown promising results, especially when the treatment is started early. This does involve, however, motivation and casting skills on the part of the physician and "buying in" by the family. Surgical options for patients who progress despite casting or for those who are not candidates for casting include distraction-based growing rods or expansion thoracoplasty, compression-based anterior tether, or guided-growth systems. Sturm and colleagues review the recent advances in the field of early-onset scoliosis and discuss the pros and cons of all different treatment options. These current trends in management and their results are important to understand to advance toward the ultimate goal of fusionless correction of early-onset scoliosis.

Shital N. Parikh, MD
Pediatric Orthopaedic Sports Medicine
Cincinnati Children's Hospital Medical Center
University of Cincinnati School of Medicine
530 Walnut Street
Philadelphia, PA 19106, USA

E-mail address:
Shital.Parikh@cchmc.org

orthopedic.theclinics.com

Recent Advances in the Management of Early Onset Scoliosis

Peter F. Sturm, MD[a,*], Jennifer M. Anadio, MA[a],
Ozgur Dede, MD[a,b]

KEYWORDS

- Early onset scoliosis • Casting • Growing rods • Shila • Nitinol staple • Expansion thoracoplasty

KEY POINTS

- Current literature supports the use of serial casting for most progressive early onset spinal deformities as either a definitive or a surgical delay treatment.
- If and when surgery is required for early onset scoliosis treatment, the most commonly used system is growing rods, but this may change in the future with other viable options undergoing research, including magnetically controlled growing rods, nitinol staples, tethering, and the Shilla procedure.
- Expansion thoracoplasty is generally recommended for patients with thoracic insufficiency syndrome.
- Future goals include scoliosis treatment methods that involve less complications and to successfully treat patients with "fusionless" methods.

INTRODUCTION

Early onset scoliosis (EOS), as defined by Dickson,[1] is severe spinal deformity of any cause affecting children less than 5 years of age. This definition is different from the standard definition of infantile scoliosis, taking into consideration the unique and profound respiratory consequences associated with moderate to severe curves in this age group. Spinal growth peaks by the age of 5; however, pulmonary development continues until the age of 8.[2,3] A severe scoliotic spine in this young population impedes the multiplication of pulmonary alveoli, which are supposed to reach near adult numbers (300 million) by 8 years of age, thus restricting overall pulmonary development.[4]

EOS curves can be broadly categorized based on their cause, including idiopathic, neuromuscular, syndromic, and congenital. Idiopathic scoliosis is a diagnosis of exclusion, defined as scoliosis that is not associated with any other abnormality. Neuromuscular scoliosis patients have innate abnormalities of the neuromuscular system. Common examples are cerebral palsy, spinal muscular atrophy, and muscular dystrophies. Syndromic scoliosis is a broad term that defines scoliotic curves associated with syndromes such as Marfan, Ehlers-Danlos, Pierre Robin, and velocardiofacial syndromes. Congenital scoliosis is classified either by a failure of vertebral formation or by segmentation. If left untreated, EOS curves can likely cause cosmetic disfigurement, rib-cage

Disclosures: None.
[a] Department of Pediatric Orthopaedic Surgery, Cincinnati Children's Hospital Medical Center, 3333 Burnet Avenue, MLC 2017, Cincinnati, OH 45229, USA; [b] Department of Orthopaedic Surgery, Children's Hospital of Pittsburgh of University of Pittsburgh Medical Center, Pittsburgh, PA 15224, USA
* Corresponding author. 3333 Burnet Avenue, MLC 2017, Cincinnati, OH 45229.
E-mail address: Peter.Sturm@cchmc.org

Orthop Clin N Am 45 (2014) 501–514
http://dx.doi.org/10.1016/j.ocl.2014.06.010

orthopedic.theclinics.com

distortion, dyspnea, and cardiorespiratory failure in early adult life.[5]

The previous standard of care for these children was early definitive anterior and posterior spinal fusion. Complications of this method, including crank shaft phenomenon and thoracic insufficiency, led to very modest results.[6] Today "a short but straight spine" is no longer considered to be a good outcome for the treatment of EOS[7] and providers have moved toward strategies for avoiding curve progression while still allowing for spine and thorax growth, and unrestricted multiplication of the pulmonary alveoli.[5,6] The quest for "fusionless scoliosis correction" started to gain momentum in the previous decade.[8] Nonsurgical and surgical treatment options continue to evolve as the understanding of the pathologic abnormality continues to improve and results of current treatment methods become available.[9]

CURRENT TREATMENT AND TRENDS

Mehta[10] developed a method to distinguish progressive from spontaneously resolving EOS, creating a means of early detection of curves that requirement treatment. This method uses the rib vertebral angle of difference (RVAD) between the apical vertebra and the corresponding concave and convex side ribs. The RVAD in resolving curves is typically less than 20° on initial radiograph and decreases on subsequent radiographs taken 2 or 3 months apart. The RVAD in progressive curves is typically greater than 20° on initial radiograph and either remains unchanged or increases on subsequent radiographs. In Mehta's study,[10] this pattern was noted in 83% of children with progressive scoliosis. Following this method, those patients who are diagnosed with progressive EOS should begin treatment immediately.

Nonoperative Treatment

Currently, the only widely accepted nonoperative management method that has shown effectiveness in the EOS population is serial casting. Bracing is often used as an adjunct to serial casting, but there is not enough evidence to support the use of bracing as a sole management method. A retrospective review by Smith and colleagues[11] showed that bracing was the only treatment (compared with casting and expansion thoracoplasty [ET]) in their study that did not provide adequate curve control. In addition, the authors note that the patients for whom bracing treatment was effective had spontaneously resolving curves that may have improved despite bracing due to their significantly smaller RVAD and Cobb measurements. Another consideration in bracing

treatment is brace-wear compliance. There is no study specifically on compliance in EOS patients, but compliance has been shown to be challenging in other patient populations; it may be inferred that the EOS population would encounter some of the same issues.[11]

In contrast to bracing reports in the EOS population, casting has been thoroughly evaluated and has shown very good results. There are numerous earlier reports of casting present in orthopedic literature, but the serial corrective casting technique for EOS, as used today, was first described by Cotrel and Morel in 1964.[12] Forty years passed until results from this technique were reported and gained acceptance as a definitive treatment method for certain deformities.[10] As subsequent clinical results became available, serial casting became a well-accepted method for the management of EOS as both a definitive treatment and a surgical delay tactic.[13,14]

Serial casting harnesses the patient's own growth as a corrective force. An infant grows almost twice as fast during their first year, and as fast during their second year as adolescents do during their growth spurt. Mehta[10] reports that harnessing the rigorous growth of infancy can straighten progressive curves that would otherwise develop into severe deformities. Historically, Risser casting was a popular method of scoliosis casting but, due to chest and abdominal expansion restriction and decreased chest wall compliance, it has since become nearly extinct in this capacity. Modern forms of casting are referred to as EDF casting: elongation, derotation, and flexion. Spinal deformities are 3-dimensional (3D) deformities, and EDF casts are able to address all dimensions. During the casting application, the patient is put in traction to "elongate" and gently derotate the spinal deformity; the corrected position is then held by the applied cast. Risser casts were only able to straighten the spine in one plane, allowing the deformity continued development. Mehta[10] explains that the shape of an organ or part determines the direction of its continued growth; "if the direction remains constant, growth will simply perpetuate and enlarge its existing shape." If a curved spine is left untreated, it will grow more curved, but with the external force of the cast, especially during a period of rapid growth, the spine will continue to grow in the corrected position and the final shape can be altered. In addition, EDF casts use a large "mushroom"-shaped cutout on the front of the cast to allow for proper chest expansion, as well as a smaller cutout on the back over the concavity to allow for rib-cage expansion, which better aligns the spine and corrects rotation (**Fig. 1**).

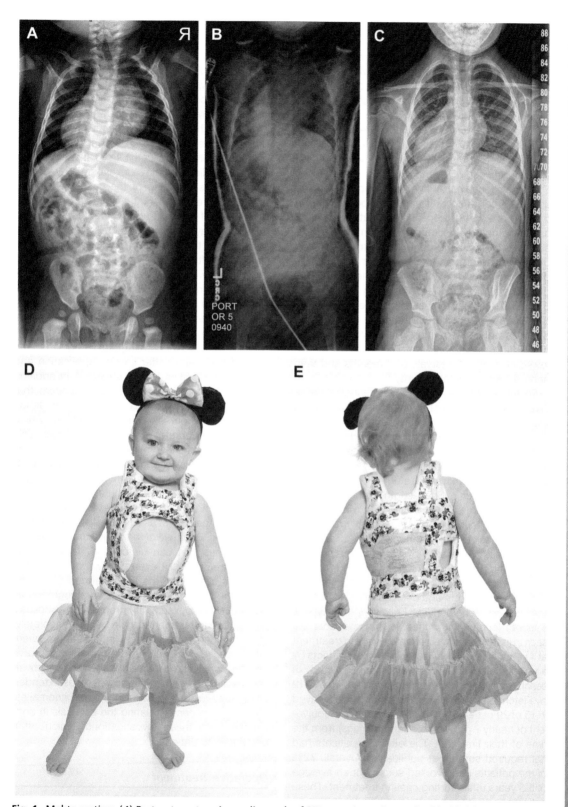

Fig. 1. Mehta casting. (*A*) Pretreatment supine radiograph of 37° curve in an 8-month-old girl. (*B*) Radiograph of patient in applied cast. (*C*) Radiograph of 13° curve in same patient at 37 months from initial cast. (*D*) Clinical photo of patient in cast (front). (*E*) Clinical photo of patient in cast (back).

For those patients whose scoliosis is completely or "definitively" corrected via serial casting, success is correlated with treatment beginning during the first 2 years of rapid growth (ie, before the age of 2). In Mehta's study,[10] all curves in patients (with syndromic or idiopathic scoliosis) who began casting between 15 and 21 months old with Cobb angles between 27° and 35° resolved; conversely, curves in patients who began their treatment between 27 and 34 months old with Cobb angles between 47° and 53° did not resolve. Further evidence has shown that idiopathic curves up to 60° can resolve if treatment begins before the age of 2.[13] In the definitive treatment group, casting is usually discontinued when radiographs show restoration of rib-cage symmetry, derotation of apical vertebra, and complete, or nearly complete, correction of the curve. These patients are generally prescribed a bracing regimen for 6 months to a year to ensure that the spine stabilizes in its new position. If the spine continues to show complete correction, brace wear may be ceased at this time and the patient should be followed clinically at intervals of 6 months and then annually until skeletal maturity.[10]

For those patients whose curves cannot be definitively treated with serial casting, this treatment can still serve as a means to delay surgical intervention and its associated complications, including wound-healing problems, infection, premature fusion, implant failure, and many others.[13,15] Furthermore, the concept of "diminished returns," or the progressive decrease in spinal length gained at each lengthening surgery, is of great concern in these patients. This phenomenon is presumably related to spinal autofusion and, according to Sankar and colleagues,[16] is especially notable after the seventh lengthening procedure. Their study found that the average distraction gained at the initial lengthening surgery was 1.04 cm and decreased to 0.41 cm by the seventh lengthening. Following the typical 6-month lengthening schedule, these effects are seen in just 3.5 years. A patient beginning treatment at 4 years of age would experience these effects by age of 7, before full lung development. In a study of serial casting outcomes conducted in 2012 by Fletcher and colleagues,[15] surgery was delayed in 15 of 29 patients by 39 ± 25 months (the equivalent of nearly 7 growing rod lengthenings) from the time of their first cast. The other 14 patients had not required surgery at publication. Overall, 72% of the patients had avoided surgery at an average of 5.5 years after starting casting treatment. These patients had both congenital and neuromuscular diagnoses with Cobb angles greater than 50° and did not begin their casting treatment until an average age of 4.4.[15] Surgical intervention may even be delayed until final fusion is indicated, bypassing any need for growth-friendly surgical techniques.

Although casting prevents most complications associated with surgery, it does come with its own set of complications. Most are minor skin problems; however, a case report of lateral subclavian vein thrombosis in a patient with a Cotrel cast suggests that casting treatment is not free of more severe complications.[17] This serious potential complication may be avoided by careful and generous trimming of the cast at the groin and axillary regions. Another concern is that the application of the rigid and molded cast over the chest wall may impair ventilation.[13] A recent study investigating the change in pulmonary pressures during and after the application of scoliosis casts in children with EOS reported increased peak inspiratory pressures during the application of the cast, with a decrease (but still higher than the baseline) after casting windows were cut out. They reported difficulty in maintaining ventilation in two procedures, one hypotensive episode, one case of hypoxemia after casting application and breathing difficulties in one patient.[18] In addition to medical complications, there is concern that casts and braces restrict a child's interaction with their environment and with others, which may, in turn, create psychological stigma and impede social development.[19]

In conclusion, nonoperative treatment of EOS patients is available in the form of serial casting. It may serve as definitive treatment (generally for idiopathic and syndromic curves that are treated before the age of 2) or as a means to delay surgical intervention. Because of the significant differences in outcomes that can be caused by a delay in casting treatment of even a few months, Mehta suggests confirming the EOS diagnosis by measuring the RVAD on 2 successive radiographs as previously discussed. If progressive scoliosis is diagnosed, treatment should begin immediately. Mehta found that delays in treatment were often caused by physicians who monitored curve progression over too long a period. At times, physicians stated the monitoring process was extended while they were investigating other anomalies; Mehta recommends treating the scoliosis in conjunction with these investigations, which often occur in EOS patients.[10]

Operative Treatment

Surgical indications for EOS patients may still greatly vary between providers, but a survey of the Growing Spine Study Group found that surgery was often recommended when curves progressed to 60° in patients younger than 8 to 10 years of age.[20] Historically, definitive fusion was the only reliable surgical treatment for these patients, but outcomes were less than desirable with continued deformity, low rates of circumferential fusion, and poor pulmonary function and cosmesis.[15] In light of these poor outcomes, there has been a transition to growth-friendly surgery. This transition has also been encouraged by considerable advances in growth-friendly instrumentation and techniques, which are resulting in better outcomes.[21-30] Recently, Skaggs and colleagues[31] proposed a classification of these techniques to create common terminology and to facilitate comparative studies. According to this classification, currently available techniques fall into 3 categories: distraction-based, compression-based, and guided growth systems.

DISTRACTION-BASED SYSTEMS
Growing Rods

Currently, growing rods are probably the most commonly used surgical management method for EOS in North America.[32] This technique has existed for nearly 2 decades, promoted first by Paul Harrington, who began with a single growing rod construct. This single growing rod has been replaced with a dual rod technique due to evidence of better correction, increased stability, and a greater proportion of expected spinal growth.[33] Although the technique has changed, the premise has remained the same: provide distraction between the ends of a scoliotic curve by anchoring instrumentation to the spine proximally and to the spine or pelvis distally, avoiding instrumentation in the intervening spinal segment (**Fig. 2**).[34] The rods are composed of 2 sections joined by a tandem connector. As the spine grows, the distraction needs to be "reset" by surgically lengthening the rods (typically every 6 months). The goal is to provide distraction through the early adolescent growth period until sufficient vertebral column growth is achieved. Generally, at the termination of growing rod treatment, they are replaced with a permanent rod system during a definitive fusion.[25,28,33,35]

It has been established by numerous studies that repeated growing rod distractions provide maintenance of deformity correction and promote spinal growth, possibly even greater than normal growth rates.[16,25,35] The Hueter-Volkmann law states that spinal distraction may promote growth of individual vertebral bodies. This theory is supported by the findings of a recent study that found there was considerably more growth per vertebra within the instrumented zone compared with the vertebra outside the instrumented zone.[36] Other studies have concluded that patients lengthened at intervals of less than 6 months have a higher annual growth rate than those lengthened between 9 and 20 months (1.8 cm and 1.0 cm, respectively).[25]

In a study of general growing rod outcomes in 23 patients with idiopathic, congenital, and syndromic scoliosis, Akbarnia[35] reported a curve reduction from an average of 82° preoperatively to 36° at final follow-up and an average of almost 9 cm in growth from T1-S1. Patients underwent an average of 6.3 lengthening procedures and had a 48% complication rate. Spinal elongation from T1-S1 averaged 10.7 cm after final fusion. In addition, Elsebai and colleagues[26] were also able to confirm that growing rods are able to improve the space available for lung (SAL). Overall advantages of distraction-based systems are regeneration of disks by relieving surrounding pressure and restoration in the decrease of disk height and vascular channel volume in the endplates caused by compression.[37-39]

Growing rod complications include high rates of implant breakage and pull-out and wound complications.[40] As previously discussed, there appears to be a phenomenon of "diminishing returns" with multiple lengthenings. Diminishing returns with multiple lengthenings is thought to be due to increasing spine stiffness, but whether it represents autofusion or ankylosis of the instrumented segment is unclear. Numerous studies report a complication rate of 40% to 60%,[15,26,34,41] with chances increasing with each additional surgical procedure by as much as 24%.[41] Although there is a high rate of complications, most are addressed during planned lengthening surgeries and the occurrence of major complications is rare. Regarding neurologic safety, growing rod placement and lengthening procedures are extremely safe with an overall neuromonitoring change incidence of 0.9%.[42]

Magnetically Controlled Growing Rod System

There have been major advances toward the clinical use of a magnetically controlled growing rod (MCGR) in the past few years. The implant includes a telescopic actuator that contains a small internal magnet; otherwise, the construct is the same as traditional growing rods.[43,44] The internal magnet is rotated by an electrically powered remote control, which is placed externally over the spine to lengthen or shorten the rod.[45] Lengthenings can be performed in an outpatient setting without anesthesia or analgesia. Because of the inverse relationship between growth rate and lengthening intervals and the relative ease of

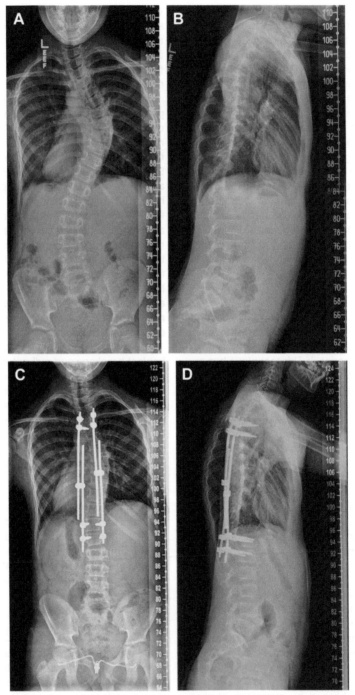

Fig. 2. Growing rods. (*A*) Preoperative posterior anterior (PA) radiograph of an 8-year-old boy. (*B*) Preoperative lateral (LAT) radiograph. (*C*) Postoperative PA radiograph of same patient 30 months from initial surgery. (*D*) Postoperative LAT radiograph.

lengthenings, 3-month lengthening intervals are recommended to optimize spinal growth.

Dannawi and colleagues[45] released findings on the largest series of MCGR use in humans. Thirty-four patients, diagnosed with EOS of any

cause, received either a single or a dual MCGR (mean age at implant was 8). Their goal was to distract the rod faster than the rate of predicted growth to allow for better curve correction. At follow-up, they reported a mean of 4.8 distractions (minimum of 3), a mean of 66 days to first distraction, and a mean of 87 days between distractions. Both groups showed significant reduction in mean Cobb angles from preoperative to immediate postoperative; a significant difference between mean preoperative, immediate postoperative, and final distance between T1 and S1; a significant increase in the mean distance between T1 and S1 from preoperative to immediate postoperative; and an overall significant difference between the mean preoperative, immediate postoperative, and final Cobb angles. Although both constructs showed significant results, the dual rod improved the Cobb angle significantly better than the single rod.

Like growing rods, the MCGR construct also comes with complications. In Dannawi's study,[45] one patient in each group had a superficial wound infection and a broken rod requiring revision. Two single rods lost distraction, which was rectified by subsequent lengthening. However, there were no spontaneous fusions or neurologic deficits and, in comparison with traditional growing rods, these patients experienced less wound infections[35,41,46] and broken rods.[24] It should be noted that this study had a shorter follow-up period than most growing rods studies. In addition, it is likely that stiffness, spontaneous fusions, and "diminished returns" will also be observed with this technique, but avoidance of multiple surgeries is a colossal advantage over conventional growing rods. The numerous complications associated with surgical lengthenings, including wound infection, rod breakage, autofusion, anchor failure, and implant prominence, should be greatly reduced. There is no evidence that the electromagnetic field causes any persistent or major side effect with repeated distraction.[47] Although these results are promising, longer follow-up is necessary to clarify the effectiveness and the complication rates of this exciting device. MCGR was approved for use in the United States in February 2014.

ET, Vertical, Expandable, Prosthetic Titanium Rib, and Hybrid Rib to Spine Devices

In contrast to growing rods, which focus on the spinal deformity, Expansion Thoracoplasty (ET) focuses on the thoracic deformity.[48] Typical constructs use a proximal rib anchor (hook or a rib cradle) and connect to either another rib, to the lumbar spine, or to the posterior iliac crest. Vertical, expandable, prosthetic titanium rib (VEPTR) is an instrument specifically developed for this purpose and is the most commonly used construct for ET. As with growing rods, the construct is surgically lengthened at 6-month intervals (**Fig. 3**).[49] The deformed thoracic segment is not exposed and there is no intervention in the spinal column.[50,51] The expansion of the chest indirectly provides correction of the thoracic spinal deformity.

ET is primarily indicated in children with thoracic insufficiency syndrome (TIS) and spinal deformity.[49] Studies have demonstrated the positive effects of ET on pulmonary function and volumes[52,53] and have also shown that the spinal deformity is corrected and maintained similar to growing rods. The indications have expanded from TIS to EOS, older children with complex spine deformities, congenital scoliosis (including fused ribs), myelomeningocele, kyphosis, and neuromuscular scoliosis.[54–57] Interestingly, these studies reported spinal growth rates similar to normal values, even in congenital deformities.[58] Another instrumentation construct used rib hooks as proximal anchors to the thoracic wall, instead of the spine. This method, introduced by Skaggs,[59] may have utility in EOS cases with cervicothoracic curves and/or very dysplastic pedicles. Although this technique provides an alternative fixation method in children with EOS, currently there is not enough clinical evidence supporting its routine use.

ET complications include skin problems, soft tissue scarring, infection, rib drift, rib breakage, thoracic outlet syndrome, and brachial plexus palsy.[41,42,50,60,61] Possibly because of the overlying implant or spontaneous rib fusions, increased chest stiffness as a function of decreased respiratory system compliance has also been reported.[53] Furthermore, although the hope was that this technique would eliminate autofusion, a recent study[48] of 5 patients who underwent ET with non-VEPTR implants demonstrated spontaneous fusions at the convexity of the deformity apex, which was neither exposed nor instrumented, in all 5 patients. Spontaneous autofusion has also been reported by others.[62,63] In addition, there is a concern of increased proximal thoracic kyphosis and loss of spinal balance with repeated lengthenings.[63] Secondary to these changes, final arthrodesis of the spine may become very challenging.

Despite these concerns, the efficacy of ET instrumentation in increasing lung capacity and SAL, and maintaining spinal deformity, has been shown repeatedly. It is unknown if the increase in lung volume is a result of the treatment or part of the normal growth, but radiographically, the chest does appear to benefit from ET treatment.[53,57,64,65] Another proven benefit is weight gain.[66] Failure to thrive and increased energy expenditure due to difficulty breathing is a major problem in children with TIS. The documented weight gain following ET treatment can probably be taken as a proxy to the pulmonary benefits of this technique.

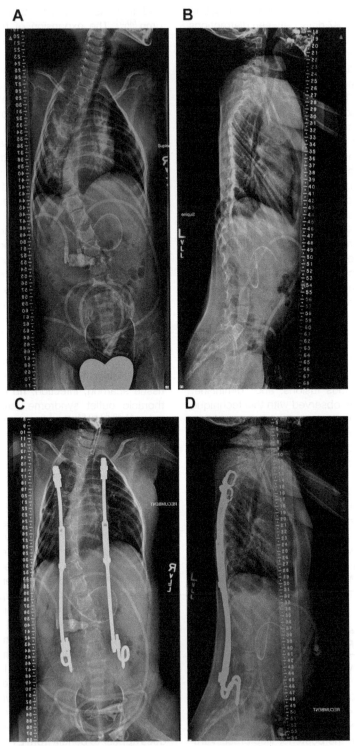

Fig. 3. VEPTR. (*A*) Preoperative PA radiograph of a bilateral rib to pelvis structure in a 4-year-old girl with spinal muscular atrophy type I. (*B*) Preoperative LAT radiograph. (*C*) Postoperative PA radiograph. (*D*) Postoperative LAT radiograph.

COMPRESSION-BASED SYSTEMS
Anterolateral Staple/Tether

Tethering and stapling methods aim to achieve hemiepiphysiodesis to correct or control the progress of spinal deformity. The first study on spine stapling was published in 1951 by Nachlas and Borden,[67] who used a canine model to produce evidence of successful spinal growth modulation. This study was followed by another study with disappointing results in 3 human patients by Smith and colleagues[68] in 1954; all 3 patients progressed despite stapling. Even with the disappointing results, much information was gained on the utility of the staple; specifically, the entire curve should be stapled and that it was more effective for moderate versus severe curves. Many of the first staples were unsuccessful because they pulled out of the spine. From that time, the nitinol staple, a shape memory alloy, was developed by Medtronic (Minneapolis, MN, USA) for fixation of hand and foot osteotomies. The prongs are straight when cooled, but bend into a "c" shape when they reach body temperature. The "c" shape ensures that the staple clamps into the bone and provides secure fixation. These staples are inserted across the end plates on the convex side of the spine, compressing the growth and allowing for the concave side of the spine to "catch up" through growth plate modulation (**Fig. 4**).[69]

In a study of 28 patients, Betz and colleagues[70] reported that stapling was successful for treating thoracic curves less than 35° (77.7% success), curves that reached less than or equal to 20° on the first erect radiograph (85.7% success), and flexible curves that showed greater than 50% correction on bending films (71.4% success). Overall, lumbar curves demonstrated a success rate of 86.7%. There were 3 broken staples but no dislodgements (none required removal). One patient, who underwent stapling at the age of 6, overcorrected and required a definitive fusion. From these findings, the authors recommend waiting until patients are at least 8 years of age before considering stapling.

With the limited data available, general consensus is that vertebral stapling may be a treatment option for idiopathic curves with mild severity (flexible lumbar curves less than 45° and thoracic curves less than 35°) in children with substantial remaining growth.[70–72] Vertebral stapling would require surgical intervention earlier than traditional EOS surgery, which is generally indicated at 60°. Complications can include broken and/or dislodged staples, but Lavelle and colleagues[69] reported that with placement of more than 1400 staples they have only encountered 2

staples that moved and subsequently had to be removed. Thoracic kyphosis is a contraindication because anterior growth modulation may increase kyphosis.

In addition to staples, a new device was recently introduced that consists of anterolateral screws that are inserted into the vertebral bodies with a propylene connector in between, providing a tethering effect.[73] Recent animal studies using anterolateral spinal tethering have been encouraging, showing that tethering may be a nonfusion option for larger curves that promotes correction to 3D alignment.[74,75] This technique is experimental and will require rigorous testing to determine specific indications and applicable patient populations. No testing has been completed in the EOS population.

Overall complications of compression-based systems are reported to be intervertebral disk compression leading to degeneration, a decrease in vascular channel volume in the endplates, and ossification of the cartilaginous endplates.[76] At this time, indications remain limited and the role of compression-based systems and their potential advantages over serial casting and bracing remain to be defined. Theoretically, it is a surgical option with a low complication rate that could spare patients a definitive fusion, but future research is needed to determine beneficial patient populations.

GUIDED-GROWTH SYSTEMS
Luque-Trolley and Shilla

Growth-guided or self-lengthening systems were developed to provide surgical treatment that does not require repeated operative lengthenings or a definitive fusion, leaving the patient free of implants at the termination of their treatment. These systems use the inherent growth potential of the child's vertebral column, allowing the spine to gradually correct itself. The first growth-guided system created was the Luque-Trolley. This technique used multiple levels of bilateral sublaminar wires linked to parallel longitudinal rods. This technique required extensive subperiosteal dissection, causing interlaminar ankylosis and autofusion, thus limiting spinal growth. Because of these complications, the Luque-Trolley system is considered a historical technique.[8,77,78]

More recently, 2 devices have been introduced that function somewhat similar to the Luque-Trolley, following the self-lengthening concept with anchors gliding over the rods as the spine grows.[78,79] Of these, the Shilla system seems to be more popular and is undergoing extensive research. During this procedure, the apex of the curve undergoes a limited fusion (3 to 4 segments).

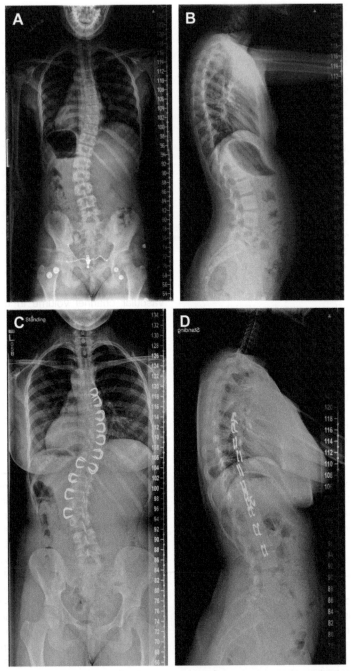

Fig. 4. Staples. (*A*) Preoperative PA radiograph of an 11–year-old girl with juvenile-onset idiopathic scoliosis. (*B*) Preoperative LAT radiograph. (*C*) Final postoperative PA radiograph 7 years from initial placement showing a stable curve after the onset of skeletal maturity at the age of 18. (*D*) Postoperative LAT radiograph.

Dual stainless steel rods are then fixed to the corrected apex with pedicle screws. Four to 6 extraperiosteally gliding pedicle screws are placed at each end of the construct and vertebral growth occurs in a cephalad and caudad direction through these screws. The use of these screws as an anchor instead of the wires used in the Luque-

Trolley allows for continued spine growth without the complications of ankylosis and autofusion.[19,34]

In the longest follow-up series to date, McCarthy et al[19] provided results for 10 patients (average age at surgery was 7.5 years) with 2 years (average of 28 months) of follow-up data. The average preoperative curve of 70.5° was reduced to 27° at

6 weeks of follow-up and was maintained at an average of 34° at 2-years of follow-up. SAL improved an average of 13% and truncal height (C7-S1) increased an average of 12%. Growth occurred at both ends equally on both sides and no change in kyphosis was noted (an important consideration as proximal junctional kyphosis has been noticed in distraction based systems). No neuromonitoring changes were noted. Although these statistics appear significant, further information is needed to delineate the amount of growth achieved during the treatment period.

Complications included one rod revision due to growth off the ends of the rods, one rod replacement due to a smaller size, one broken rod requiring replacement, and 2 low-grade infections in neuromuscular patients. Although spontaneous autofusion can still occur, careful placement without disruption of the periosteum may decrease the probability. The number of unplanned procedures was comparable to distraction methods; however, if these same patients had received growing rods, they would have undergone an additional 49 scheduled procedures.[25,35,80] The other "Modern Luque-Trolley" method was developed by Ouellet[78] and differs from the Shilla technique in the placement of the "gliding anchors"; Shilla technique uses proximal and distal gliding sites, whereas Ouellet's method uses the apex of the deformity as the gliding site. Preliminary results are similar to Shilla outcomes.

Because of the limited number of additional surgeries required for these techniques, it may be an especially attractive option for use in patients with complex medical histories that would preclude them from being good candidates for multiple surgeries. In comparison with traditional growing rods, better coronal deformity correction is achieved, but requires more levels of anchor placement.[19,78] In addition, both systems will likely require rod exchanges due to growth, but this should not occur for years after the index surgery. Also of note, although one of the main goals of using the growth-guided techniques is to leave the patients implant free at treatment end, it has not yet been determined if these implants can be removed at maturity or if a definitive fusion will be required.

SUMMARY

EOS continues to be a major challenge to the pediatric spine surgeon but, with recent advances, physicians are one step closer to the ultimate goal of fusionless and lasting scoliosis correction. With the evolving technology and better understanding of the pathologic abnormality, more progress is on the way. Current literature supports the use of serial casting for most progressive early onset spinal deformities as either a definitive or a surgical delay treatment. If casting is not an option or it did not control the deformity, a growth-friendly surgical option is generally recommended. Currently, the most commonly used system is growing rods, but this may change in the future with other viable options undergoing research, including MCGRs, nitinol staples, tethering, and the Shilla procedure. Generally, ET is recommended for those patients with TIS. As innovation and technology advance, so do alternative methods of scoliosis treatment. Future goals will continue to include creating methods that involve fewer complications and to treat patients successfully with EOS with "fusionless" methods.

REFERENCES

1. Dickson R. Early-onset idiopathic scoliosis. In: Weinstein S, editor. The pediatric spine: principles and practice. New York: Raven Press, Ltd; 1994. p. 421–9.
2. Davies G, Reid L. Effect of scoliosis on growth of alveoli and pulmonary arteries and on right ventricle. Arch Dis Child 1971;46:623–32.
3. Muirhead A, Conner AN. The assessment of lung function in children with scoliosis. J Bone Joint Surg Br 1985;67:699–702.
4. Reid L. Lung growth. In: Zorab PA, editor. Scoliosis and growth: proceedings of a third symposium. London: Churchill Livingstone; 1971. p. 117–21.
5. Branthwaite MA. Cardiorespiratory consequences of unfused idiopathic scoliosis. Br J Dis Chest 1986;80:360–9.
6. Williams BA, Asghar J, Matsumoto H, et al. More experienced surgeons less likely to fuse: a focus group review of 315 hypothetical EOS cases. J Pediatr Orthop 2013;33:68–74.
7. Karol LA, Johnston C, Mladenov K, et al. Pulmonary function following early thoracic fusion in non-neuromuscular scoliosis. J Bone Joint Surg Am 2008;90:1272–81.
8. Gomez JA, Lee JK, Kim PD, et al. "Growth friendly" spine surgery: management options for the young child with scoliosis. J Am Acad Orthop Surg 2011;19:722–77.
9. Akbarnia BA, Campbell RM, Dimeglio A, et al. Fusionless procedures for the management of early-onset spine deformities in 2011: what do we know? J Child Orthop 2011;5:159–72.
10. Mehta MH. Growth as a corrective force in the early treatment of progressive infantile scoliosis. J Bone Joint Surg Br 2005;87:1237–47.
11. Smith JR, Samdani AF, Pahys J, et al. The role of bracing, casting, and vertical expandable

prosthetic titanium rib for the treatment of infantile idiopathic scoliosis: a single-institution experience with 31 consecutive pateitns. J Neurosurge Spine 2009;11:3–8.

12. Cotrel Y, Morel G. The elongation-derotation-flexion technic in the correction of scoliosis. Rev Chir Orthop Reparatrice Appar Mot 1964;50:59–75 [in French].

13. Sanders JO, D'Astous J, Fitzgerald M, et al. Derotational casting for progressive infantile scoliosis. J Pediatr Orthop 2009;29:581–7.

14. Baulesh DM, Huh J, Judkins T, et al. The role of serial casting in early-onset scoliosis (EOS). J Pediatr Orthop 2012;32:658–63.

15. Fletcher ND, McClung A, Rathjen KE, et al. Serial casting as a delay tactic in the treatment of moderate-to-severe early-onset scoliosis. J Pediatr Orthop 2012;32:664–71.

16. Sankar WN, Skaggs DL, Yazici M, et al. Lengthening of dual growing rods and the law of diminishing returns. Spine (Phila Pa 1976) 2011;36:806–9.

17. Badlani N, Korenblit A, Hammerberg K. Subclavian vein thrombosis after application of body cast. J Pediatr Orthop 2013;33:e1–3.

18. Dhawale AA, Shah SA, Reichard S, et al. Casting for infantile scoliosis: the pitfall of increased peak inspiratory pressure. J Pediatr Orthop 2013;33: 63–7.

19. McCarthy RE, Luhmann S, Lenke L, et al. The Shilla growth guidance technique for early-onset spinal deformities at 2-year follow-up: a preliminary report. J Pediatr Orthop 2014;34:1–7.

20. Yang JS, McElroy MJ, Akbarnia BA, et al. Growing rods for spinal deformity: characterizing consensus and variation in current use. J Pediatr Orthop 2010; 30:264–70.

21. Moe JH, Kharrat K, Winter RB, et al. Harrington instrumentation without fusion plus external orthotic support for the treatment of difficult curvature problems in young children. Clin Orthop Relat Res 1984;(185):35–45.

22. Tello CA. Harrington instrumentation without arthrodesis and consecutive distraction program for young children with severe spinal deformities. Experience and technical details. Orthop Clin North Am 1994;25:333–51.

23. Blakemore LC, Scoles PV, Poe-Kochert C, et al. Submuscular Isola rod with or without limited apical fusion in the management of severe spinal deformities in young children: preliminary report. Spine (Phila Pa 1976) 2001;26:2044–8.

24. Mineiro J, Weinstein SL. Subcutaneous rodding for progressive spinal curvatures: early results. J Pediatr Orthop 2002;22:290–5.

25. Akbarnia BA, Breakwell LM, Marks DS, et al. Dual growing rod technique followed for three to eleven years until final fusion: the effect of

frequency of lengthening. Spine (Phila Pa 1976) 2008;33:984–90.

26. Elsebai HB, Yazici M, Thompson GH, et al. Safety and efficacy of growing rod technique for pediatric congenital spinal deformities. J Pediatr Orthop 2011;31:1–5.

27. Karatas AF, Dede O, Rogers K, et al. Growth-sparing spinal instrumentation in skeletal dysplasia. Spine (Phila Pa 1976) 2013;38:1517–26.

28. Klemme WR, Denis F, Winter RB, et al. Spinal instrumentation without fusion for progressive scoliosis in young children. J Pediatr Orthop 1997;17: 734–42.

29. McElroy MJ, Sponseller PD, Dattilo JR, et al. Growing rods for the treatment of scoliosis in children with cerebral palsy: a critical assessment. Spine (Phila Pa 1976) 2012;37:1504–10.

30. McElroy MJ, Shaner AC, Crawford TO, et al. Growing rods for scoliosis in spinal muscular atrophy: structural effects, complications, and hospital stays. Spine (Phila Pa 1976) 2011;36:1305–11.

31. Skaggs DL, Akbarnia BA, Flynn JM, et al. A classification of growth friendly spine implants. J Pediatr Orthop 2014;34:260–74.

32. Fletcher ND, Larson AN, Richards BS, et al. Current treatment preferences for early onset scoliosis: a survey of POSNA members. J Pediatr Orthop 2011;31:326–30.

33. Thompson GH, Akbarnia BA, Kostial P, et al. Comparison of single and dual growing rod techniques followed through definitive surgery: a preliminary study. Spine (Phila Pa 1976) 2005;30:2039–44.

34. Tis JE, Karlin LI, Akbarnia BA, et al. Early onset scoliosis: modern treatment and results. J Pediatr Orthop 2012;32:647–57.

35. Akbarnia BA, Marks DS, Boachie-Adjei O, et al. Dual growing rod technique for the treatment of progressive early-onset scoliosis: a multicenter study. Spine (Phila Pa 1976) 2005;30(17 Suppl): S46–57.

36. Olgun ZD, Ahmadjadlj H, Alanay A, et al. Vertebral body growth during growing rod instrumentation: growth preservation or stimulation? J Pediatr Orthop 2012;32:184–9.

37. Kroeber M, Unglaub F, Guehring T, et al. Effects of controlled dynamic disc distraction on degenerated intervertebral discs: an in vivo study on the rabbit lumbar spine model. Spine (Phila Pa 1976) 2005;30:181–7.

38. Kroeber MW, Unglaub F, Wang H, et al. New in vivo animal model to create intervertebral disc degeneration and to investigate the effects of therapeutic strategies to stimulate disc regeneration. Spine (Phila Pa 1976) 2002;27:2684–90.

39. Guehring T, Unglaub F, Lorenz H, et al. Intradiscal pressure measurements in normal discs, compressed discs and compressed discs treated

with axial posterior disc distraction: an experimental study on the rabbit lumbar spine model. Eur Spine J 2006;15:597–604.

40. Cahill PJ, Marvil S, Cuddihy L, et al. Autofusion in the immature spine treated with growing rods. Spine (Phila Pa 1976) 2010;35:E1199–203.

41. Bess S, Akbarnia BA, Thompson GH, et al. Complications of growing-rod treatment for early-onset scoliosis: analysis of one hundred and forty patients. J Bone Joint Surg Am 2010;92:2533–43.

42. Sankar WN, Skaggs DL, Emans JB, et al. Neurologic risk in growing rod spine surgery in early onset scoliosis: is neuromonitoring necessary for all cases? Spine (Phila Pa 1976) 2009;34:1952–5.

43. Akbarnia BA, Mundis GM Jr, Salari P, et al. Innovation in growing rod technique: a study of safety and efficacy of a magnetically controlled growing rod in a porcine model. Spine (Phila Pa 1976) 2012;37:1109–14.

44. Miladi L, Dubousset JF. Magnetic powered extensible rod for thorax or spine. In: Akbarnia BA, Yazici M, Thompson GH, editors. The growing spine: management of spinal disorders in young children. Berlin; Heidelberg (Germany): Springer; 2010. p. 585–91.

45. Dannai Z, Altaf F, Harshavardhana NS, et al. Early results of a remotely-operated magnetic growth rod in early-onset scoliosis. Bone Joint J 2013; 95-B:75–80.

46. Farooq N, Garrido E, Altaf F, et al. Minimizing complications with single submuscular growing rods: a review of technique and results on 88 patients with minimum two-year follow-up. Spine (Phila Pa 1976) 2010;35:2252–8.

47. Yamaguchi-Sekino S, Sekino M, Ueno S. Biological effects of electromagnetic fields and recently updated safety guidelines for strong static magnetic fields. Magn Reson Med Sci 2011;10:1–10.

48. Yilgor C, Demirkiran G, Ayvaz M, et al. Is expansion thoracoplasty a safe procedure for mobility and growth potential of the spine? Spontaneous fusion after multiple chest distractions in young children. J Pediatr Orthop 2012;32:483–9.

49. Campbell RM Jr, Smith MD, Hell-Vocke AK. Expansion thoracoplasty: the surgical technique of opening-wedge thoracostomy. Surgical technique. J Bone Joint Surg Am 2004;86-A(Suppl 1):51–64.

50. Hell AK, Campbell RM, Hefti F. The vertical expandable prosthetic titanium rib implant for the treatment of thoracic insufficiency syndrome associated with congenital and neuromuscular scoliosis in young children. J Pediatr Orthop B 2005;14:287–93.

51. Hasler CC, Mehrkens A, Hefti F. Efficacy and safety of VEPTR instrumentation for progressive spine deformities in young children without rib fusions. Eur Spine J 2010;19:400–8.

52. Campbell RM, Smith MD, Mayes TC, et al. The effect of opening wedge thoracostomy on thoracic insufficiency syndrome associated with fused ribs and congenital scoliosis. J Bone Joint Surg Am 2004;86-A:1659–74.

53. Motoyama EK, Yang CI, Deeney VF. Thoracic malformation with early-onset scoliosis: effect of serial VEPTR expansion thoracoplasty on lung growth and function in children. Paediatr Respir Rev 2009;10:12–7.

54. Samdani AF, St. Hilaire T, Emans JB, et al. The usefulness of VEPTR in the older child with complex spine and chest deformity. Clin Orthop Relat Res 2010;468:700–4.

55. Smith JT. The use of growth-sparing instrumentation in pediatric spinal deformity. Orthop Clin North Am 2007;38:547–52.

56. Smith JT. Bilateral rib-to-pelvis technique for managing early-onset scoliosis. Clin Orthop Relat Res 2011;469:1349–55.

57. White KK, Song KM, Frost N, et al. VEPTR growing rods for early-onset neuromuscular scoliosis: feasible and effective. Clin Orthop Relat Res 2011; 469:1335–41.

58. Flynn JM, Emans JB, Smith JT, et al. VEPTR to treat nonsyndromic congenital scoliosis: a multicenter, mid-term follow-up study. J Pediatr Orthop 2013; 33:679–84.

59. Skaggs DL. Hybrid distraction-based growing rods. In: Akbarnia BA, Yazici M, Thompson GH, editors. The growing spine: management of spinal disorders in young children. Berlin; Heidelberg (Germany): Springer; 2010. p. 601–12.

60. Ramirez N, Flynn JM, Serrano JA, et al. The vertical expandable prosthetic titanium rib in the treatment of spinal deformity due to progressive early onset scoliosis. J Pediatr Orthop B 2009;18:197–203.

61. Yazici M, Emans J. Fusionless instrumentation systems for congenital scoliosis: expandable spinal rods and vertical expandable prosthetic titanium rib in the management of congenital spine deformities in the growing child. Spine (Phila Pa 1976) 2009;34:1800–7.

62. Groenefeld B, Hell AK. Ossifications after vertical expandable prosthetic titanium rib treatment in children with thoracic insufficiency syndrome and scoliosis. Spine (Phila Pa 1976) 2013;38: E819–23.

63. Lattig F, Taurman R, Hell AK. Treatment of Early Onset Spinal Deformity (EOSD) with VEPTR: A challenge for the final correct spondylodesis: a case series. J Spinal Disord Tech 2012. [Epub ahead of print].

64. Campbell RM Jr. VEPTR: past experience and the future of VEPTR principles. Eur Spine J 2013; 22(Suppl 2):S106–17.

65. Motoyama EK, Deeney VF, Fine GF, et al. Effects on lung function of multiple expansion thoracoplasty in children with thoracic insufficiency syndrome: a

longitudinal study. Spine (Phila Pa 1976) 2006;31: 284–90.

66. Skaggs DL, Sankar WN, Albrekston J, et al. Weight gain following vertical expandable prosthetic titanium ribs surgery in children with thoracic insufficiency syndrome. Spine (Phila Pa 1976) 2009;34: 2530–3.

67. Nachlas IW, Borden JN. The cure of experimental scoliosis by directed growth control. J Bone Joint Surg Am 1951;33:24–34.

68. Smith AD, Von Lackum WH, Wylie R. An operation for stapling vertebral bodies in congenital scoliosis. J Bone Joint Surg Am 1954;36:342–8.

69. Lavelle WF, Samdani AF, Cahill PJ, et al. Clinical outcomes of nitinol staples for preventing curve progression in idiopathic scoliosis. J Pediatr Orthop 2011;31(Suppl 1):S107–13.

70. Betz RR, Ranade A, Samdani AF, et al. Vertebral body stapling: a fusionless treatment option for a growing child with moderate idiopathic scoliosis. Spine (Phila Pa 1976) 2010;35:169–76.

71. O'Leary PT, Sturm PF, Hammerberg KW, et al. Convex hemiepiphysiodesis: the limits of vertebral stapling. Spine (Phila Pa 1976) 2011;36:1579–83.

72. Trobisch PD, Samdani A, Cahill P, et al. Vertebral body stapling as an alternative in the treatment of idiopathic scoliosis. Oper Orthop Traumatol 2011; 23:227–31.

73. Crawford CH 3rd, Lenke LG. Growth modulation by means of anterior tethering resulting in progressive correction of juvenile idiopathic scoliosis: a case report. J Bone Joint Surg Am 2010;92:202–9.

74. Chay E, Patel A, Ungar B, et al. Impact of unilateral corrective tethering on the histology of the growth plate in an established porcine model for thoracic scoliosis. Spine (Phila Pa 1976) 2012;37:E883–9.

75. Moal B, Schwab F, Demakakos J, et al. The impact of a corrective tether on a scoliosis porcine model: a detailed 3D analysis with a 20 week follow-up. Eur Spine J 2013;22:1800–9.

76. Hee HT, Chuah YJ, Tan BH, et al. Vascularization and morphological changes of the endplate after axial compression and distraction of the intervertebral disc. Spine (Phila Pa 1976) 2011;36:505–11.

77. Mardjetko SM, Hammerberg KW, Lubicky JP, et al. The Luque trolley revisited. Review of nine cases requiring revision. Spine (Phila Pa 1976) 1992;17: 582–9.

78. Ouellet J. Surgical technique: modern Luque trolley, a self-growing rod technique. Clin Orthop Relat Res 2011;469:1356–67.

79. McCarthy RE. Growth guided instrumentation: Shilla procedure. In: Akbarnia BA, Yazici M, Thompson GH, editors. The Growing spine: management of spinal disorders in young children. Berlin; Heidelberg (Germany): Springer; 2010. p. 593–600.

80. Thompson GH, Akbarnia BA, Campbell RM. Growing rod techniques in early onset scoliosis. J Pediatr Orthop 2007;27:354–61.

Upper Extremity

Preface
Upper Extremity

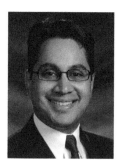

Asif M. Ilyas, MD
Editor

In this issue of the *Orthopedic Clinics of North America*, we present several interesting articles in the Upper Extremity section reviewing a broad range of topics.

Wong and Abraham present a detailed review of musculoskeletal neoplasms of the upper extremity. Biopsy principles and the differential diagnosis of common lesions in the shoulder, elbow, wrist, and hand are discussed. Moreover, surgical considerations are also presented relative to the type of neoplasm and location.

Horneff and colleagues discuss *Propionibacterium acnes* infections in shoulder surgery. *P acnes* infections are common gram-positive bacteria endemic on our skin that can complicate shoulder surgery. Diagnosis, prevention, and treatment for *P acnes* infections are reviewed.

Patel and colleagues discuss the management of shoulder instability associated with glenohumeral bone loss. In particular, instability associated with Hill-Sachs and bony Bankart defects can pose a unique challenge. Their diagnosis, evaluation, and surgical treatment, including soft tissue and bony reconstruction, are discussed.

Miller and colleagues present several cases and a review of the literature on "Thrower's Fractures." These fractures represent spiral fractures of the humerus caused by forceful throwing, most commonly associated with baseball pitching. A review of three cases, the phases of throwing, diagnosis, the possible relationship with a preceding stress fracture, and their management are discussed in detail.

Following the theme of throwing injuries, Kancherla et al review thrower's injuries to the elbow. The elbow is exposed to high valgus and extension loads with throwing that can lead to a number of chronic and acute pathologies. A detailed review of the pathomechanics, physical exam findings, applicable diagnostic studies, and treatment options is presented.

Asif M. Ilyas, MD
Rothman Institute
Thomas Jefferson University
925 Chestnut Street
Philadelphia, PA 19107, USA

E-mail address:
asif.ilyas@rothmaninstitute.com

Orthop Clin N Am 45 (2014) xix
http://dx.doi.org/10.1016/j.ocl.2014.07.004
0030-5898/14/$ – see front matter © 2014 Published by Elsevier Inc.

Propionibacterium acnes Infections in Shoulder Surgery

John G. Horneff, MD, Jason E. Hsu, MD,
G. Russell Huffman, MD, MPH*

KEYWORDS

- *Propionibacterium acnes* • Shoulder joint • Infection • Revision surgery

KEY POINTS

- *Propionibacterium acnes* is a common cause of bacterial infection postoperatively in patients who have undergone shoulder surgery.
- *P acnes* is a common gram-positive bacteria found commonly in the hair follicles and sebaceous glands that are abundantly common in the shoulder region.
- The key to characterize a *P acnes* infection is to have a high clinical suspicion in a patient who continues to complain of pain and stiffness even if the other prototypical signs of infection are absent. A comprehensive physical examination, radiographs, and prolonged culture times are often necessary to accurately diagnose a *P acnes* infection.
- Proper preventive care with the use of sterile techniques in the operating room is often not as effective in the treatment of *P acnes* as they are for other common orthopedic infections. When an infection with *P acnes* does occur, treatment options include antibiotics, surgical debridement, and revision surgery.

INTRODUCTION

Propionibacterium acnes is a gram-positive anaerobic bacillus bacterium that is found to preferentially colonize the neck, chest, and shoulder region. In years past this slow-growing, indolent bacterium was considered a contaminant of many intraoperative cultures taken at the time of shoulder surgery. Recently, however, there have been a growing number of reports in the literature that *P acnes* is an organism capable of colonizing the shoulder joint and causing disorder in the perioperative period. Although indolent in its course, *P acnes* infection of the shoulder can lead to failure of surgery including rotator cuff repair and arthroplasty. Most of the literature has described such infection in the setting of joint replacement, but *P acnes* colonization of the skin in the shoulder region certainly places all patients undergoing shoulder surgery at risk.

Patients with postoperative *P acnes* shoulder infection often describe substantial pain and limitation of range of motion in active and passive shoulder function. When a patient presents with continued difficulty of the shoulder even years after the operative procedure, the index of suspicion for infection should increase and proper intervention should be initiated. Unfortunately, the evaluation and treatment of a *P acnes* infection is not as well described and can often be subtle in its presentation. The determination of an infection with *P acnes*

Funding Sources/Conflicts of Interest: None.
Department of Orthopedic Surgery, Hospital of University of Pennsylvania, 2 Silverstein, 3400 Spruce Street, Philadelphia, PA 19104, USA
* Corresponding author.
E-mail address: Russell.huffman@uphs.upenn.edu

Orthop Clin N Am 45 (2014) 515–521
http://dx.doi.org/10.1016/j.ocl.2014.06.004

orthopedic.theclinics.com

requires a comprehensive physical examination, and often includes the need for radiographic imaging and laboratory studies. Treatment options include antibiotic therapy, debridement surgery, and, in the case of arthroplasty, revision surgery. Perhaps even more important to the treatment of *P acnes* infection in the shoulder is the practice of prevention via proper preparation of the surgical site.

INFECTIONS OF THE SHOULDER JOINT
Common Pathogens

Many of the bacteria responsible for infection in patients who undergo shoulder surgery are the same organisms that can cause an infection in any orthopedic patient. Typically, bacteria that are normally found as skin flora are most likely to invade the shoulder joint following any procedure that violates the skin barrier. *Staphylococcus aureus, Staphylococcus epidermidis,* and other coagulase-negative *Staphylococcus* species are the most common potential pathogens that colonize human skin.[1–3] In several case series, *S aureus* has been found to account for as much as 60% of native joint infections.[4–6] Similarly, when it comes to prosthetic joint infections *S aureus* and coagulase-negative *Staphylococcus* have been found to be responsible for as much as 23% and 43% of cases, respectively.[7] These pathogens, however, are not unique to the shoulder and are usually the first targets of directed antibiotic therapy when an infection following orthopedic surgery is suspected. More unique to the shoulder is *P acnes*, which has been found to be responsible for as much as 51.3% of postoperative shoulder infections.[8,9] A study by Patel and colleagues[1] looked to characterize the colonization of bacteria at various sites common for orthopedic surgery, and found that although the burden of *S aureus* was increased at hip, knee, and shoulder compared with *P acnes*, the burden of *P acnes* was significantly greater for the shoulder region than for the lower extremity. This higher concentration of *P acnes* in the shoulder region has even led some to speculate that the bacterium is responsible for shoulder abnormality even before surgical treatment. Levy and colleagues[10] collected shoulder aspirates and tissue samples from 55 consecutive patients before primary joint replacement, and found that 41.8% of patients were positive for *P acnes* colonization.

MICROBIOLOGY

P acnes is a non–spore-forming, gram-positive anaerobic bacillus. Although it is considered as part of the normal superficial skin flora, *P acnes*

tends to live deep in the hair follicles and sebaceous pores of the skin rather than on the surface. The metabolic by-products found in the oily sebum produced by sebaceous glands serve as a source of energy for the bacteria. The neck, axilla, and chest wall each have an increased number of these glands and follicles in comparison with other regions of the body. For this reason, *P acnes* is often found in increased numbers in these areas of the body compared with other anatomic regions common for orthopedic surgery such as the hip or knee.[1,11,12] Male patients tend to have an even higher concentration of hair follicles and sebaceous glands, placing them at further risk.[11,12] Similarly, patients with excess activity in these glands who are sufferers of dermatologic acne can have an elevated number of colonies of the bacteria living on their skin. In most cases, however, *P acnes* tends to be isolated from healthy moist skin that would not be expected to have any sort of colonization.[13] *P acnes* has also been found to colonize other regions of the body, including eye mucosa and layers of the respiratory and digestive tracts. Given these numerous regions of colonization, *P acnes* has been implicated as a pathogen in infections including endocarditis, meningitis, conjunctivitis, and various abscesses. For many years its implication as an infective agent in shoulder surgery had been ignored or, when present in cultures, assumed to be a contaminant. This historical perspective was mostly propagated by the indolent course of *P acnes* infections and the organism's slow growth cycle. Over the past few decades, however, its role in shoulder infections has become more recognized.

PROPHYLACTIC TREATMENT OF INFECTION

One of the best ways to treat a potential surgical-site infection is to prevent it from ever occurring. There are certain strategies to decrease the chance of infection that can be performed in the preoperative and perioperative periods. Many of these strategies have become the standard of care for orthopedic surgical care.

Surgical-Site Preparation

Preoperative surgical-site preparation with an antiseptic solution is often performed in the operating room just before incision. Various iodine and alcohol-based solutions are available that have been shown to have varying efficacy. Saltzman and colleagues[14] performed a randomized prospective study of 3 commercially available solutions: ChloraPrep (2% chlorhexidine gluconate and 70% isopropyl alcohol; ChloraPrep, Leawood, KS, USA), DuraPrep (iodine povacrylex and 74% isopropyl alcohol; 3M, Minneapolis, MN, USA), and Betadine (Purdue Pharma, Stamford, CT, USA). The investigators found ChloraPrep solution to be significantly more effective than the other 2 solutions in eliminating coagulase-negative *Staphylococcus.* However, no solution was found to be superior in eliminating *P acnes.*[14] Similarly, a randomized controlled trial that compared patients who used 2% chlorhexidine gluconate cloths at home before surgery with those who washed with standard soap and water found the positive culture rate for coagulase-negative *Staphylococcus* and overall positive culture rate to be lower in the patients who used the chlorhexidine cloths.[2] A trend toward a lower positive culture rate was also observed for *P acnes,* but this was not a significant reduction.[2] Given the tendency of *P acnes* to colonize the hair follicles and sebaceous glands deep to the skin surface, it is not surprising that these solutions are less effective in decreasing its numbers.

Given the ineffectiveness of surface cleaning solutions on *P acnes,* other methods of reducing infection are encouraged.

Shaving, Draping, Incision

Many techniques necessary for decreasing the rate of *P acnes* infection are implemented in the operating room at the time of surgery. Like the clinical guidelines used by orthopedic surgeons in other subspecialties, the use of proper hair clipping and draping of the surgical site are encouraged to reduce infection rates.[12,15] In addition, the use of proper ventilation flows, reduced operating theater traffic, and sterile autoclaving of surgical instruments and equipment should always be implemented.[9,13] Some investigators have advocated the use of separate surgical knives for skin and deeper tissues to avoid possible seeding of the deeper surgical planes.[16] A study that used separate knives for the skin and deeper layers found that the rate of contamination of the skin blades with *P acnes* (among other flora) was more than twice that of the inside blades.[16] As *P acnes* is often found in the deeper layers of the skin that are untouched by surface-cleaning solutions, the idea of using a separate knife blade for shoulder surgery certainly seems a cheap and efficient way to reduce deep-tissue contamination. Such a simple technique can easily be added to the normal sterile precautions used in orthopedic operating rooms worldwide.

EVALUATION OF THE *P ACNES* INFECTION

Infection following shoulder surgery should be worked up in the same manner as for any other concerning infection surrounding an orthopedic surgery. A thorough infection diagnostic workup requires multiple modalities including physical examination, imaging, blood work with a white cell (WBC) count, erythrocyte sedimentation rate (ESR), C-reactive protein (CRP), and shoulder aspiration culture with cell count.

Physical Examination

P acnes infections of the shoulder are difficult to assess on physical examination because of the indolent nature of the bacteria. Unlike an infection with *Staphylococcus* species, patients with *P acnes* infections do not tend to present with the classic signs of inflammation such as erythema, fever, micromotion tenderness, or swelling. The most common complaint of postoperative patients harboring a *P acnes* infection tends to be persistent shoulder pain.[13] In a retrospective review of 10 patients diagnosed with a *P acnes* deep shoulder infection, 9 patients had only a chief complaint of pain for a mean duration of about 3 months.[13] The remaining patient also presented with pain with the additional prototypical infection symptoms of fever, swelling, and wound drainage. In a patient population that presents preoperatively with shoulder pain, it is easy for the treating clinician to disregard infection in the differential in favor of normal postoperative pain or adhesive capsulitis as the offending cause. However, there should be earnest concern for infection when a patient continues to complain of a painful motion arc postoperatively.

In some instances, symptoms do not even occur until years after surgery. Zeller and colleagues[17] studied *P acnes* infections in 50 patients who underwent arthroplasty for various joints including the hip, knee, and shoulder, and found that patients could be divided into two groups: those who developed symptoms within 2 years of their index operation and those who developed symptoms more than 2 years after their operation. The most common symptoms were pain and limited range of motion. Symptoms of infection were significantly more frequent in the group that had an asymptomatic interval of less than 2 years; however, positive intraoperative cultures were significantly greater in those patients with a longer asymptomatic interval. This finding led the investigators to suggest that different pathophysiologic mechanisms of infection can occur. In the former group a more acute *P acnes* infection is manifested, whereas in the latter group a colonization of the arthroplasty occurs first, which later leads to symptomatic infection.[17] If a patient does develop the prototypical symptoms of infection, these will tend to manifest sooner in the postoperative period rather than later. Fever, local inflammation, and sinus tract formation was seen in 18 of 35 patients within 2 years of surgery, compared with only 1 of 15 patients who developed symptoms beyond 2 years.[17]

The shoulder surgery patient who presents postoperatively with continued difficulty should always be approached in a similar manner, with the treating physician having concern for infection even years after surgery. Physical assessment should include a thorough examination of the patient's surgical incisions to assess for any erythema, swelling, or drainage. In the setting of a *P acnes* infection, incisions are likely to appear normal. However, there is the possibility of a multiple organism infection, and treatment should be tailored to account for all organisms. In addition, the patient should have a complete examination of shoulder range of motion and pain level. Stiffness and continued pain are the most likely symptoms to present in the *P acnes*–infected patient. Dictating thorough physical examinations in the patient's medical record are essential for comparison, and may reveal a decreasing range of motion arc or increased pain levels. Documenting a worsening examination allows the patient and physician to recall prior presentations and guide further evaluation if deemed necessary.

Imaging

Evaluation of the painful postoperative shoulder should always include plain radiographs (anterior-posterior view, scapular-Y view, and axillary view). Radiographs are important to rule out subluxation of the humeral head, heterotopic ossification, hardware failure, or joint arthrosis or other mechanical causes that contribute to joint pain and stiffness in the postoperative patient. With early pyogenic infection, radiographic findings are typically normal.[12] By contrast, radiographs in subacute and delayed cases of pyogenic infections may show osteopenia, lucencies around a prosthetic component, and pseudosubluxation of a prosthetic humeral head.[12,18] Most *P acnes* infections tend to fit into this latter category of indolence. A retrospective study of 52 patients with *P acnes* infections of various orthopedic implants divided patients into 3 categories: definite infection (based on local signs and at least 2 *P acnes*–positive isolates), probable infection (based on local signs and one positive *P acnes* isolate), and possible infection (based on no signs of infection but signs of prosthetic dysfunction or arthrosis and one positive *P acnes* isolate).[19] Of note, all 15 patients found to have changes on plain radiographs were in the possible infection group (n = 17). None of the patients in the more clinically concerning infection groups were found to have radiographic changes.[19]

The divergence between clinical and radiographic presentation in cases of *P acnes* creates a challenge for the treating physician. On one hand, a patient who appears to have an infection of the postoperative shoulder on physical examination may not have any infectious signs on radiography; conversely, a patient with signs of infection on radiography may not present with the most concerning physical examination. Pottinger and colleagues[11] prospectively followed patients undergoing revision arthroplasty of the shoulder, and found that patients with evidence of humeral component osteolysis radiographically had a 10-fold increase in the prognosis of a *P acnes* infection ($P<.01$), whereas those with evidence of humeral component loosening in the absence of osteolysis had a 3-fold increase ($P<.01$). Similarly, evidence of glenoid loosening was also found to significantly correlate with a positive *P acnes* culture ($P<.01$).[11] For the treating orthopedic surgeon, these studies show that one should maintain a high index of suspicion for infection when either the physical examination or radiographic imaging is concerning. In patients without visible hardware (ie, synthetic polymer anchors) or no implants, plain radiographs are most often unremarkable. Advanced imaging techniques, such as magnetic resonance (MR) imaging or computed tomography, are often unnecessary unless a raised clinical suspicion on physical examination or plain radiographs requires further investigation. In the absence of cystic absorption around anchor material, no clear MR imaging findings have been observed in patients with *P acnes* infections in the native shoulder joint.

Laboratory Evaluation

Peripheral blood tests are often an element of the infection workup. ESR and CRP are 2 of the most common inflammatory markers obtained along with a peripheral leukocyte count. These tests are nonspecific and are normally elevated even after an uncomplicated surgical procedure.[12] After an uneventful operation, the ESR will slowly decline while the CRP level declines more rapidly, normalizing within about 2 weeks.[12,20] In cases of acute purulent infections with virulent organisms, these inflammatory markers can be significantly elevated and can help reveal an infectious process. Unfortunately, they are typically within the range of normal values in the setting of a *P acnes* infection.[3,10–13,17,21–23] In a retrospective study of

107 patients undergoing revision shoulder arthroplasty who were found to have unexpected positive cultures, 88% of patients had all blood test results (WBC, ESR, CRP) within normal reference ranges.[22] Similarly, a prospective examination of 108 revision shoulder arthroplasty cases associated with positive cultures found no significant association with the WBC, ESR, or CRP values.[11] Zeller and colleagues[17] found a small correlation between positive *P acnes* cultures and elevated ESR/CRP values, but only in one-third of cases. Lastly, a comparison of definite prosthetic shoulder infections with cultures positive for *P acnes* versus those with cultures positive for other microorganisms showed a trend of the former group being less likely to have elevated ESR or CRP counts in contrast to the latter.[3] In short, peripheral blood tests for inflammatory markers are often unremarkable in the setting of *P acnes* infection. Regardless of the observed low sensitivity and specificity of general inflammatory markers, such laboratory measures should still be obtained if a patient has an indolent or early infection from another microorganism that could possibly elevate their levels.

Culture

The culturing of *P acnes* is a difficult process in comparison with that of other microorganisms responsible for orthopedic infections. The growth cycle of *P acnes* is inherently slow. Many laboratories routinely discard culture samples after 3 to 5 days.[21] Most bacterial species responsible for orthopedic infections, such as *Staphylococcus* species, are identified within this time frame, but the slow growth of *P acnes* requires further incubation. Studies have placed the average incubation time for a positive *P acnes* culture at between 9 and 15 days.[11,12,21,24,25] In 108 revision shoulder arthroplasties performed for increased pain and stiffness, positive *P acnes* cultures taken at the time of surgery went from 45% within 1 week to 100% within 4 weeks.[11] This finding indicates that more than half of potential *P acnes* infections can be missed within the typical hospital laboratory incubation time and that a large false-negative rate can occur. Some investigators argue that this increased incubation time is not required as long as proper handling of the culture samples is carried out to encourage *P acnes* growth. Shannon and colleagues[24] performed multiple broth and plate culture of 14 subjects who had more than 1 positive shoulder culture for *P acnes*, and found that 52 of 53 broth and 27 of 28 plate cultures were positive within 7 days of sampling. The investigators argued that the difference in their results in comparison with those in most of the literature is that the collection and transportation of their samples were under anaerobic conditions, unlike in prior studies. Typically, hospital laboratories place initial culture specimens under both aerobic and anaerobic conditions, although the latter is sometimes not strictly devoid of oxygen when performed.

It is important for the treating orthopedic surgeon to be familiar with the practices of the microbiology laboratory to determine the most accurate culturing of a suspected shoulder infection. The need for extended incubation times can be impractical for many laboratories because of increased labor costs and the costs associated with increased recovery of nondiagnostic isolates.[25] A 7-day incubation period seems to be sufficient time for *P acnes* growth if an institution's microbiology laboratory is able to perform all the tasks of collection and preparation of culture samples under ideal anaerobic conditions; however, if exposure to aerobic conditions is used, the incubation time should last at least 2 weeks. Regardless of preparation protocols, it is best for multiple culture samples to be taken in the operating room at the time of surgery, as multiple cultures positive for *P acnes* at the time of surgery appear to correlate more convincingly with true infection than with a contaminant.[22]

TREATMENT

The treatment of a *P acnes* postsurgical shoulder infection that involves the bone, joint, or implants is typical of any infection seen in orthopedic surgery. Typically the treatment of a deep infection in the shoulder requires a multimodal approach with antibiotics, surgical debridement, and potential revision surgery. In the setting of infected arthroplasty or fracture nonunions, a staged surgical approach may be best.

Antibiotic Therapy

Intravenous antibiotics remain the mainstay of treating any deep musculoskeletal infection. The typical antibiotic course for osteomyelitis is 4 to 6 weeks of intravenous dosing. Intravenous administration allows for better penetrance of the antibiotic into the deep tissue, as opposed to first being absorbed through the digestive tract as is the case with oral dosing. Although oral dosing is an option, the length and success of treatment is more variable.[12]

In the case of *P acnes*, the choice of antibiotic is variable. *P acnes* is often susceptible to penicillin, tetracyclines, vancomycin, and erythromycin.[13] Typically penicillin and other β-lactam antibiotics are the first choice for antibiotic coverage. In a series of 10 surgical shoulder patients that included rotator cuff repair, arthroplasty, and open reduction and internal fixation, the use of intravenous penicillin or ampicillin-sulbactam was sufficient for treatment of the cultured *P acnes* isolates.[13] However, as in many of the pathogens responsible for infection, *P acnes* resistance is steadily increasing. Sixty percent to 65% of *P acnes* isolates are found to be resistant to at least 1 antibiotic.[13,26,27] The cause for this increased resistance mostly stems from the antibiotic regimens used to treat dermatologic *P acnes* in cases of acne vulgaris.[13,26–29] As in *Staphylococcus* species, the development of β-lactamase enzyme in resistant strains of *P acnes* infections has led to the need for alternative antibiotics such as vancomycin. In the case of polymicrobial infection, the use of more than 1 antibiotic may be required.

The key to using antibiotic therapy effectively against *P acnes* shoulder infections is to properly culture tissue or fluid taken from the shoulder and to test that sample for various antibiotic resistances. A consultation with the Infectious Disease department should be performed for every infected patient to ensure that the correct agent, dosing, and duration of therapy are chosen. Collaboration with infectious disease physicians also ensures that the antibiotics chosen are nontoxic for the patient with regard to the kidney and liver function required for proper excretion.

Surgical Debridement or Revision

The use of antibiotic therapy, although a necessary component of treating the *P acnes* shoulder infection, is often not sufficient as a lone means of treatment, and this holds especially with regard to shoulder surgery that involves the use of implants. In a biomaterials study of polymethylmethacrylate cement and titanium alloy implants, investigators found that *P acnes* isolates allowed to grow in a biofilm environment were considerably more resistant to antibiotics such as cefamandole, ciprofloxacin, and vancomycin.[29] Once bacteria have developed biofilm on foreign material, antibiotic penetration and efficacy to work against the offending pathogen are impeded. In these instances, little information is available to guide clinical decision making. In the case of an obvious infected shoulder arthroplasty, treatment options for infection include 1- or 2-stage exchange, resection arthroplasty, irrigation and debridement, antibiotic suppression, and arthrodesis.[23] This approach is in compliance with the standard guidelines of orthopedic care for an infected arthroplasty. In the case of a *P acnes* infection

whereby the infection can have a more indolent course, the choice of operative treatment is not as easily discerned, as the diagnosis is often elusive. A retrospective study of 17 patients undergoing revision of a failed shoulder arthroplasty with 1-stage revision surgery and no antibiotic treatment reported only a 5.9% recurrence rate of infection, suggesting a low risk for recurrent infection with surgery alone.[23] However, most practicing orthopedic surgeons agree on a multimodal approach with antibiotics and surgical treatment, as the external validity guiding treatment algorithms from small case series is questionable.[12,13]

SUMMARY

P acnes infection of the shoulder presents the orthopedic surgeon with unique diagnostic and treatment challenges. Unlike other common infectious microorganisms, *P acnes* can be very subtle in its presentation, with no constitutive patient symptoms and often negative inflammatory markers. Proper standards in prepping and draping are mandatory in preventing infection, but may be uniquely inadequate for this pathogen given the location of *P acnes* in the deep dermal layer. Successful treatment of *P acnes* infection includes a high clinical suspicion in the postsurgical patient with continuing complaints. Diagnosis requires careful attention to the patient's history and physical examination, most notably for increasing pain and decreasing range of motion. The addition of imaging and peripheral blood tests has been shown to offer little additional information to aid in making a definitive diagnosis. Culturing of shoulder aspiration fluid can also prove to be difficult, but prolonged incubation and proper specimen handling are necessary to minimize false-negative cultures when *P acnes* infection is suspected. Multiple surgical tissue specimens remain the gold standard when aspirates are negative and clinical concern is present. When appropriately identified and treated, A 7-day incubation period seems to be sufficient for *P acnes* growth. A shoulder infected by *P acnes* can be successfully treated with antibiotics, surgical debridement, or revision surgery.

REFERENCES

1. Patel A, Calfee RP, Plante M, et al. *Propionibacterium acnes* colonization of the human shoulder. J Shoulder Elbow Surg 2009;18(6):897–902.
2. Murray MR, Saltzman MD, Gryzlo SM, et al. Efficacy of preoperative home use of 2% chlorhexidine

gluconate cloth before shoulder surgery. J Shoulder Elbow Surg 2011;20(6):928–33.

3. Piper KE, Jacobson MJ, Cofield RH, et al. Microbiologic diagnosis of prosthetic shoulder infection by use of implant sonication. J Clin Microbiol 2009; 47(6):1878–84.

4. Ryan MJ, Kavanaugh R, Wall PG, et al. Bacterial joint infections in England and Wales: analysis of bacterial isolates over four years. Br J Rheumatol 1997;36(3):370–3.

5. Morgan DS, Fisher D, Merianos A, et al. An 18 year clinical review of septic arthritis from tropical Australia. Epidemiol Infect 1996;117(3):423–8.

6. Gupta MN, Sturrock RD, Field M. Prospective comparative study of patients with culture proven and high suspicion of adult onset septic arthritis. Ann Rheum Dis 2003;62(4):327–31.

7. Zimmerli W, Trampuz A, Ochsner PE. Prosthetic-joint infections. N Engl J Med 2004;351(16):1645–54.

8. Levy PY, Fenollar F, Stein A, et al. *Propionibacterium acnes* postoperative shoulder arthritis: an merging clinical entity. Clin Infect Dis 2008;46(12): 1884–6.

9. Athwal GS, Sperling JW, Rispoldi DM, et al. Deep infection after rotator cuff repair. J Shoulder Elbow Surg 2007;16(3):306–11.

10. Levy O, Iyer S, Atoun E, et al. *Propionibacterium acnes*: an underestimated etiology in the pathogenesis of osteoarthritis? J Shoulder Elbow Surg 2013; 22(4):505–11.

11. Pottinger P, Butler-Wu S, Neradilek MB, et al. Prognostic factors for bacterial cultures positive for *Propionibacterium acnes* and other organisms in a large series of revision shoulder arthroplasties performed for stiffness, pain, or loosening. J Bone Joint Surg Am 2012;94(22):2075–83.

12. Saltzman MD, Marecek GS, Edwards SL, et al. Infection after shoulder surgery. J Am Acad Orthop Surg 2011;19(4):208–18.

13. Millett PJ, Yen YM, Price CS, et al. *Propionibacterium acnes* infection as an occult case of postoperative shoulder pain: a case series. Clin Orthop Relat Res 2011;469(10):2824–30.

14. Saltzman MD, Nuber GW, Gryzlo SM, et al. Efficacy of surgical preparation solutions in shoulder surgery. J Bone Joint Surg Am 2009;91(8):1949–53.

15. Bosco JA 3rd, Slover JD, Haas JP. Perioperative strategies for decreasing infection: a comprehensive evidence-based approach. Instr Course Lect 2010;59:619–28.

16. Schindler OS, Spencer RF, Smith MD. Should we use a separate knife for the skin? J Bone Joint Surg Br 2006;88(3):382–5.

17. Zeller V, Ghorbani A, Strady C, et al. *Propionibacterium acnes*: an agent of prosthetic joint infection and colonization. J Infect 2007;55(2):119–24.

18. Brems JJ. Complications of shoulder arthroplasty: Infections, instability, and loosening. Instr Course Lect 2002;51:29–39.

19. Lutz MF, Berthelot P, Fresard A, et al. Arthroplastic and osteosynthetic infections due to *Propionibacterium acnes*: a retrospective study of 52 cases, 1995-2002. Eur J Clin Microbiol Infect Dis 2005; 24(11):739–44.

20. Niskanen RO, Korkala O, Pammo H. Serum C-reactive protein levels after total hip and knee arthroplasty. J Bone Joint Surg Br 1996;78(3):431–3.

21. Dodson CC, Craig EV, Cordasco FA, et al. *Propionibacterium acnes* infection after shoulder arthroplasty: a diagnostic challenge. J Shoulder Elbow Surg 2010;19(2):303–7.

22. Foruria AM, Fox TJ, Sperling JW, et al. Clinical meaning of unexpected positive cultures (UPC) in revision shoulder arthroplasty. J Shoulder Elbow Surg 2013;22(5):620–7.

23. Grosso MJ, Sabesan VJ, Ho JC, et al. Reinfection rates after 1-stage revision shoulder arthroplasty for patients with unexpected positive intraoperative cultures. J Shoulder Elbow Surg 2012;21(6):754–8.

24. Shannon SK, Mandrekar J, Gustafson DR, et al. Anaerobic thioglycolate broth culture for recovery of *Propionibacterium acnes* from shoulder tissue and fluid specimens. J Clin Microbiol 2013;51(2):731–2.

25. Butler-Wu SM, Burns EM, Pottinger PS, et al. Optimization of periprosthetic culture for diagnosis of *Propionibacterium acnes* prosthetic joint infection. J Clin Microbiol 2011;49(7):2490–5.

26. Nord CE, Oprica C. Antibiotic resistance in *Propionibacterium acnes*. Microbiological and clinical aspects. Anaerobe 2006;12(5–6):207–10.

27. Eady EA, Gloor M, Leyden JJ. *Propionibacterium acnes* resistance: a worldwide problem. Dermatology 2003;206(1):54–6.

28. Cooper AJ. Systematic review of *Propionibacterium acnes* resistance to systemic antibiotics. Med J Aust 1998;169(5):259–61.

29. Ramage G, Tunney MM, Patrick S, et al. Formation of *Propionibacterium acnes* biofilms on orthopaedic biomaterials and their susceptibility to antimicrobials. Biomaterials 2003;24(19):3221–7.

Management of Bone Loss in Glenohumeral Instability

Ronak M. Patel, MD*, Nirav H. Amin, MD,
T. Sean Lynch, MD, Anthony Miniaci, MD

KEYWORDS

- Glenohumeral instability • Hill-Sachs • Bankart lesion • Latarjet

KEY POINTS

- With anterior dislocations, bony defects of the anterior glenoid and posterosuperior aspect of the humeral head occur with relative frequency.
- In shoulders sustaining a Hill-Sachs lesion at the initial dislocation, there exists a statistically significant association with recurrent dislocation.
- When a patient has symptomatic anterior instability associated with an engaging Hill-Sachs lesion with an articular arc deficit, treatment must be directed at both repairing the Bankart lesion, if present, and preventing the Hill-Sachs lesion from engaging the anterior glenoid.
- Glenoid bone loss often requires bone-block transfers using the coracoid (Bristow/Latarjet) or iliac crest autograft.
- Humeral bone loss can be addressed through a variety of surgical options, including humeroplasty, remplissage, partial resurfacing, allograft transfers, and total shoulder arthroplasty.

INTRODUCTION

The human shoulder is the most mobile joint in the body and consequently the glenohumeral joint is one of the most commonly dislocated joints in the body.[1] Glenohumeral instability affects approximately 2% of the general population, with anterior dislocations occurring 95% to 98% of the time.[2,3] With anterior dislocations, bony defects of the anterior glenoid and posterosuperior aspect of the humeral head occur with relative frequency (**Fig. 1**). These osseous injuries directly affect recurrent instability by altering joint-contact area, congruency, and function of the static restraints.[4–8] Thus, restoration of normal articular geometry should be considered when critical bone loss exists, especially in cases of failed soft-tissue stabilization procedures.

This review presents the epidemiology and pathophysiology of bone loss relevant to anterior shoulder instability, and summarizes the evaluation and management of this problem.

HUMERAL BONE LOSS

One of the first descriptions of the lesions found on the humeral head was by Flower in 1861, with many subsequent investigators reporting on these bony defects.[9,10] In 1940, 2 radiologists, Hill and Sachs, reported that these defects were actually compression fractures produced when the posterolateral humeral head impinged against the

The authors have nothing to disclose.
Sports Health, Department of Orthopaedic Surgery, Cleveland Clinic Foundation, 5555 Transportation Boulevard, Garfield Heights, Cleveland, OH 44125, USA
* Corresponding author.
E-mail address: Rmpatel7@gmail.com

Orthop Clin N Am 45 (2014) 523–539
http://dx.doi.org/10.1016/j.ocl.2014.06.005

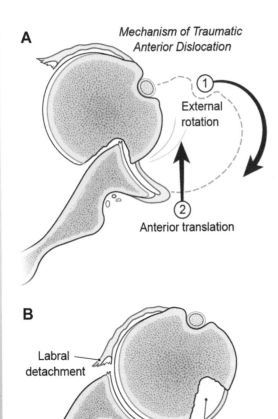

A Mechanism of Traumatic Anterior Dislocation

① External rotation

② Anterior translation

B

Labral detachment

Posterolateral head defect

BG
©CCF 2012

Fig. 1. Mechanism of traumatic anterior shoulder dislocation. (*A*) Combined forces in external rotation and anterior translation overcome internal restraints, resulting in anterior dislocation. (*B*) This process results in compression of the posterolateral aspect of the humeral head onto the anterior glenoid rim. (*Courtesy of Cleveland Clinic Foundation, Cleveland, OH.*)

anterior rim of the glenoid.[11] In their series of recurrent anterior glenohumeral instability, these lesions were found in 74% of patients. The true incidence of Hill-Sachs lesions is unknown; however, they are associated with approximately 40% to 90% of initial anterior glenohumeral dislocations.[12–16] The incidence in recurrent instability can vary from 70% up to 100%, with arthroscopy often identifying lesions not appreciated on imaging.[11,14] The management of Hill-Sachs lesions depends mainly on the size of the lesion and whether it is engaging.[17] Most lesions are small and clinically insignificant. Often, lesions that are clinically relevant may be indirectly managed with procedures aimed at addressing primary instability at the glenoid (ie, Bankart repair, glenoid reconstruction, and so forth).

GLENOID BONE LOSS

The characteristic anteroinferior capsulolabral injury (ie, Bankart lesion) associated with an acute anterior shoulder dislocation has been termed the essential lesion. Rowe and colleagues[13] first described glenoid bone loss as a "rim fracture" following anterior instability. Rowe's key finding was the importance of the anterior glenoid rim in providing anterior shoulder stability, by creating a deepened concave surface of the glenoid and increased articular coverage. The importance of the rim fracture is shown in multiple studies by analyzing the relationship of the glenoid and humerus, especially in external rotation and abduction. Bigliani and colleagues[18] provided the first detailed description of osseous glenoid rim injuries, which included rim fractures and erosions (**Fig. 2**). In a radiographic study of patients with recurrent instability, 87% of shoulders involved the presence of either a glenoid rim fracture or erosion.[19] Griffith and colleagues[20] used 2-dimensional (2D) computed tomography (CT) to find glenoid bone loss in 41% of 66 patients with a first-time dislocation and 86% of 137 patients with recurrent instability. The predominant pattern of injury was attritional bone loss, with glenoid rim fractures reported in only 21% of 233 dislocated shoulders. However, using 3-dimensional (3D) CT to assess glenoid bone loss in 100 patients with recurrent instability, Sugaya and colleagues[21] found that only 40% of patients had erosive or attritional bone loss.

BIPOLAR BONE LOSS

The literature investigating osseous lesions of both the glenoid and humeral head is limited. The prevalence of combined bone defects is reported to be 64% to 70% in first-time anterior dislocations and 79% to 84% in recurrent anterior glenohumeral instability.[20,22]

PATHOPHYSIOLOGY

Knowledge of the pathoanatomy and biomechanics of glenohumeral bone loss and instability is crucial in the appropriate management to prevent recurrent instability. The most common mechanism of traumatic anterior shoulder dislocation occurs with an indirect force on the abducted and externally rotated arm. The humeral head externally rotates relative to the glenoid while translating anteriorly. The static glenohumeral restraints (ie, capsule, ligaments, labrum) are stretched or torn with further anterior translation, and dislocation, of the humeral head. The posterosuperolateral aspect of the humeral head then

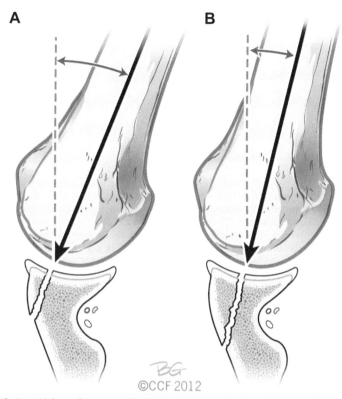

Fig. 2. Mechanism of glenoid fossa fractures. The force vector at the time of impact between the humeral head and glenoid fossa determines the morphology of the glenoid fracture. (*A*) Small rim-type fracture. (*B*) Larger fracture extending into the glenoid vault. (*Courtesy of* Cleveland Clinic Foundation, Cleveland, OH.)

impacts on the anterior aspect of the glenoid rim and can create a Hill-Sachs lesion and/or a bony Bankart lesion.

Richards and colleagues[23] investigated the location and depth of 28 arthroscopically confirmed Hill-Sachs lesions. On an axial view with 0° representing direct anterior, the typical Hill-Sachs lesion lies between 170° and 260° with a midpoint at 209°.[23] Saito and colleagues[24] used axial CT imaging to demonstrate that the normal bare area of the humeral head was located deeper than a typical posterolateral humeral head Hill-Sachs defect, allowing differentiation between the two.

Palmer and Widen[25] and Burkhart, Danaceau, and De Beer[17,26] described an "engaging" Hill-Sachs lesion as one that encounters the anterior glenoid rim with the arm in the "active" position of abduction (90°) and external rotation (0°–135°) and can lever the humerus from the glenoid concavity (**Fig. 3**).[17,25,26] These humeral head defects are parallel to the surface of the anterior glenoid when the arm is abducted and externally rotated.[27] This defect has been termed an articular arc deficit, as there is disruption of the glenohumeral articulation on motion.[17] Lesions that are not parallel to the glenoid rim in the active or athletic

position do not engage, and are termed nonengaging lesions.[17,26] The Hill-Sachs defect passes diagonally across the anterior glenoid with external rotation; therefore, there is continual contact of the articulating surfaces and no engagement of the Hill-Sachs lesion by the anterior glenoid.[28]

Cho and colleagues[29] looked at 3D CT scans of 107 shoulders undergoing surgery for recurrent anterior instability to preoperatively predict engagement of a Hill-Sachs lesion. The mean width was 52% (range, 27%–66%) and depth 14% (range, 8%–20%) of the humeral head diameter on axial images. The magnitude of bone loss that coincides with a Hill-Sachs lesion depends on multiple factors including dislocation frequency, chronicity, and force. Cetik and colleagues[30] found an increasing percentage of articular surface involvement with increasing frequency of dislocations. Intraoperative assessment revealed an average involvement of 26% of the articular head in patients with greater than 20 dislocations. The size of the humeral head defect is also directly related to dislocations of longer duration, as seen with neglected and locked shoulder dislocations.[31–33]

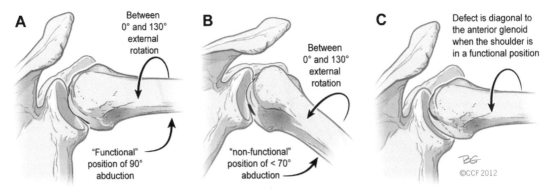

Fig. 3. Engaging and nonengaging Hill-Sachs lesions. (*A*) An engaging lesion is parallel to the anterior glenoid rim when the shoulder is in a functional position. (*B*) The "engagement point" of a nonengaging lesion occurs with the arm in a nonfunctional position. (*C*) In a functional position, a nonengaging lesion is diagonal and nonparallel to the anterior glenoid rim. (*Adapted from* Burkhart SS, De Beer JF. Traumatic glenohumeral bone defects and their relationship to failure of arthroscopic Bankart repairs: significance of the inverted-pear glenoid and the humeral engaging Hill-Sachs lesion. Arthroscopy 2000;16:677–94; *Courtesy of* Cleveland Clinic Foundation, Cleveland, OH.)

The critical limit or threshold of humeral bone loss on glenohumeral stability has been investigated in many ways. In a cadaveric study, Sekiya and colleagues[34] found that defects that were 25% of the humeral head diameter or larger revealed significantly ($P<.05$) less anterior translation before dislocation, and decreased stability ratios (displacing force divided by compressive load) when compared with the intact specimens. Furthermore, Kaar and colleagues[35] noted that defects that were greater or equal to five-eighths of the humeral head radius lead to decreased glenohumeral stability when tested in the functional position of abduction and external rotation.

Hill-Sachs lesions typically are accompanied with other abnormality including soft-tissue and/or bony Bankart lesions and anterior glenohumeral ligament disruption. In the clinical setting, there are essentially 2 types of anterior glenoid defects that occur after an instability event: rim fracture or avulsion, and compression fracture or erosive bone loss. The angle of the humeral head and shaft relative to the glenoid fossa, along with the energy, determine the extent of the resulting glenoid rim fracture (see **Fig. 2**). Recurrent or repetitive subluxations may have more shear and less axial load, leading to attritional bone loss rather than a large rim fracture that may accompany a high-energy axial load. When viewing the glenoid en face, the area of bone defect is nearly parallel to the long axis of the glenoid fossa. Saito and colleagues[36] found the average osseous glenoid injury to range from 12:08 to 6:32 on the clockface scheme with the midpoint in line with 3:01. However, clinical bone loss can still occur in more anterior-inferior locations.

Glenoid defects are typically classified with large lesions accounting for greater than 20% of the glenoid fossa, medium lesions ranging from 5% to 15%, and small lesions usually less than 5% of the glenoid fossa.[21,37] Itoi and colleagues[38] performed a biomechanical analysis on amount of glenoid defect and force required to translate the humeral head to dislocation. The investigators made sequentially larger glenoid defects in the anterior-inferior glenoid (45° from the longitudinal axis) and found that stability progressively decreased as the size of the glenoid defect increased. Specifically, defects at least 21% of the glenoid length led to instability and limited the range of motion of the shoulder. Similarly, Yamamoto and colleagues[39] looked at anterior glenoid rim defects and found that the stability ratio significantly decreased with defects that were 20% or greater of the glenoid length. Optimal surgical management requires addressing these lesions and management of the clinically significant Hill-Sachs lesion.

The concept of the glenoid track was proposed by Yamamoto and colleagues in 2007 (**Fig. 4**), and serves to illustrate the dynamic of glenohumeral instability in cases of combined defects. The glenoid track represents the pattern of articular contact between the humeral head and the glenoid with the arm in a position of vulnerability for anterior dislocation. The width of the glenoid track was found to be 84% of the inferior glenoid surface. When a glenoid defect exists, the resulting glenoid width is multiplied by 0.84 to calculate the new glenoid track width. If a humeral head defect exists and remains within the glenoid track, there will be no engagement with the anterior glenoid rim.

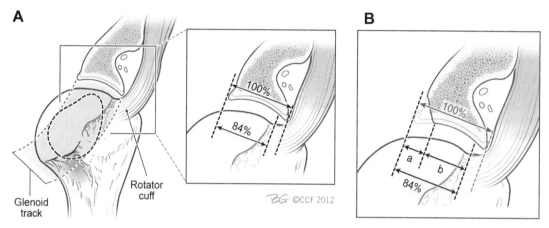

Fig. 4. Glenoid track concept. (*A*) In extremes of external rotation and abduction, the glenoid displaces the cuff tendon close to its footprint, creating a glenoid track that is close to 84% of the glenoid width. (*B*) When a glenoid defect exists, the defect width is subtracted from the 84% width obtained from the normal glenoid to calculate the true glenoid track width. (*Adapted from* Yamamoto N, Itoi E, Hidekazu A, et al. Contact between the glenoid and the humeral head in abduction, external rotation, and horizontal extension: a new concept of glenoid track. J Shoulder Elbow Surg 2007;16:649–56; *Courtesy of* Cleveland Clinic Foundation, Cleveland, OH.)

However, if even a margin of the humeral head defect extends beyond the glenoid track, there is a risk that it will engage the glenoid rim. This concept has proved valuable in understanding the clinical significance of bipolar bone loss.

NATURAL HISTORY

Hovelius and colleagues[40] prospectively followed 229 shoulder dislocations for 25 years. All patients were treated nonoperatively initially and prognostic factors, recurrence, and surgical intervention were monitored. At 10 years, 99 of 185 (53.5%) shoulders that were evaluated with radiographs had evidence of a Hill-Sachs lesion; of these 99 shoulders, 60 redislocated at least once and 51 redislocated at least twice during the 10-year follow-up,[41] compared with 38 (44%) of the 86 shoulders that did not have such a lesion documented (*P*<.04). However, at 25 years, the investigators concluded that a small humeral impression fracture at the time of initial dislocation did not influence the recurrence rate. Rowe and colleagues[13] analyzed the long-term results of Bankart repairs for recurrent instability, and found an overall recurrence rate of 3.4% (5 of 145); the recurrence rates were 4.7% and 6% for patients with moderately severe and severe Hill-Sachs lesions, respectively. Whereas Rowe and colleagues used depths of 3 mm, 5 mm, and greater than 10 mm to differentiate their size of Hill-Sachs lesions, various other methods of determining size and/or volume of the humeral head defect have been proposed without consensus; these include the Hill-Sachs quotient, articular arc circumference, and Hill-Sachs angle.[9,26,29,34,35,42–44]

Lo and colleagues[45] noted that bone loss of 25% or greater of the diameter of the inferior glenoid will create an "inverted pear" appearance, and recommended coracoid transfer when glenoid deficiency reached this magnitude. The inverted-pear glenoid had a poor prognosis in the study by Burkhart and De Beer[26] evaluating a series of 194 patients who underwent primary soft-tissue repair for anterior instability. Of the 21 patients with recurrent instability, 14 had either an engaging Hill-Sachs lesion (n = 3) or an inverted pear glenoid shape (n = 11).

HISTORY AND PHYSICAL EXAMINATION

A thorough orthopedic history must be obtained from the patient regarding shoulder instability. Specifics of the history that must be elucidated include the mechanism of instability and timing of initial symptoms. Arm position and amount of force required for instability may be an evolving process with progressively less rotation or force required for subsequent dislocations. Need and method of reduction of the glenohumeral joint may indicate the extent of laxity present. Presenting symptoms should be noted, including pain, frequency, instability, and level of function. Though infrequent, pertinent medical history including collagen disorders or epilepsy should be noted. Many patients will report a history of recurrent dislocations or multiple surgical attempts to correct the instability. All previous surgical procedures performed on the shoulder should be considered and, if possible, operative reports and photos should be obtained.

Physical examination should focus on inspection for previous scars, gross asymmetry, a thorough comparison of active and passive range of motion, strength testing, particularly evaluation of the integrity and strength of the rotator cuff, and axillary nerve function. The clinician should perform a detailed examination for glenohumeral laxity in the anterior, posterior, and inferior directions. Examination for apprehension should be performed in multiple positions (ie, sitting, standing, supine), as patients with large Hill-Sachs lesions usually exhibit apprehension that often occurs with the arm in significantly less than 90° abduction and 90° external rotation.[9,28] A positive anterior apprehension will be associated with anterior labral injuries. Moreover, apprehension with fewer degrees of abduction may indicate a significant and symptomatic bony contribution to the instability.

IMAGING AND OTHER DIAGNOSTIC STUDIES

The ideal imaging technique is easy to reproduce, with excellent reliability among physicians, and able to predict clinically significant bone defects. In addition to standard radiographs of the shoulder, specialized views allow for evaluation of bony defects of the glenoid and humeral head. Preoperative imaging includes a comprehensive radiographic evaluation with anteroposterior (AP), true AP, axillary, West Point axillary, and Stryker notch views of the involved shoulder (**Fig. 5**).

The Stryker notch view, in addition to AP internal rotation views, has been found to be most sensitive in detecting humeral head lesions on plain radiographs.[19,46] Based on these views, various quantification methods have been described (**Fig. 6**). However, Bois and colleagues[47] note that no method has been universally accepted because of the learning curve required to obtain

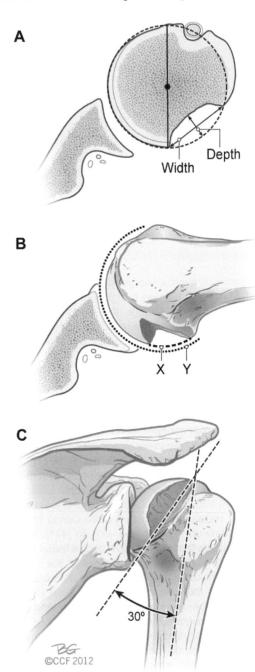

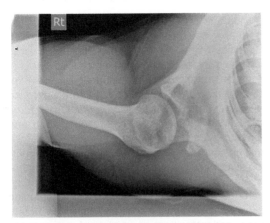

Fig. 5. Axillary view of the right shoulder shows congruency of the glenohumeral joint. This view also allows for evaluation of bone loss and glenoid version.

Fig. 6. Methods used to quantify Hill-Sachs lesions. Such defects may be quantified using (*A*) depth or width measurements, (*B*) percentage of humeral head involvement [(*X/Y*) × 100], and/or (*C*) measurement of the Hill-Sachs angle. (*Courtesy of* Cleveland Clinic Foundation, Cleveland, OH.)

these radiographic projections and the inconsistency often seen in special radiographic views.

Multiple variations of the axillary lateral view have been proposed to evaluate for glenoid defects on plain radiographs (ie, West Point, Bernageau, Garth, and Didiee).[46,48–50] The West Point view has been found to be the most accurate for demonstrating glenoid bone loss.[38]

Despite the vast array of radiographic views available, bone loss may often go undetected on plain radiographs. Preoperative advanced imaging study (CT and/or magnetic resonance imaging [MRI]) are obtained to better define the bony architecture of the glenoid and humeral head (**Fig. 7**). CT can offer the added value of providing better bony detail, with 1-mm slices and 3D reconstructions improving the accuracy of determining the true location and size of the defect.[47] Kodali and colleagues[51] investigated the reliability and accuracy of making width and depth measurements of different-sized Hill-Sachs lesions using axial, sagittal, and coronal 2D CT images. Measurements by 5 physicians were compared with measurements from a 3D laser scanner, and were found to be reproducible and most accurate in the sagittal and axial planes. However, on the glenoid side, in a study performed by Bois and colleagues[52] comparing various 2D and 3D methods of measurement of glenoid bone loss, there was variable agreement and inaccuracy for all 6 observers using 2D CT in measuring defect length and calculating the width/length ratio. Rather, 3D reconstruction is the most reliable and accurate imaging modality for the assessment of glenoid bone loss, and can be a useful tool to more clearly define the size and location of the defect and to estimate the amount of articular surface involved. Quantification of glenoid bone loss can be

performed via either a linear method or measurement of surface area. Again, various methods of quantification for both the glenoid and humeral head have been described as being useful in preoperative planning, without universal acceptance.[51,53,54]

Despite the known advantages of 3D CT imaging techniques, the disadvantages include the financial burden to the institution and possibly the patient, the need for specialized computer software to quantify bone loss, and the lack of awareness in the orthopedic and radiology communities of the multiple measurement methods available and their general validity.[47]

Dynamic arthroscopy remains the gold standard for evaluation of bone loss, and can be useful for the preoperative planning of patients undergoing open osteoarticular allograft reconstruction to address bony deficiency.[29]

CLASSIFICATION OF BONE LOSS

Ideally classification schemes incorporate clinical, radiographic, and prognostic factors. In bone loss with anterior glenohumeral instability, few studies have validated classification schemes (**Table 1**). On the humeral side, Burkhart and De Beer[26] differentiated between engaging and nonengaging defects; clinically, patients with engaging lesions had a higher failure rate with soft-tissue stabilization procedures. This diagnostic sign has since been adopted by most investigators and surgeons as the method of classifying Hill-Sachs lesions. Glenoid defects were classified by Bigliani and colleagues[18] into 3 main types based on the nature of the rim fracture. This classification was later modified after the work of Boileau and colleagues[55] demonstrated a 75% recurrence rate in patients with a glenoid compression fracture and a stretched inferior glenohumeral ligament (**Fig. 8**).

SURGICAL INDICATIONS

Algorithms for the treatment of glenohumeral bone loss associated with anterior instability currently stem from clinical evidence levels IV and V. The lack of quality (level I or II) research limits the validity and generalizability of proposed treatment techniques. Traditionally, direct osseous injuries in instability were addressed with soft-tissue procedures; however, the negative biomechanical effects of bone loss have been correlated with failure and recurrence rates in soft-tissue stabilization procedures. Thus, recent trends toward addressing osseous defects on the glenoid and humeral head have led to greater discussion

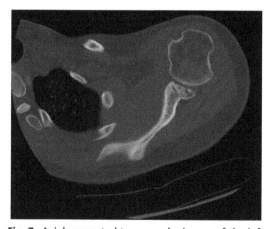

Fig. 7. Axial computed tomography image of the left shoulder showing anterior glenoid bone loss in addition to a large Hill-Sachs defect on the humeral head.

Table 1
Classification schemes in bone loss associated with anterior glenohumeral instability

Authors,[Ref.] Year	Basis	Classification		
Humeral Head				
Rowe et al,[42] 1984	Size (length and depth)	Mild 2 × 0.3 cm	Moderate 4 × 0.5 cm	Severe ≥4 × 1.0 cm
Bigliani et al,[99] 1996	Percentage of head involvement	Mild <20%	Moderate 20%–45%	Severe >45%
Glenoid				
Bigliani et al,[18] 1998	Size of rim	Type I A displaced avulsion fracture with attached capsule	Type II A medially displaced fragment malunited to the glenoid rim	Type III Erosion of the glenoid rim with <25% (type IIIA) or >25% (type IIIB) bone loss

among surgeons managing these problems. The following are considered general indications for bone-augmentation procedures in anterior instability, but are neither validated nor widely accepted.

Humeral Head Bone Loss

- Absolute:
  - Displaced humeral head fracture with humeral fracture-dislocation and associated Hill-Sachs injury
  - Lesion greater than 30% to 40% of the humeral head with chronic dislocation or recurrent anterior instability
- Relative:
  - Engaging lesion greater than 20% to 25% of the humeral head

- Lesion greater than 10% to 25% of the humeral head that does not remain well-centered in the glenoid fossa after arthroscopic instability repair

Glenoid Bone Loss

In most cases of glenoid bone loss, surgery is indicated when nonsurgical management or soft-tissue stabilization has failed to prevent instability and restore function.

- Absolute:
  - Active patients with acute fractures constituting greater than 30% loss of glenoid
- Relative:
  - Young (<25–30 years of age), active (overhead, contact) patients/athletes with bone loss greater than 25% to 30%

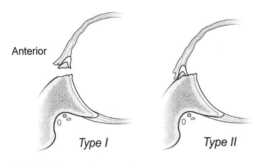
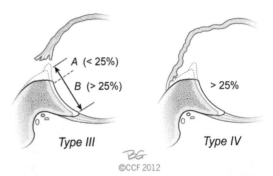

Anterior

Type I   Type II

A (< 25%)
B (> 25%)
Type III

> 25%
Type IV

Posterior

©CCF 2012

Fig. 8. Glenoid rim lesion types associated with anterior glenohumeral instability. Type I, a displaced avulsion fracture with attached capsule; type II, a medially displaced fragment malunited to the glenoid rim; type III, erosion of the glenoid rim with less than 25% (type IIIA) or greater than 25% (type IIIB) deficiency; type IV, erosion of the glenoid rim with greater than 25% deficiency combined with a stretched inferior glenohumeral ligament. (*Courtesy of* Cleveland Clinic Foundation, Cleveland, OH.)

HUMERAL HEAD TREATMENT OPTIONS
Nonoperative Treatment

Small osseous lesions and nonengaging Hill-Sachs lesions can be managed nonoperatively. Often, combined humeral head and glenoid injuries may be treated by addressing the primary defect alone (ie, Bankart, humeral avulsion of the glenohumeral ligament, or glenoid bone loss). A monitored rehabilitation program focusing on strengthening the dynamic stabilizers (deltoid, rotator cuff, and periscapular muscles) of the shoulder should be started after an initial brief period of immobilization.

Operative Treatment

Several techniques have been described in the literature to address symptomatic engaging Hill-Sachs lesions. Some of these techniques are considered historical and are performed infrequently (rotational osteotomies and east-west plications). Rotational proximal humeral osteotomies externally rotate the proximal humerus, reducing humeral retroversion and minimizing the potential for the defect to engage the anterior glenoid on internal rotation.[27] This technique is essentially of historical interest given the risk of complications and more successful alternatives.[13,17,26,56,57] Open anterior procedures, such as an east-west plication or capsulorrhaphy, shift the glenoid track medially and superiorly to limit external rotation, preventing the humeral head defect from engaging.[17,26] These soft-tissue-only techniques may not be adequate in the setting of a large humeral head defect; furthermore, concerns with restricted motion in young patients may prevent return to function and cause late arthrosis.[58]

Most surgical bone-augmentation procedures include the following:

1. Humeroplasty or disimpaction may be possible in the acute (<3 weeks) setting
2. Remplissage: Transfer of the infraspinatus into the defect to render the lesion essentially extra-articular[59,60]
3. Humeral head augmentation using either osteochondral bone plugs or size-matched bulk allograft transfers can be used to restore native anatomy
4. Humeral head augmentation with a prosthetic cap matched to defect size
5. In severe or failed reconstructive cases, prosthetic replacement using a hemiarthroplasty or total shoulder arthroplasty may become necessary[61]
6. Reconstruction of the anterior glenoid, even in cases without bone loss, to lengthen the glenoid articular arc to prevent engagement[62,63]

Bone-augmentation procedures have typically been performed as open surgery; however, the role of arthroscopic examination of the joint can prove vital in addressing associated disorder, particularly in cases of recurrent instability.

In acute injuries (<3 weeks) humeroplasty, or humeral head disimpaction, may be an option. Although this is a relatively new technique that requires further clinical and biomechanical research, it may be able to restore anatomy in cases with less than 40% of articular surface involved. The procedure can be performed in open fashion or, more commonly, percutaneously, and involves using a tamp or kyphoplasty balloon (Kyphon, Sunnyvale, CA, USA) to disimpact the humeral head lesion. Early results have shown promise. Stachowicz and colleagues[64] performed percutaneous balloon humeroplasties in 18 cadaveric shoulder Hill-Sachs lesions and regained 99.3% of the volume of initial defect. Kazel and colleagues[65] performed humeroplasties with tamps in cadaveric humeri in which they created Hill-Sachs lesions, and were able to reduce the lesions from -1755 mm^3 to -50 mm^3.

In French *remplissage* means "to fill." In shoulder instability with humeral bone loss, this term means to transfer a tendon into the humeral head defect, effectively turning the defect into an extra-articular defect with soft-tissue coverage to prevent engagement with the anterior glenoid rim (**Fig. 9**). Remplissage was originally described by Connolly as an open procedure by filling the Hill-Sachs lesion via transfer of the infraspinatus tendon with a portion of greater tuberosity.[60] An all-arthroscopic technique was first described by Wolf and Pollack,[66] which involved a posterior capsulodesis and infraspinatus tenodesis with transfer into the humeral head defect in conjunction with standard anteroinferior glenoid repair. This procedure is typically reserved for large Hill-Sachs lesions defects with associated glenoid loss of less than 25%; larger glenoid defects would require a conversion to open Latarjet. This approach was modified by Koo and colleagues[67] by using a double-pulley technique whereby 2 anchors were used to insert the infraspinatus tendon into the humeral head defect. This method allowed for the sutures to be tied over the tendon rather than through the tendon or on the muscle belly, allowing a more anatomic and tissue-preserving construct that is biomechanically stronger. Elkinson and colleagues[68] studied the effect of different anchor positions with the remplissage technique in a cadaveric model. Their biomechanical analysis showed that of the various suture techniques, medial suture passage through the infraspinatus muscle belly consistently had the greatest mean

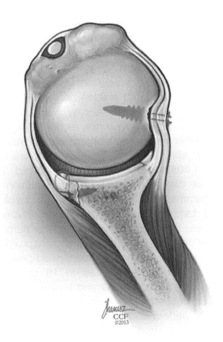

Fig. 9. Remplissage technique for humeral bone loss. The infraspinatus tendon is transferred into the humeral head defect, effectively turning the defect into an extra-articular defect with soft-tissue coverage to prevent engagement with the anterior glenoid rim. (*Courtesy of* Cleveland Clinic Foundation, Cleveland, OH.)

restriction of range of motion and highest stiffness value.

Despite criticism for the technique's nonanatomic nature and potential for loss of motion and subsequent revision surgery, clinical outcomes have been relatively successful. Early studies reported a 7% (2 of 24) incidence of recurrent instability with no loss of motion in any plane at 2-year follow-up.[56] Zhu and colleagues[69] evaluated 49 consecutive patients with a minimum 2-year follow-up. Patients had an increased mean of 8° of forward elevation with only an average loss of 1.9° of external rotation. Boileau and colleagues[70] studied 47 patients with a mean of 24-month follow-up who underwent arthroscopic remplissage. There was an average deficit of 8° (±7°) of external rotation and 9° (±7°) abduction, which was not functionally limiting. Of the 41 patients who participated in athletics before surgery, 37 (90%) returned to sport with 28 (68%) returning to the same level of sport, including overhead sports. A systematic review evaluated 7 studies (levels II, III, IV) of combined arthroscopic remplissage with Bankart repair with an average 26 month follow-up and a pooled rate of recurrent dislocation of 3.4%.[71] The investigators concluded there was no clinically significant loss of range of motion

after remplissage. Furthermore, in 4 of the 7 studies postoperative imaging showed high rates of healing and tissue filling at the infraspinatus tenodesis. Similarly, an MRI investigation of 11 patients at an average follow-up of 18 months found evidence of tendon incorporation into humeral head defect as early as 8 months.[72]

Restoring the articular arc through anatomic allograft reconstruction has been described in young patients without osteoporosis or degenerative joint disease who meet the surgical indications.[28] There are 2 main categories of allograft reconstructions: osteochondral plug transfer and size-matched bulk graft. Only 2 case reports exist in the literature describing the technique of osteochondral plug transfer into the base of a humeral defect, both reporting good results after 12 months of follow-up.[73,74] The bulk graft reconstruction requires a size- and side-matched osteoarticular humeral head allograft, preferably a fresh-frozen cryopreserved graft, for optimal recreation of the radius of curvature of the humeral head (±2 mm). An extended deltopectoral approach and capsulotomy is made to expose, inspect, and address any abnormality at the anteroinferior capsulolabral complex and glenoid. The Hill-Sachs lesion is identified and osteotomized in a chevron fashion (**Fig. 10**). The matching allograft is then cut to fit the site of the humeral head osteotomy and is secured with countersunk screws in lag fashion.

Miniaci and Gish[9] and Miniaci and Martineau[28] reviewed 18 patients who underwent this procedure (16 fresh-frozen grafts, 2 irradiated grafts) after failing previous attempts at surgical stabilization, with an average follow-up of 50 months (range 24–96 months). There were no episodes of recurrent instability, and 16 of 18 (89%) patients returned to work. The average Constant score was 78.5 postoperatively while the WOSII, a validated quality-of-life scale specific to shoulder instability, decreased, indicating improvement. Complications included radiographic evidence of partial graft collapse in 2 of 18 patients, early evidence of osteoarthritis in 3 patients (marginal osteophytes), and 1 mild subluxation (posterior).[9,28] Furthermore, 2 patients required reoperation within 2 years to remove irritable screws. Diklic and colleagues[75] treated 13 patients with fresh-frozen femoral head allograft reconstructions for Hill-Sachs lesions between 25% and 50% of the humeral head. At an average of 54 months postoperatively, the mean Constant score for the cohort was 86.8. Twelve patients had stable shoulders and 1 patient had evidence of osteonecrosis. More long-term and higher-quality research is needed with allograft reconstructions, but may be limited because of the

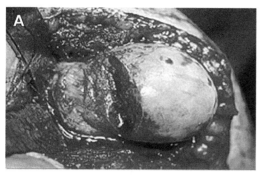

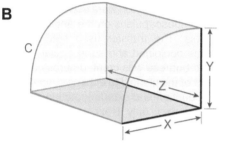

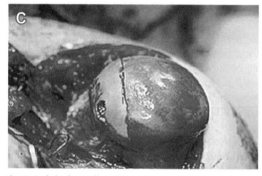

Fig. 10. (*A*) The Hill-Sachs lesion is identified and osteotomized in a chevron fashion. (*B*) The osteotomy is sized in a 3-dimensional pattern. (*C*) The matching allograft is then cut to fit the humeral head osteotomy site and secured with screws.

narrow indications and the required technical expertise.

Reconstituting the articular arc with prosthetic surface implants is another option. This technique uses a round cap-like cobalt-chrome articular component that fills the Hill-Sachs lesion on the posterosuperior humeral head (**Fig. 11**). The technique requires technical expertise and accuracy similar to those of allograft reconstruction without the associated potential complications of disease transmission, nonunion, and graft resorption.[27] Though not described in the limited literature, the use of prosthetic components potentially introduces elements of adverse reactions, hardware loosening, and glenoid wear. Moros and Ahmad[76] described a case report of a 50-year-old man with recurrent anterior shoulder instability and an engaging Hill-Sachs lesion. A Latarjet coracoid transfer and a partial humeral head resurfacing were performed with a successful result at 10-year follow-up. In another case series, Grondin and Leith[77] reported on 2 cases whereby a bony Bankart and a large Hill-Sachs were treated with a Latarjet procedure and partial humeral head resurfacing. In these 2 cases instability was reduced with the procedure, but only short-term follow-up was provided. In 2009, Raiss and colleagues[78] performed uncemented resurfacing arthroplasty in a series of 10 patients with chronic locked anterior shoulder dislocations with large Hill-Sachs defects. At mean follow-up of 24 months, the Constant score increased from 20 points preoperatively to 61 postoperatively (*P*<.007). There were 2 reoperations: one patient developed glenoid erosion and the other had a dislocation. Postoperative radiographs showed the humeral head centered on the glenoid in 9 of the 10 cases, and there were no signs of loosening appreciated.

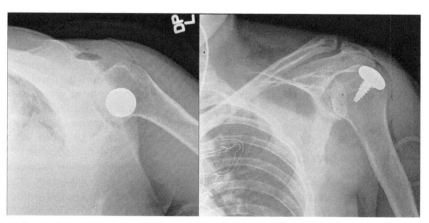

Fig. 11. Two radiographic views of prosthetic implant filling the void created by a large posterosuperior Hill-Sachs defect.

Partial resurfacing may be contraindicated in patients with osteoporosis or deficient bone stock. Scalise and colleagues[79] recommend sufficient quantity and quality of bone in the epiphyseal portion of the humerus to allow stable fixation of the implant, and suggest caution for its use in patients with severe Hill-Sachs lesions associated with chronic locked dislocations. Moreover, Copeland and colleagues[80] suggest a minimum of 60% of normal bone stock for a humeral resurfacing procedure. Elderly patients with osteoporotic bone and large defects (>40% of the humeral head) may have better outcomes with a stemmed prosthesis regardless of a degenerative joint.[32,81] Similarly, Armitage and colleagues[27] recommend a partial resurfacing in small to moderate lesions, but cautioned that future studies are needed.

As stated earlier, complete humeral head resurfacing or isolated humeral head arthroplasty (hemiarthroplasty) is an option in patients with Hill-Sachs defects greater than 40% of the articular surface.[61] Hemiarthroplasty or total shoulder arthroplasty (TSA) (if there is concomitant glenoid wear/erosion) may be particularly beneficial in elderly patients or those who are of low demand; however, indications are not well defined. In younger or more active patients, hemiarthroplasty or TSA should be used with caution because the likelihood of revision increases secondary to glenoid erosion, component wear, and loosening.[82] Pritchett and Clark[61] reported their outcomes of hemiarthroplasty and TSA in 7 patients with chronic dislocations and significant Hill-Sachs lesions. The average patient age was 55 years (range, 36–67 years) and average follow-up was only 2 years. Five of the 7 patients had good results, and there were no recurrent dislocations. These procedures should be reserved for older or less active patients with defects involving greater than 40% of the articular surface and/or significant degeneration of articular cartilage. Further research is needed to outline indications for age and activity levels.

Reconstruction of the anterior glenoid with bone augmentation has been used as the primary procedure for treatment of a Hill-Sachs lesion in recurrent anterior instability. The concept is to lengthen the glenoid articular arc to prevent engagement with the humeral head defect.[62,63]

GLENOID DEFECT TREATMENT OPTIONS
Nonoperative Treatment

As discussed earlier, small osseous lesions may be treated with monitored therapy focusing on strengthening the dynamic stabilizers. Hovelius and colleagues[40] followed the natural history of 229 shoulder dislocations for 25 years, and found that half of the patients between the ages of 12 to 25 years did not experience recurrent instability. Operative treatment of anterior shoulder instability has typically been reserved for large glenoid defects, extending past 25% of the surface area.[40,83,84]

Operative Treatment

Helfet[85] initially described a procedure known as the Bristow, whereby 1 cm of the distal coracoid and the conjoined tendon were transferred through a slit in the subscapularis on the anterior neck of the scapula. The transfer used suture fixation through the conjoined and subscapular tendons. A dynamic buttress was created across the anterior aspect of the glenoid to enhance shoulder stability in abduction and external rotation. Of the 30 patients reported, only 1 experienced continued instability after the coracoid bone-block transfer.[85] Schroder and colleagues[86] reported their findings on 52 Bristow procedures at an average follow-up of 26.4 years. In this cohort, 5 shoulders subsequently had dislocations, with 3 additional shoulders experiencing recurrent instability. Overall, 70% of the patients showed good to excellent results. However, the study only had 10 patients with clinical and radiographic follow-up, and found high rates of glenohumeral arthritis and loss of external rotation in 4 of 11 patients. Schauder and Tullos[87] reported that isolated Bristow results have been only 50% successful at preventing shoulder instability. Therefore, continued modifications to the Bristow procedure have been suggested and made to improve stability and decrease the rate of glenohumeral arthritis.

A similar bone-block technique was described by Latarjet to provide stability for anterior shoulder instability. The coracoid was secured to the anterior glenoid at the medial scapular neck using screw fixation. Since the early studies on bone block for anterior instability, several techniques have emerged for the Latarjet harvest, alignment, and fixation. Regardless of these techniques, Patte[88] described the location of the bone block being flush with the anterior glenoid rim as being a critical element in stabilization. To restore the articular concavity and contact pressures of the glenohumeral joint while avoiding ongoing instability and/or arthrosis, placement of the bone block at the level of the native glenoid fossa is necessary.[89]

Nevertheless, few high-quality studies have reported the results of Latarjet procedures. Allain and colleagues[90] found no instability at 14.3 years of follow-up in a series of 95 cases, but did note that 34 (37%) patients had glenohumeral arthritis.

Based on these findings they concluded that lateral placement of the bone block was a risk factor for higher rates of osteoarthritis. Walch and colleagues[91] found similar results on 160 patients who underwent a Latarjet with minimum 3-year follow-up. The investigators reported persistent instability at only 1%, but found that a laterally displaced coracoid graft led to higher rates of osteoarthritis.

In a study assessing clinical instability without radiographic review, Burkhart and colleagues[92] reported their findings on a modification of the original Latarjet by using the inferior surface of the coracoid in 102 patients, and found recurrent instability in 5 patients with a mean follow-up of 59 months. Hovelius and colleagues[93] reported outcomes of 118 patients at 15-year follow-up. One patient had recurrent shoulder instability within 2 years of follow-up; however, at final follow-up 14 patients had a dislocation or subluxation event. Nevertheless, 98% of the patients were very satisfied and/or satisfied with their results.

In 1948, Palmer and Widen reported their outcomes on the Hybbinette-Eden anterior bone-block procedure that used iliac crest autografting to prevent engagement of the Hill-Sachs lesion and recurrent instability. The idea of using the inner table of the iliac crest was that it would better match the articular contour and better restore the contact pressures within the glenohumeral joint.[94] Niskanen and colleagues[95] described a modification to the iliac crest technique, known as the Alvik glenoplasty, using press fixation at the anterior glenoid. Although the recurrence rate was 21%, there were degenerative changes within 52% of the shoulders. This finding demonstrates the importance of graft fixation and location on restoring the biomechanics of the glenohumeral joint in long-term outcomes.

Warner and colleagues[96] analyzed 11 cases with bony reconstruction for anterior glenoid bone loss at a mean follow-up of 33 months. CT scans with 3D reconstructions were obtained at 4 to 6 months postoperatively to demonstrate union of the bone graft. American Shoulder and Elbow Surgeons scores improved from 65 to 94, University of California Los Angeles scores improved from 33 to 18, and Rowe scores improved from 28 to 94. Two patients had pain with overhead activities, with no cases of recurrent instability.

However, Moroder and colleagues[97] studied the clinical and radiologic outcome of iliac crest autograft for anterior shoulder instability with glenoid bone loss in 9 patients with a mean follow-up of 34.6 months. Two patients reported the recurrence

of instability and demonstrated a positive apprehension test. The overall glenoid surface increased 6.4% compared with preoperative findings, leading the investigators to suspect graft osteolysis and subsequent clinical instability. Moroder and colleagues[98] used a J-bone graft in 20 patients with a CT evaluation at 1-year follow-up, noting that the J-bone graft overcorrected the glenoid concavity and subsequently normalized as a result of remodeling processes.

Investigators continue to explore different types of bone blocks and fixation methods to restore optimal glenohumeral biomechanics. Further biomechanical and long-term follow-up studies are needed to not only reduce anterior shoulder instability but also decrease glenohumeral arthritis.

REFERENCES

1. Zacchilli MA, Owens BD. Epidemiology of shoulder dislocations presenting to emergency departments in the United States. J Bone Joint Surg Am 2010; 92(3):542–9.
2. Hovelius L. Incidence of shoulder dislocation in Sweden. Clin Orthop Relat Res 1982;(166):127–31.
3. Mazzocca AD, Cote MP, Solovyova O, et al. Traumatic shoulder instability involving anterior, inferior, and posterior labral injury: a prospective clinical evaluation of arthroscopic repair of 270 degrees labral tears. Am J Sports Med 2011;39(8):1687–96.
4. Bollier MJ, Arciero R. Management of glenoid and humeral bone loss. Sports Med Arthrosc 2010; 18(3):140–8.
5. Ghodadra N, Gupta A, Romeo AA, et al. Normalization of glenohumeral articular contact pressures after Latarjet or iliac crest bone-grafting. J Bone Joint Surg 2010;92(6):1478–89.
6. Greis PE, Scuderi MG, Mohr A, et al. Glenohumeral articular contact areas and pressures following labral and osseous injury to the anteroinferior quadrant of the glenoid. J Shoulder Elbow Surg 2002; 11(5):442–51.
7. Matsen F 3rd, Chebli C, Lippitt S, American Academy of Orthopaedic Surgeons. Principles for the evaluation and management of shoulder instability. J Bone Joint Surg Am 2006;88:648–59.
8. Montgomery WH Jr, Wahl M, Hettrich C, et al. Anteroinferior bone-grafting can restore stability in osseous glenoid defects. J Bone Joint Surg 2005; 87(9):1972–7.
9. Miniaci A, Gish MW. Management of anterior glenohumeral instability associated with large Hill–Sachs defects. Tech Shoulder Elbow Surg 2004;5(3):170–5.
10. Flower WH. On the pathological changes produced in the shoulder-joint by traumatic dislocation: as derived from an examination of all the

specimens illustrating this Injury in the Museums of London. Trans Pathol Soc London 1861;12:179.

11. Hill HA, Sachs MD. The grooved defect of the humeral head a frequently unrecognized complication of dislocations of the shoulder joint. Radiology 1940;35(6):690–700.

12. Calandra JJ, Baker CL, Uribe J. The incidence of Hill-Sachs lesions in initial anterior shoulder dislocations. Arthroscopy 1989;5(4):254–7.

13. Rowe CR, Patel D, Southmayd WW. The Bankart procedure: a long-term end-result study. J Bone Joint Surg Am 1978;60(1):1–16.

14. Saupe N, White LM, Bleakney R, et al. Acute traumatic posterior shoulder dislocation: MR findings. Radiology 2008;248(1):185–93.

15. Taylor DC, Arciero RA. Pathologic changes associated with shoulder dislocations. Arthroscopic and physical examination findings in first-time, traumatic anterior dislocations. Am J Sports Med 1997;25(3):306–11.

16. Yiannakopoulos CK, Mataragas E, Antonogiannakis E. A comparison of the spectrum of intra-articular lesions in acute and chronic anterior shoulder instability. Arthroscopy 2007;23(9):985–90.

17. Burkhart SS, Danaceau SM. Articular arc length mismatch as a cause of failed Bankart repair. Arthroscopy 2000;16(7):740–4.

18. Bigliani LU, Newton PM, Steinmann SP, et al. Glenoid rim lesions associated with recurrent anterior dislocation of the shoulder. Am J Sports Med 1998;26(1):41–5.

19. Edwards TB, Boulahia A, Walch G. Radiographic analysis of bone defects in chronic anterior shoulder instability. Arthroscopy 2003;19(7):732–9.

20. Griffith JF, Antonio GE, Yung PS, et al. Prevalence, pattern, and spectrum of glenoid bone loss in anterior shoulder dislocation: CT analysis of 218 patients. AJR Am J Roentgenol 2008;190(5):1247–54.

21. Sugaya H, Moriishi J, Dohi M, et al. Glenoid rim morphology in recurrent anterior glenohumeral instability. J Bone Joint Surg Am 2003;85-A(5): 878–84.

22. Widjaja AB, Tran A, Bailey M, et al. Correlation between Bankart and Hill-Sachs lesions in anterior shoulder dislocation. ANZ J Surg 2006;76(6): 436–8.

23. Richards RD, Sartoris DJ, Pathria MN, et al. Hill-Sachs lesion and normal humeral groove: MR imaging features allowing their differentiation. Radiology 1994;190(3):665–8.

24. Saito H, Itoi E, Minagawa H, et al. Location of the Hill-Sachs lesion in shoulders with recurrent anterior dislocation. Arch Orthop Trauma Surg 2009; 129(10):1327–34.

25. Palmer I, Widen A. The bone block method for recurrent dislocation of the shoulder joint. J Bone Joint Surg Br 1948;30B(1):53–8.

26. Burkhart SS, De Beer JF. Traumatic glenohumeral bone defects and their relationship to failure of arthroscopic Bankart repairs: significance of the inverted-pear glenoid and the humeral engaging Hill-Sachs lesion. Arthroscopy 2000; 16(7):677–94.

27. Armitage MS, Faber KJ, Drosdowech DS, et al. Humeral head bone defects: remplissage, allograft, and arthroplasty. Orthop Clin North Am 2010; 41(3):417–25.

28. Miniaci A, Martineau PA. Humeral head bony deficiency (large Hill-Sachs). In: El Attrache NS, editor. Surgical Techniques in Sports Medicine. Philadelphia: Lippincott Williams & Wilkins; 2006.

29. Cho SH, Cho NS, Rhee YG. Preoperative analysis of the Hill-Sachs lesion in anterior shoulder instability: how to predict engagement of the lesion. Am J Sports Med 2011;39(11):2389–95.

30. Cetik O, Uslu M, Ozsar BK. The relationship between Hill-Sachs lesion and recurrent anterior shoulder dislocation. Acta Orthop Belg 2007; 73(2):175–8.

31. Loebenberg MI, Cuomo F. The treatment of chronic anterior and posterior dislocations of the glenohumeral joint and associated articular surface defects. Orthop Clin North Am 2000;31(1):23–34.

32. Flatow EL, Miller SR, Neer CS 2nd. Chronic anterior dislocation of the shoulder. J Shoulder Elbow Surg 1993;2(1):2–10.

33. Kirtland S, Resnick D, Sartoris DJ, et al. Chronic unreduced dislocations of the glenohumeral joint: imaging strategy and pathologic correlation. J Trauma 1988;28(12):1622–31.

34. Sekiya JK, Wickwire AC, Stehle JH, et al. Hill-Sachs defects and repair using osteoarticular allograft transplantation biomechanical analysis using a joint compression model. Am J Sports Med 2009; 37(12):2459–66.

35. Kaar SG, Fening SD, Jones MH, et al. Effect of humeral head defect size on glenohumeral stability a cadaveric study of simulated Hill-Sachs defects. Am J Sports Med 2010;38(3):594–9.

36. Saito H, Itoi E, Sugaya H, et al. Location of the glenoid defect in shoulders with recurrent anterior dislocation. Am J Sports Med 2005;33(6):889–93.

37. d'Elia G, Di Giacomo A, D'Alessandro P, et al. Traumatic anterior glenohumeral instability: quantification of glenoid bone loss by spiral CT. Radiol Med 2008;113(4):496–503 [in English, Italian].

38. Itoi E, Lee SB, Amrami KK, et al. Quantitative assessment of classic anteroinferior bony Bankart lesions by radiography and computed tomography. Am J Sports Med 2003;31(1):112–8.

39. Yamamoto N, Itoi E, Abe H, et al. Effect of an anterior glenoid defect on anterior shoulder stability: a cadaveric study. Am J Sports Med 2009;37(5): 949–54.

40. Hovelius L, Olofsson A, Sandstrom B, et al. Nonoperative treatment of primary anterior shoulder dislocation in patients forty years of age and younger. a prospective twenty-five-year follow-up. J Bone Joint Surg Am 2008;90(5):945–52.

41. Hovelius L, Augustini BG, Fredin H, et al. Primary anterior dislocation of the shoulder in young patients. A ten-year prospective study. J Bone Joint Surg Am 1996;78(11):1677–84.

42. Rowe C, Zarins B, Ciullo J. Recurrent anterior dislocation of the shoulder after surgical repair. Apparent causes of failure and treatment. J Bone Joint Surg Am 1984;66(2):159.

43. Kralinger FS, Golser K, Wischatta R, et al. Predicting recurrence after primary anterior shoulder dislocation. Am J Sports Med 2002;30(1):116–20.

44. Chen AL, Hunt SA, Hawkins RJ, et al. Management of bone loss associated with recurrent anterior glenohumeral instability. Am J Sports Med 2005;33(6):912–25.

45. Lo IKY, Parten PM, Burkhart SS, et al. The inverted pear glenoid: an indicator of significant glenoid bone loss. Arthroscopy 2004;20:169–74.

46. Pavlov H, Warren RF, Weiss CB Jr, et al. The roentgenographic evaluation of anterior shoulder instability. Clin Orthop Relat Res 1985;(194):153–8.

47. Bois AJ, Walker RE, Kodali P, et al. Imaging instability in the athlete: the right modality for the right diagnosis. Clin Sports Med 2013;32(4):653–84.

48. Garth WP Jr, Slappey CE, Ochs CW. Roentgenographic demonstration of instability of the shoulder: the apical oblique projection. A technical note. J Bone Joint Surg Am 1984;66(9):1450–3.

49. Bernageau J, Patte D, Debeyre J, et al. Value of the glenoid profile in recurrent luxations of the shoulder. Rev Chir Orthop Reparatrice Appar Mot 1976;62(2 suppl):142–7 [in French].

50. Rokous JR, Feagin JA, Abbott HG. Modified axillary roentgenogram. A useful adjunct in the diagnosis of recurrent instability of the shoulder. Clin Orthop Relat Res 1972;82:84–6.

51. Kodali P, Jones MH, Polster J, et al. Accuracy of measurement of Hill-Sachs lesions with computed tomography. J Shoulder Elbow Surg 2011;20(8):1328–34.

52. Bois AJ, Fening SD, Polster J, et al. Quantifying glenoid bone loss in anterior shoulder instability: reliability and accuracy of 2-dimensional and 3-dimensional computed tomography measurement techniques. Am J Sports Med 2012;40(11):2569–77.

53. Baudi P, Righi P, Bolognesi D, et al. How to identify and calculate glenoid bone deficit. Chir Organi Mov 2005;90(2):145–52 [in English, Italian].

54. Burkhart SS, Debeer JF, Tehrany AM, et al. Quantifying glenoid bone loss arthroscopically in shoulder instability. Arthroscopy 2002;18(5):488–91.

55. Boileau P, Villalba M, Hery JY, et al. Risk factors for recurrence of shoulder instability after arthroscopic Bankart repair. J Bone Joint Surg Am 2006;88(8):1755–63.

56. Purchase RJ, Wolf EM, Hobgood ER, et al. Hill-Sachs "remplissage": an arthroscopic solution for the engaging hill-sachs lesion. Arthroscopy 2008;24(6):723–6.

57. Weber B, Simpson L, Hardegger F, et al. Rotational humeral osteotomy for recurrent anterior dislocation of the. J Bone Joint Surg Am 1984;66:1443–50.

58. Bigliani LU, Weinstein DM, Glasgow MT, et al. Glenohumeral arthroplasty for arthritis after instability surgery. J Shoulder Elbow Surg 1995;4(2):87–94.

59. Yagishita K, Thomas BJ. Use of allograft for large Hill-Sachs lesion associated with anterior glenohumeral dislocation: a case report. Injury 2002;33(9):791–4.

60. Connolly RS. Humeral head defects associated with shoulder dislocations: their diagnostic and surgical significance. Instr Course Lect 1972;21:42–54.

61. Pritchett JW, Clark JM. Prosthetic replacement for chronic unreduced dislocations of the shoulder. Clin Orthop Relat Res 1987;216:89–93.

62. Balg F, Boileau P. The instability severity index score. A simple pre-operative score to select patients for arthroscopic or open shoulder stabilisation. J Bone Joint Surg Br 2007;89(11):1470–7.

63. Millett PJ, Clavert P, Warner JJ. Open operative treatment for anterior shoulder instability: when and why? J Bone Joint Surg Am 2005;87(2):419–32.

64. Stachowicz RZ, Romanowski JR, Wissman R, et al. Percutaneous balloon humeroplasty for Hill-Sachs lesions: a novel technique. J Shoulder Elbow Surg 2013;22:e7–13.

65. Kazel MD, Sekiya JK, Greene JA, et al. Percutaneous correction (humeroplasty) of humeral head defects (Hill-Sachs) associated with anterior shoulder instability: a cadaveric study. Arthroscopy 2005;21(12):1473–8.

66. Wolf EM, Pollack ME. Hill-Sachs "remplissage": an arthroscopic solution for the engaging Hill-Sachs lesion. Arthroscopy 2004;20(Suppl 1):e14–5.

67. Koo SS, Burkhart SS, Ochoa E. Arthroscopic double-pulley remplissage technique for engaging Hill-Sachs lesions in anterior shoulder instability repairs. Arthroscopy 2009;25(11):1343–8.

68. Elkinson I, Giles JW, Boons HW, et al. The shoulder remplissage procedure for Hill-Sachs defects: does technique matter? J Shoulder Elbow Surg 2013;22(6):835–41.

69. Zhu YM, Lu Y, Zhang J, et al. Arthroscopic Bankart repair combined with remplissage technique for the treatment of anterior shoulder instability with

engaging Hill-Sachs lesion: a report of 49 cases with a minimum 2-year follow-up. Am J Sports Med 2011;39(8):1640–7.

70. Boileau P, O'Shea K, Vargas P, et al. Anatomical and functional results after arthroscopic Hill-Sachs remplissage. J Bone Joint Surg Am 2012; 94(7):618–26.

71. Leroux T, Bhatti A, Khoshbin A, et al. Combined arthroscopic Bankart repair and remplissage for recurrent shoulder instability. Arthroscopy 2013; 29:1693–701.

72. Park MJ, Garcia G, Malhotra A, et al. The evaluation of arthroscopic remplissage by high-resolution magnetic resonance imaging. Am J Sports Med 2012;40(10):2331–6.

73. Chapovsky F, Kelly JD 4th. Osteochondral allograft transplantation for treatment of glenohumeral instability. Arthroscopy 2005;21(8):1007.

74. Kropf EJ, Sekiya JK. Osteoarticular allograft transplantation for large humeral head defects in glenohumeral instability. Arthroscopy 2007;23(3): 322.e1–5.

75. Diklic ID, Ganic ZD, Blagojevic ZD, et al. Treatment of locked chronic posterior dislocation of the shoulder by reconstruction of the defect in the humeral head with an allograft. J Bone Joint Surg Br 2010; 92(1):71–6.

76. Ahmad CS, Moros C. Partial humeral head resurfacing and latarjet coracoid transfer for treatment of recurrent anterior glenohumeral instability. Orthopaedics 2009;32(8):602.

77. Grondin P, Leith J. Combined large Hill–Sachs and bony Bankart lesions treated by Latarjet and partial humeral head resurfacing: a report of 2 cases. Can J Surg 2009;52(3):249.

78. Raiss P, Aldinger PR, Kasten P, et al. Humeral head resurfacing for fixed anterior glenohumeral dislocation. Int Orthop 2009;33(2):451–6.

79. Scalise JJ, Miniaci A, Iannotti JP. Resurfacing arthroplasty of the humerus: Indications, surgical technique, and clinical results. Tech Shoulder Elbow Surg 2007;8:152–60.

80. Copeland S. The continuing development of shoulder replacement: "reaching the surface". J Bone Joint Surg Am 2006;88:900–5.

81. Flatow EL, Warner JI. Instability of the shoulder: complex problems and failed repairs: Part I. Relevant biomechanics, multidirectional instability, and severe glenoid loss. Instr Course Lect 1998;47: 97–112.

82. Denard PJ, Raiss P, Sowa B, et al. Mid- to long-term follow-up of total shoulder arthroplasty using a keeled glenoid in young adults with primary glenohumeral arthritis. J Shoulder Elbow Surg 2013; 22(7):894–900.

83. Hovelius L, Sandstrom B, Olofsson A, et al. The effect of capsular repair, bone block healing, and position on the results of the Bristow-Latarjet procedure (study III): long-term follow-up in 319 shoulders. J Shoulder Elbow Surg 2012;21(5): 647–60.

84. Hovelius L, Sandstrom B, Saebo M. One hundred eighteen Bristow-Latarjet repairs for recurrent anterior dislocation of the shoulder prospectively followed for fifteen years: study II-the evolution of dislocation arthropathy. J Shoulder Elbow Surg 2006;15(3):279–89.

85. Helfet AJ. Coracoid transplantation for recurring dislocation of the shoulder. J Bone Joint Surg Br 1958;40-B(2):198–202.

86. Schroder DT, Provencher MT, Mologne TS, et al. The modified Bristow procedure for anterior shoulder instability: 26-year outcomes in Naval Academy midshipmen. Am J Sports Med 2006;34(5): 778–86.

87. Schauder KS, Tullos HS. Role of the coracoid bone block in the modified Bristow procedure. Am J Sports Med 1992;20(1):31–4.

88. Patte D, Debeyre J. Luxations recidivantes de l'epaule. Encycl Med Chir Paris. Tech Chir Orthop 1980;44265. 4.4–02 [in French].

89. Lynch JR, Clinton JM, Dewing CB, et al. Treatment of osseous defects associated with anterior shoulder instability. J Shoulder Elbow Surg 2009;18(2): 317–28.

90. Allain J, Goutallier D, Glorion C. Long-term results of the Latarjet procedure for the treatment of anterior instability of the shoulder. J Bone Joint Surg Am 1998;80(6):841–52.

91. Walch G, Boileau P. Latarjet-Bristow procedure for recurrent anterior instability. Tech Shoulder Elbow Surg 2000;1:256–61.

92. Burkhart SS, De Beer JF, Barth JR, et al. Results of modified Latarjet reconstruction in patients with anteroinferior instability and significant bone loss. Arthroscopy 2007;23(10):1033–41.

93. Hovelius L, Sandstrom B, Sundgren K, et al. One hundred eighteen Bristow-Latarjet repairs for recurrent anterior dislocation of the shoulder prospectively followed for fifteen years: study I–clinical results. J Shoulder Elbow Surg 2004;13(5): 509–16.

94. Hutchinson MR, Dall BE. Midline fascial splitting approach to the iliac crest for bone graft. A new approach. Spine 1994;19(1):62–6.

95. Niskanen RO, Lehtonen JY, Kaukonen JP. Alvik's glenoplasty for humeroscapular dislocation. 6-year follow-up of 52 shoulders. Acta Orthop Scand 1991;62(3):279–83.

96. Warner JJ, Gill TJ, O'Hollerhan JD, et al. Anatomical glenoid reconstruction for recurrent anterior glenohumeral instability with glenoid deficiency using an autogenous tricortical iliac crest bone graft. Am J Sports Med 2006;34(2):205–12.

97. Moroder P, Blocher M, Auffarth A, et al. Clinical and computed tomography-radiologic outcome after bony glenoid augmentation in recurrent anterior shoulder instability without significant glenoid bone loss. J Shoulder Elbow Surg 2014;23:420–6.

98. Moroder P, Hitzl W, Tauber M, et al. Effect of anatomic bone grafting in post-traumatic recurrent anterior shoulder instability on glenoid morphology. J Shoulder Elbow Surg 2013;22(11):1522–9.

99. Bigliani LU, Flatow EL, Pollock RG. Fractures of the proximal humerus. In: Rockwood CA, Green DP, Bucholz RW, et al, editors. Fractures in adults. 4th edition. Philadelphia: Lippincott-Raven; 1996. p. 1055–107.

Upper Extremity Considerations for Oncologic Surgery

Justin C. Wong, MD[a], John A. Abraham, MD[b],*

KEYWORDS

- Upper extremity • Sarcoma • Reconstruction • Endoprosthesis • Allograft

KEY POINTS

- Nearly 30% of soft tissue sarcomas occur in the upper extremity.
- Elements of the patient's history that would warrant a higher level of suspicion for malignancy include change in size of a mass, presence of night pain, and constitutional symptoms such as fevers, chills, and night sweats.
- Diagnostic imaging is a crucial component of the workup of a patient with a musculoskeletal tumor and should proceed in an organized fashion.
- Soft tissue masses that are larger than 5 cm or deep to the investing fascia have a high increased chance of being a sarcoma and should be referred on to an orthopedic oncologist before obtaining biopsy.
- Current grading and staging systems for musculoskeletal tumors are designed to guide treatment, provide prognostic information for patients, and standardize research.

BACKGROUND

According to the National Cancer Institute estimates, more than 3000 people would be diagnosed with primary bone or joint malignancy and more than 11,000 people would be diagnosed with a soft tissue sarcoma in 2013.[1] A large report on more than 1000 soft tissue sarcomas treated at Memorial Sloan Kettering Cancer Center showed that the upper extremity was involved in approximately 29% of cases.[2] Although primary bone and soft tissue tumors of the upper extremity are infrequent, it is imperative that the clinician be familiar with a systematic approach to the diagnosis and treatment of these conditions to prevent inadvertently compromising patient outcome. With advances in chemotherapy, radiotherapy, tumor imaging, and surgical reconstructive options, limb salvage surgery is estimated to be feasible in 95% of extremity bone or soft tissue sarcomas.

APPROACH TO THE PATIENT WITH AN UPPER EXTREMITY TUMOR
Presentation

A thorough history and physical examination remain the cornerstone for the diagnosis of musculoskeletal malignancy. A patient with a bone tumor may have pain in the extremity, or the tumor may be discovered as an incidental finding. In contrast, patients with soft tissue tumors often present with a painless mass. Elements of the patient's history that would warrant a higher level of suspicion for malignancy include change in size of a mass,

Each author has contributed substantially to the research, preparation, and production of the article and approves of its submission to the journal.

[a] Department of Orthopaedic Surgery, Thomas Jefferson University, 1025 Walnut Street, Room 516, College Building, Philadelphia, PA 19107, USA; [b] The Rothman Institute of Orthopaedics, Thomas Jefferson University Hospital, 925 Chestnut Street, 5th Floor, Philadelphia, PA 19107, USA

* Corresponding author.

E-mail address: John.abraham@rothmaninstitute.com

Orthop Clin N Am 45 (2014) 541–564
http://dx.doi.org/10.1016/j.ocl.2014.06.007

presence of night pain, and constitutional symptoms such as fevers, chills, and night sweats.[3] In the setting of a pathologic fracture, history of antecedent pain may be a clue to a more aggressive process. Although sarcoma metastasis to regional lymph nodes is uncommon, it may be seen in certain subtypes of soft tissue sarcoma. The clinician should always remember that metastases are more common than primary sarcomas, and therefore, history should include asking about common primary carcinoma sources, such as lung, kidney, breast, thyroid, and prostate.

Workup

Diagnostic imaging is a crucial component of the workup of a patient with a musculoskeletal tumor and should proceed in an organized fashion. Initial imaging often includes radiographs in orthogonal planes to localize and characterize a lesion. Although soft tissue lesions may not be seen on plain radiographs, at least 1 set is usually taken to look for calcifications, erosion into adjacent bone, or other features (**Fig. 1**: Soft tissue tumor radiograph and magnetic resonance imaging [MRI]). Bone lesions must be evaluated for location of lesion within the bone, size, margin, zone of transition, periosteal reaction, mineralization, and number of lesions.[4] For lytic bone lesions, the Lodwick classification[5] is commonly used. Lesions may be described as geographic, moth-eaten, or permeative. Geographic lesions with sclerotic or well-defined borders tend to be benign, whereas more aggressive lesions may have a moth-eaten or permeative appearance and a wide zone of transition to normal bone. Cortical destruction, periosteal reaction, and the presence of soft tissue mass are typical of more pathologic processes. Radiographic matrix, when present, may give clues to the diagnosis; for example, fibrous dysplasia has a typical ground-glass appearance,

and chondroid matrix may often present with calcified rings, arcs, and stippling.

Although ultrasonography is generally not used for bone tumors, it may be useful in evaluation of soft tissue mass to determine if a structure is cystic. Clinical scenarios in which ultrasonography might be useful include a superficial soft tissue mass or one adjacent to a joint.

Cross-sectional imaging is able to provide crucial information regarding size, tissue characteristics, and anatomic relationship to other structures of a lesion. Computed tomography (CT) is ideally suited for evaluation of the characteristics of a bony lesion, but may have some usefulness in evaluating soft tissue masses, particularly if there is periosteal reaction or osseous erosions adjacent to the soft tissue mass. MRI of the involved area is useful for both soft tissue and bony lesions and should be performed before any biopsy procedure. The basic imaging sequences used are T1-weighted and T2-weighted images. T1-weighted imaging has a higher signal-to-noise ratio, which makes it useful for defining anatomy and the spatial relationship between the lesion and surrounding tissue, whereas T2-weighted images are fluid sensitive and enable detection of fluid or edema. Fat-suppressed T2-weighted imaging provides improved contrast in detecting edema. For bony lesions, MRI may be helpful in showing extent of marrow replacement or soft tissue mass. Gadolinium may be used as an intravenous contrast agent to determine if a mass is solid with a blood supply.

Whole-body bone scintigraphy can be used to determine if a bony lesion is singular or multifocal. The uptake on bone scintigraphy may also correlate with the aggressiveness of the lesion, except in the case of myeloma, which often has limited bony uptake. For soft tissue tumors, bone scintigraphy may show areas of bony metastases.[6] In the case of multifocal lesions, bone scintigraphy may

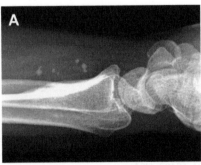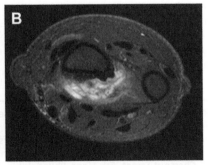

Fig. 1. Radiograph and magnetic resonance imaging (MRI) of soft tissue mass. (A) Lateral radiograph of distal radius shows phleboliths in soft tissue volar to distal radius; bone changes include scalloping and sclerosis of volar distal radius cortex. (B) Axial T2-weighted MRI of distal radius soft tissue mass in pronator quadratus. (*Courtesy of* W. Morrison, MD, Philadelphia, PA.)

show a lesion that is more easily accessible for biopsy than the originally detected lesion.[7]

Because bone and soft tissue sarcomas have a tendency to metastasize to the lungs, CT of the thorax is imperative in the evaluation of these patients, although it does not need to be performed before biopsy. In the case of a metastatic lesion from an unknown source, chest, abdomen, and pelvis CT should be obtained in addition to common laboratory studies (**Table 1**). Approximately 85% of skeletal metastases of unknown origin may be identified with inclusion of these imaging modalities.[7]

Positron emission tomography (PET) is an imaging modality that detects localization of radiolabeled tracers, such as fluorodeoxyglucose (FDG), and is commonly used for evaluation of metastases of carcinomas and lymphomas. In a recent meta-analysis, FDG-PET has been shown to have high sensitivity and specificity for diagnosis of soft tissue or mixed soft tissue and osseous lesions and may be able to differentiate between benign and malignant lesions.[8] However, its role in the routine staging of soft tissue and osseous sarcomas continues to be investigated.

Biopsy

Often the clinical history, patient age, and radiographic features of a bony lesion are helpful in determining a differential diagnosis for bone tumors, and in the case of lesions that are benign and appear latent, they may obviate biopsy.

However, in aggressive appearing bone lesions and most soft tissue masses, a histologic specimen should be obtained for diagnosis. The importance of obtaining a biopsy in the appropriate manner cannot be overemphasized, because of the potential for compromising the definitive surgical treatment as well as patient outcome.[9,10] For this reason, suspected primary malignancies should be referred to the surgeon who will be providing definitive management. Soft tissue masses that are larger than 5 cm or deep to the investing fascia have a high increased chance of being a sarcoma and should be referred on to an orthopedic oncologist before obtaining biopsy.[11]

Biopsy may be performed by either open or closed technique. Closed techniques such as fine-needle aspiration and core needle biopsy have the advantage of being performed outside an operating room, but in some cases, they may not yield sufficient tissue. Open biopsy has the advantage of providing more tissue for pathology evaluation and should be performed in accordance with standard principles (**Table 2**).[12]

Grading and Staging

Current grading and staging systems for musculoskeletal tumors are designed to guide treatment, provide prognostic information for patients, and standardize research. Tumor grade refers to the histologic appearance of a tumor and is determined based on cellular anaplasia, mitotic activity, presence or absence of abnormal mitotic figures,

Table 1
Diagnostic laboratory and imaging workup

Study	Rationale	Examples
Imaging Tests		
CT of chest	Evaluate for pulmonary metastases or primary carcinoma	Lung CA
CT of abdomen/pelvis	Evaluate for primary carcinoma	Renal, prostate CA
Laboratory Tests		
Complete blood count	Evaluate for anemia or leukocytosis	Infection, myeloma
Erythrocyte sedimentation rate	Evaluate for inflammatory reaction	Infection, myeloma
Complement reactive protein	Evaluate for inflammatory reaction	Infection
TSH, FT4	Evaluate for thyroid cancer	
Basic metabolic panel	Evaluate electrolytes and renal function	Renal CA
Urinalysis	Evaluate for microhematuria	Renal CA
Prostate-specific antigen	Evaluate for prostate CA	Prostate CA
SPEP/UPEP	Evaluate for multiple myeloma	Myeloma

Abbreviations: CA, Cancer; FT4, free T4; SPEP, serum protein electrophoresis; TSH, thyroid-stimulating hormone; UPEP, urine protein electrophoresis.

Table 2
Biopsy principles

Principle	Rationale
Longitudinal incision	Permits extensile exposure, less likely to compromise reconstructive options
Limited dissection through muscle	Dissection through muscle instead of around muscle limits local contamination
Hemostasis (use of tourniquet and meticulous dissection)	Limits hematoma formation and local contamination; if tourniquet is used, exsanguination should not be performed to limit tumor embolism
Send specimen for culture and pathology	Infection may mimic tumor
Circular cortical window	Limit stress risers in bone
Drain site close to and in line with incision	Drain site is considered contaminated and requires excision if pathology is malignant; drain site away from incision may compromise reconstructive options

amount of necrosis, and growth pattern. Low-grade lesions are generally well differentiated and show few mitoses and a moderate cellular atypia, whereas high-grade lesions may show a higher mitotic activity, poorly differentiated cells, evidence of microvascular invasion, and increased cellularity.

Staging incorporates the tumor grade along with factors such as tumor size, depth, and presence or absence of regional or distant metastases to better define a patient's prognosis. For malignant tumors, Enneking and colleagues[13] proposed a staging system, which was later adopted by the Musculoskeletal Tumor Society (MSTS), which is based on 3 factors: low or high tissue grade, whether or not the tumor is confined to an anatomic compartment, and presence or absence of metastasis (**Table 3**). Benign bone tumors are staged separately, based on the biological activity of the tumor (**Table 4**). Stage 1 benign bone tumors, such as nonossifying fibroma, are termed latent and remain static or are replaced spontaneously. Stage 2 benign lesions, such as an aneurysmal bone cyst or chondroblastoma, are termed active and show progressive growth but are limited by anatomic barriers. Stage 3 benign lesions, such as giant cell tumor of bone, are termed aggressive and show progressive growth not limited by anatomic barriers and may have potential for systemic metastases.

For soft tissue sarcomas, staging systems that use tumor size and depth as opposed to intracompartmental or extracompartmental status have been suggested to be more useful for prediction of systemic recurrence and death from sarcoma.[14,15] The Fifth edition of the American Joint Committee on Cancer (AJCC) staging system is

1 such staging system used for soft tissue sarcomas (**Table 5**).[16]

DIFFERENTIAL DIAGNOSIS OF BENIGN AND MALIGNANT TUMORS OF THE UPPER EXTREMITY

A variety of benign and malignant bone or soft tissue tumors may arise in the upper extremity (**Table 6**).

Common Bone-Forming Tumors

Osteoid osteomas represent approximately 10% of all benign bone tumors and may be found in the upper extremity in 19% to 31% of cases.[17] These

Table 3
Enneking sarcoma staging

Stage	Grade (G)	Site (T)	Regional or Distant Metastasis (M)
IA	Low (G1)	Intracompartmental (T1)	No
IB	Low (G1)	Extracompartmental (T2)	No
IIA	High (G2)	Intracompartmental (T1)	No
IIB	High (G2)	Extracompartmental (T2)	No
III	Any	Any	Yes

Adapted from Enneking WF, Spanier SS, Goodman MA. A system for the surgical staging of musculoskeletal sarcoma. Clin Orthop Relat Res 1980;153:111; with permission.

Table 4
Enneking benign bone lesion staging

Stage	Definition	Behavior	Example
1	Latent	Remains static, heals spontaneously	Inactive simple bone cyst
2	Active	Progressive growth, limited by natural barriers	Nonossifying fibroma
3	Aggressive	Progressive growth, NOT limited by natural barriers	Giant cell tumor

Adapted from Enneking WF, Spanier SS, Goodman MA. A system for the surgical staging of musculoskeletal sarcomas. Clin Orthop Rel Res 1980;153:106–20.

lesions commonly present with well-localized pain in the second to third decade of life. History of night pain and pain relief with use of aspirin or nonsteroidal antiinflammatory medications is common. From a radiographic perspective, there is a characteristic intracortical radiolucent nidus surrounded by a rim of dense reactive bone, which may be best appreciated on CT scan. Bone scan can show intense isotope uptake in these lesions. Although some cases are self-limiting, surgical treatment options include radiofrequency ablation or intralesional curettage. Radiofrequency ablation can be performed in the forearm, arm, and shoulder, but may be technically difficult in the hand and wrist because of proximity to neurovascular structures.[18] The recurrence rates after intralesional curettage may be as high as 25% in some studies.[19]

Osteosarcoma is a primary malignant tumor of mesenchymal origin characterized by its production of immature neoplastic osteoid.[20] When the upper extremity is affected, the humerus is the most common location, followed by lesions in the radius, ulna, metacarpals, and phalanges.[21–24] Treatment involves neoadjuvant chemotherapy,

wide resection or amputation, and postoperative chemotherapy based on tumor margins and tumor response to chemotherapy.[22,24,25] Tumors involving the phalanges and metacarpals can be successfully treated with ray resection, whereas limb salvage surgery is generally indicated for most proximal lesions.[22]

Prognostic factors for survival include tumor size and location, presence of systemic or skip metastases at the time of presentation, and response to neoadjuvant chemotherapy.[26,27] Increase of serum markers such as lactate dehydrogenase and alkaline phosphatase are also associated with risk of relapse.[27] Local recurrence is dependent on a clean tumor margin and tumor response to chemotherapy.[28]

The addition of adjuvant chemotherapy has greatly improved the survival rate of nonmetastatic osteosarcoma, with rates of disease-free survival at 2 years improving from 17% to 66% in 1 randomized controlled trial.[29] Tumor location within the extremity (proximal vs distal) may have an effect on outcome, with some investigators reporting worse outcomes for proximal humerus lesions,[26] whereas others have reported good

Table 5
AJCC *Soft Tissue Sarcoma Staging, Fifth Edition*

Stage	Pathologic Grade (G)	Primary Tumor (T)	N	M
IA (Low grade, small superficial or deep)	G1-2	T1a-1b	N0	M0
IB (Low grade, large, superficial)	G1-2	T2a	N0	M0
IIA (Low grade, large, deep)	G1-2	T2b	N0	M0
IIB (High grade, small, superficial or deep)	G3-4	T1a-1b	N0	M0
IIC (High grade, large, superficial)	G3-4	T2a	N0	M0
III (High grade, large, deep)	G3-4	T2b	N0	M0
IV (any metastasis)	Any G	Any T	N0	M1
	Any G	Any T	N1	M0

Abbreviations: G1, well differentiated; G2, moderately differentiated; G3, poorly differentiated; G4, undifferentiated; M, distant metastasis status; M0, no distant metastasis; M1, distant metastasis; N, regional lymph node status; N0, no regional lymph node metastasis; N1, regional lymph node metastasis; T1, tumor ≤5 cm in greatest diameter; T1a, superficial to fascia; T1b, deep to fascia; T2, tumor >5 cm in diameter; T2a, superficial to fascia; T2b, deep to fascia.

From Fleming ID, Cooper JS, Henson DE, et al, editors. AJCC Cancer Staging Manual. 5th edition. Philadelphia: Lippincott-Raven; 1997. p. 152.

Table 6
Benign and malignant tumors

Benign	Malignant
Osseous Lesions	
Osteoid osteoma	Osteosarcoma
Osteoblastoma	Parosteal osteosarcoma Periosteal osteosarcoma
Chondral Lesions	
Enchondroma	Primary chondrosarcoma
Osteochondroma	Secondary chondrosarcoma
Chondroblastoma	Dedifferentiated chondrosarcoma
Fibrous Lesions	
Nonossifying fibroma	Fibrosarcoma
Fibrous dysplasia	Malignant fibrous histiocytoma (undifferentiated pleomorphic sarcoma)
Cystic Lesions	
Solitary bone cyst	Telangiectatic osteosarcoma
Aneurysmal bone cyst	
Giant Cell Lesions	
Giant cell tumor	Malignant giant cell tumor

From Parsons TW 3rd, Filzen TW. Evaluation and staging of musculoskeletal neoplasia. Hand Clin 2004;20(2):137–45; with permission.

outcomes with 74% disease-free survival at 5-year.[27] Osteosarcomas arising in the hand may behave less aggressively than those in other locations, with a higher proportion of low-grade tumors and surface lesions and favorable outcomes, despite longer times between symptom onset and treatment.[21,23,24]

Common Cartilage Tumors

A spectrum of cartilage-forming tumors may present in the upper extremity. Enchondromas are one of the most common primary bone tumors in the upper extremity and typically arise in the diaphysis of the metacarpals or proximal or middle phalanges.[30] They may occur solitarily or may be multiple in certain conditions such as Ollier disease (multiple enchondromatosis) or Maffuci syndrome (multiple enchondromatosis associated with soft tissue hemangiomas). They typically are asymptomatic. Pain may be related to impending fracture

or be a sign of malignant degeneration to chondrosarcoma. Radiographically, the lesions can be expansile and lobular with endosteal scalloping and cortical thinning. MRI shows areas of multilobulated increased signal on T2-weighted imaging, interspersed with foci of low signal, representing matrix calcification. Features suggestive of malignant degeneration include progressive cortical destruction, loss of matrix mineralization, and an adjacent soft tissue mass. In certain locations, in particular the small bones of the fingers and the proximal fibula, radiographic features may appear slightly more aggressive without representing malignancy.[31] Treatment of enchondromas is dependent on symptoms and concern for malignancy. Asymptomatic lesions may be observed with serial radiographs. Pathologic fractures are generally managed with immobilization while the fracture heals, followed by biopsy and intralesional curettage with or without augmentation, such as bone graft and bone cement.[32]

Other benign cartilaginous tumors include extraskeletal chondroma, periosteal chondroma, osteochondroma, and chondroblastoma. Extraskeletal chondroma is a chondroma arising in the soft tissue and not in association with a joint, which distinguishes it from synovial chondromatosis. Periosteal chondromas arise adjacent to the bone within the periosteum and may result in scalloping of the outer cortex. MRI may confirm the characteristic appearance of cartilage in both of these lesions, and treatment with marginal excision is appropriate. Osteochondroma, as it occurs at other sites, is characterized by a bony prominence with medullary continuity to the affected bone, topped with a cartilaginous cap. Growth of the osteochondroma ceases when patients reach skeletal maturity. Multiple osteochondromas may be associated with multiple hereditary exostosis. The lesions may be observed or treated with marginal excision if symptomatic. Rarely, malignant degeneration of the cartilaginous cap may occur.

Chondrosarcomas can occur primarily or secondarily after malignant degeneration of an enchondroma or osteochondroma.[30,31] These slow-growing tumors are locally aggressive but have low metastatic potential and are not sensitive to adjuvant radiation or chemotherapy. Radiographic differentiation from enchondroma is difficult but may show significant endosteal scalloping, cortical destruction, and a soft tissue mass. Although chondrosarcoma represents one of the most common primary malignant bone tumors of the hands, its incidence is low compared with other sites such as the pelvis, femur, and humerus (**Fig. 2**).[31,33] Histologic differentiation between low-grade chondrosarcoma and enchondroma may be difficult

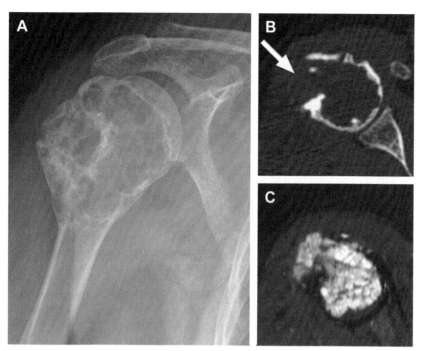

Fig. 2. Chondrosarcoma of proximal humerus. (*A*) Anteroposterior view of proximal humerus lesion with ring and arc calcifications; aggressive appearance with destruction of bony cortices. (*B*) Axial CT view of bony destruction of proximal humeral lesion; arrow points to area of cortical destruction and extracompartmental extension of tumor. (*C*) Axial T2 MRI view of proximal humeral lesion with lobulated appearance. Increased signal intensity and erosion through overlying cortex. (*Courtesy of* W. Morrison, MD, Philadelphia, PA.)

and often relies on correlation with clinical history and radiologic appearance.

Humeral lesions may be effectively treated with wide excision and limb-sparing surgery, with allograft or endoprosthetic reconstruction.[34,35] However, functional limitations in shoulder range of motion are common to both reconstructive options. Compared with chondrosarcoma at other locations, the reported overall survival for humeral lesions was better than occurrences in the pelvis or femur and equivalent to those in the tibia, with 96% survival at an average 16-year follow-up.[35] The treatment of lesions in the hand is dependent on histologic grade. Grade 1 lesions in the hand may be treated with curettage and grafting or wide excision, with similar low rate of local recurrence.[36] However, higher-grade lesions have an increased chance of local recurrence, and wide excision or amputation may be preferable.[33] Compared with high-grade lesions found in other anatomic sites, hand lesions have a lower rate of metastases.[33]

Benign but Locally Aggressive Lesions

Aneurysmal bone cyst

Aneurysmal bone cysts are benign but locally aggressive bone tumors that cause bony destruction and are seen more frequently in the lower extremities than in the upper extremities.[37–39] The humerus, radius, and ulna are more frequently involved than the smaller bones of the hand and wrist. The eccentric location of these tumors helps to distinguish them from unicameral bone cysts on plain radiographs. In addition, radiographic features of aneurysmal bone cysts include an expansile lytic lesion with cortical thinning, which in the hand may resemble giant cell tumor or enchondroma. MRI is helpful in distinguishing between these lesions and shows fluid-fluid levels in aneurysmal bone cyst. Treatment depends on the amount of bony destruction and may include curettage with or without additional bone grafting or bone cement in lesions with a stable bony architecture or excision and autograft or allograft bone reconstruction in more severely affected bone.[38]

Giant cell tumor of bone

Giant cell tumor of bone is a locally destructive neoplasm with a high recurrence rate and a small potential for distant pulmonary metastases.[37,40–42] It more commonly affects the distal femur and proximal tibia, but when it affects the upper extremity, it may involve the distal radius and proximal humerus.[40] Radiographically, it appears as an eccentric metaphyseal or epiphyseal lucency with cortical thinning. The Campanacci radiographic grading system is often used and describes the aggressiveness of the lesion. Stage I (calm) lesions do not distort the overlying cortex; stage II (active) lesions cause cortical expansion and thinning but do not perforate the overlying cortex; stage III (aggressive) lesions perforate the cortex and extend into the adjacent soft tissues.[42] MRI is useful in assessing the soft tissue component of a lesion (**Fig. 3**). The treatment of these lesions ranges from curettage and bone grafting with or without adjuvant treatments used for low-grade lesions to marginal or wide resection with autograft or allograft reconstruction for more aggressive lesions.[40,41]

Soft tissue sarcoma

Soft tissue sarcomas are a heterogeneous group of malignant tumors, with approximately 15% involving the upper extremity.[43] Some of the most common soft tissue sarcomas involving the upper extremity include epithelioid sarcoma, synovial sarcoma, and unclassified pleiomorphic sarcoma, formerly called malignant fibrous histiocytoma.[44,45] Although metastatic spread of sarcoma typically involves the lung, certain histologic subtypes such as rhabdomyosarcoma, epithelioid, clear cell, and angiosarcoma may metastasize to regional lymph nodes in 11% to 20% of cases.[46] In general, limb-sparing surgery with wide excision and adjuvant radiation therapy has shown equivalent rates of disease-free survival and improved function when compared with amputation, and it is therefore the preferred treatment strategy.[47–49] With limb-sparing surgery and adjuvant therapy, 5-year overall survival and disease-free survival

rates of 83% and 71%, respectively, have been reported.[47]

Surgical margins between 2 and 3 cm have been recommended for decreased rates of local recurrence after soft tissue sarcoma resection, but this may result in significant soft tissue defect, necessitating soft tissue reconstructive options.[44] However, with hand and wrist lesions, a clear surgical margin with local excision may be difficult, and partial amputations may sometimes be necessary to achieve local control.[50,51]

In cases of positive microscopic surgical margins, most investigators recommend reexcision to achieve a clean margin[49,50,52]; however, if reexcision or amputation would result in substantially increased morbidity, some have suggested that adjuvant therapy may be acceptable.[53–55] Although it is widely accepted that a positive microscopic margin predisposes to increased risk of local and systemic recurrence, the development of recurrent disease is not inevitable. In 1 series of 460 patients with evidence of microscopic margin after excision,[53] 72% of patients remained disease-free at more than 4-year follow-up.

SURGICAL CONSIDERATIONS
General Surgical Considerations

The goal of any surgical intervention for musculoskeletal tumors is local control. Before the 1970s, amputation was a common surgical procedure for malignant extremity tumors. Improvements in tumor imaging, adjunctive chemotherapy, radiation therapy, soft tissue coverage procedures, and reconstructive options have enabled limb salvage to be performed in 90% to 95% of upper extremity malignancies. The optimal surgical intervention is determined based on information

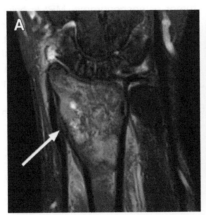
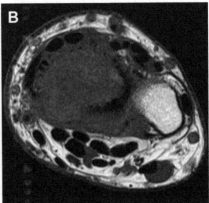

Fig. 3. MRI of giant cell tumor. (*A*) Coronal T2 MRI of giant cell tumor shows perforation of radial cortex; arrow points to area of cortical destruction and extension of tumor into soft tissue envelope. (*B*) Axial T1 MRI of giant cell tumor shows volar extension of tumor mass. (*Courtesy of* W. Morrison, MD, Philadelphia, PA.)

obtained through tumor grading and staging and tumor imaging. Enneking and colleagues[13] delineated the 4 types of surgical margins that may be achieved by excision or amputation based on the relationship of the plane of dissection to the tumor and surrounding structures. Intralesional procedures are those that dissect directly through tumor bed and result in gross contamination of the surgical field. This procedure may be acceptable for incisional biopsy or for definitive treatment of some benign tumors. Marginal procedures are those that dissect through a tumor pseudocapsule, which leaves behind residual microscopic disease. Wide excision procedures are those that avoid violating the tumor or its pseudocapsule by dissecting through a cuff of normal tissue around the tumor. Radical excision involves removing the entire bone or muscle compartment that is affected by tumor. The use of this classification for level of tumor resection facilitates comparisons in outcomes of tumor treatment among studies.

Intralesional Procedures

An intralesional procedure such as curettage and bone grafting with or without adjuvant treatments may be appropriate for aneurysmal bone cysts and giant cell tumors without soft tissue extension. The local recurrence rate of aneurysmal bone cysts treated by simple curettage with or without bone grafting varies between 10% and 60%.[56–58] Marginal resection may be considered in expendable bones to decrease the rate of local recurrence. Alternatives to marginal resection include an intralesional procedure with adjuvants such as cryosurgery with liquid nitrogen, phenol, high-speed burring, and cementation with methylmethacrylate after curettage of the lesion. The use of cryosurgery after curettage of aneurysmal bone cyst has been associated with a decreased recurrence rate between 5% and 16%.[59,60] Gibbs and colleagues[39] have advocated for high-speed burring instead of cryosurgery and had only 12% local recurrence with this technique. However, as highlighted by Athanasian,[37] cryosurgery may be technically demanding within the small bones of the hand and carries with it risks of fracture, premature physeal closure, and joint collapse.

Wide Resection

Wide resection is indicated for malignant tumors and benign but locally aggressive tumors with soft tissue extension. Although surgical resection of the tumor and secondary limb reconstruction procedures are intertwined, the primary goal of surgical intervention is to obtain local control of the tumor. Preservation of limb function should not compromise resection margins. In the preoperative planning, careful assessment of tumor involvement of neurovascular structures is critical, because this may necessitate nerve or vessel reconstruction or preclude the possibility of limb salvage.[61,62] For example, the clinical triad of intractable pain, motor deficit, and venography showing obliteration of the axillary vein has been postulated as being predictive of brachial plexus involvement.[62] During the planning for surgical resection, consideration should be given to the reconstruction of the bony, neurovascular, and soft tissue defects after tumor resection.

Nerve or Vascular Involvement

Preoperative evaluation must assess tumor involvement of peripheral neurovascular structures, because this has an impact on the feasibility of performing limb salvage surgery, reconstructive options, expected postoperative function, and potential complications. Cross-sectional imaging with MRI may show whether tumor is adjacent to or encasing nerves or vessels. Advances in microsurgery have enabled tumor resection to be carried out within the adventitial or epineural planes if tumor is lying adjacent to these critical structures.[63] However, if tumor arises from or is encasing nerves or vessels, then, they must be sacrificed at the time of resection. In general, if tumor involves 2 or more major nerves in the upper extremity or if anticipated function of the distal limb after tumor resection is predicted to be poor, then, amputation may be preferable.[64] Resection and replantation may be an alternative to amputation if tumor-free margins may be obtained.[65,66] The technique involves segmental resection of the proximal portion of the limb, including bone, soft tissue, and skin, and in some cases, nerves or vessels, with reimplantation of the distal limb to the body similar to rotationplasty described in the lower extremity.[67]

Arterial resection can often be managed well with bypass grafting using vein autografts or synthetic grafts.[68] Although not specific to the upper extremity, outcomes of limb salvage surgery in the lower extremity that required arterial reconstruction have shown higher rates of requirement of soft tissue coverage, wound complications, deep vein thrombosis, and limb edema compared with surgeries without need for vascular reconstruction.[69] In addition, the risk of progression to requiring amputation is higher when vascular reconstruction is needed. The requirement for postoperative therapeutic anticoagulation to prevent graft thrombosis may be related to the increased risk of wound complications.

In cases of single peripheral nerve resections in which motor and sensory deficits are expected, restoration of motor function has traditionally been achieved through tendon transfers. Although more commonly used in brachial plexus injuries, nerve transfers may be a promising alternative for restoring distal motor or sensory function after nerve resection.[70] Ozkan and colleagues[71] reported restoration of 10-mm 2-point discrimination in 15 of 25 hands with sensory deficits attributable to a variety of causes. To prevent contamination of the donor surgical site, tendon transfers should be performed in a delayed fashion, once negative tumor margins have been confirmed. The specific tendon transfers to be used are dependent on the expected functional deficit expected after nerve resection and should be individualized to the patient.[72]

Bone Reconstruction

The options for reconstruction of bony defects after tumor resection may be categorized based on location (diaphysis vs epiphysis) and, in the case of juxta-articular lesions, motion-preserving or arthrodesis procedures. Diaphyseal bone defects can be effectively managed with fibular bone graft. Epiphyseal bone defects of the distal radius and proximal humerus can also be managed with proximal fibular bone grafts, osteoarticular allograft, or endoprosthetic reconstruction.

Fibula Autograft

Vascularized and nonvascularized fibular autografts have a wide range of usefulness in reconstructive procedures of the upper extremity and may be used for diaphyseal defects of the humerus, radius, and ulna or as osteoarticular reconstructions of the proximal humerus, distal radius, or distal ulna.[73–77] Maruthainar and colleagues[77] reported good outcomes of 12 nonvascularized fibular autografts for reconstruction of distal radius defects. Excluding 3 patients who required forearm amputation for tumor recurrence, functional range of motion was preserved with few complications. In the proximal humerus, fibular autografts may be prone to fracture, which has been reported to occur in up to 36% of patients.[73,78] Despite this complication, which may be treated nonoperatively in some patients, quality of life and functional scores were marginally higher than in patients treated with an endoprosthesis in 1 series.[78] Hsu and colleagues[79] reviewed 30 vascularized fibula autografts for reconstruction after a variety of upper extremity and lower extremity sarcoma resections. Union rate was 90% in this series, with a 10% rate of infection and 10% rate of stress fracture. Gebert and colleagues[73] reported a higher complication rate in a series of 21 patients in whom vascularized fibula autograft was used for upper extremity reconstructions: graft fracture and pseudoarthrosis occurred in 24% and 19% of patients, respectively.

Soft Tissue Reconstruction

The importance of soft tissue reconstruction as part of the overall limb salvage procedure is critical and may involve several techniques. The spectrum of soft tissue reconstruction includes primary closure, split-thickness and full-thickness skin grafts, local or regional flaps, and free-tissue transfer. The choice of technique is dependent on tumor-related factors such as defect size, location, and involvement of neurovascular structures as well as patient-related factors such as age, health status, and functional status.[80]

The plan for soft tissue coverage should already be in place when skin incisions are made for tumor resection to prevent compromise of later reconstructive options. When primary closure would result in undue skin tension, skin grafts may be used. Full-thickness grafts are often preferable, because they do not contract and wear better than split-thickness skin grafts. Skin grafts should not be placed directly over exposed hardware, tendon, or bone and require a clean healthy wound bed to support neovascularization.

In 1 large series of 100 sarcoma resections of the upper extremity,[81] flap coverage was required in 29% of patients. In the arm and forearm, tumor sizes of 5 cm or greater are associated with need for soft tissue flap reconstruction, whereas in the hand, the tumor sizes of 2.5 cm or greater often require these complex closures.[44,81] Regional flaps commonly used in the upper extremity include the radial forearm flap, lateral arm flap, latissimus dorsi flap, and posterior interosseous flap.[80,81] Fillet flaps using the spare parts after tumor resection may be used frequently for hand lesions and can obviate other regional flaps.[44]

The radial forearm flap may be used as a free flap or pedicled reverse flap, which may reach as far distally as the webspaces and provides approximately 12 × 17 cm of tissue. It requires sacrifice of the radial artery and may be harvested as either a fascial, fasciocutaneous, or osteocutaneous flap, although fracture is a common complication if of the osteocutaneous variant. The lateral arm flap may be harvested as a fasciocutaneous flap with dimensions of 8 × 15 cm and can be used to cover the shoulder or turned down to cover the elbow. The latissimus dorsi flap, based off the thoracodorsal artery, may be used as a large (25 × 35 cm) myocutaneous flap for coverage of the shoulder, arm, and elbow. A functional reconstruction may be performed in which the latissimus dorsi is transferred to provide elbow flexion or extension in addition to soft tissue coverage.[82,83] The gracilis may be harvested as a free myocutaneous flap to cover small and medium-sized defects. Its use as a functional free-tissue transfer to the arm and forearm has been described.[83,84]

ANATOMIC CONSIDERATIONS
Shoulder

The proximal humerus is the fourth most common site for primary tumors such as osteosarcoma, high-grade chondrosarcoma, and Ewing sarcoma.[31] Resections around the shoulder may be classified as intra-articular or extra-articular and according to bony involvement (S1, scapular body; S2, glenoid-acromion complex; S3, proximal humeral epiphysis; S4, humeral metaphysis; and S5, humeral diaphysis) and the status of the abductor mechanism (deltoid and rotator cuff; A, intact; B, deficient).[85] Intra-articular tumors often require extra-articular resections to obtain tumor-free margins, which may result in compromise of the rotator cuff and axillary nerve, leading to abductor dysfunction. If the rotator cuff and deltoid are deficient after tumor resection, then arthrodesis with allograft, vascularized fibular autograft, or a combination of the 2 may be the preferred procedure (**Table 7**).[78,86]

Arthrodesis with the arm in 30° of abduction, 30° of forward flexion, and 20° to 30° of internal rotation places the distal extremity in a functional position for the hand to reach the mouth.[86] Other reconstructive options to preserve shoulder motion include prosthetic implants, osteoarticular allografts, vascularized or nonvascularized fibula transfer, clavicula pro humero procedure, or a combination of prosthetic and allograft bone, termed allograft prosthetic composite.[86,88,89,92,96] The method of reconstruction should be chosen based on the level of bony resection and the functional needs of the patient.

Osteoarticular allografts may be used in the setting of an intra-articular proximal humeral epiphysis and metaphysis resection and have the advantage of providing soft tissue attachment sites for the rotator cuff and other soft tissues.[89] However, complications such as joint instability, allograft fracture, subchondral collapse, and infection are common.[86,88,89] In 1 series of 16 proximal humeral allograft reconstructions, allograft fracture occurred in 25% of patients, and 50% of patients had sustained an episode of glenohumeral dislocation.[89] Allograft survival at 5 years was 68%, and in 44% of patients with surviving allografts, no active glenohumeral abduction was possible. Subchondral collapse is a unique complication of osteoarticular allografts and may lead to progressive decline in shoulder function. This complication has been reported in 20% to 50% of proximal humeral allografts, although not all cases are symptomatic or require revision.[86,89,97]

Endoprostheses are frequently used in the reconstruction after proximal humeral resections.[86,88,90,93] These implants are typically cemented into the distal humerus, allowing for early motion of the shoulder joint, compared with osteoarticular allograft reconstructions, which require postoperative immobilization. Although the endoprosthetic reconstruction avoids the problem of subchondral collapse seen in osteoarticular allografts, joint stability is a significant concern because of the inability to reconstruct the soft tissue attachments around the glenohumeral joint (**Fig. 4**). Some investigators have advocated using a synthetic mesh as a sleeve around the prosthesis, or suspensory Dacron tapes and muscle transfers to improve postoperative joint stability.[93,94]

Reverse total shoulder arthroplasty is a more recent reconstructive option described for some patients in whom the rotator cuff is sacrificed but deltoid function is preserved (**Fig. 5**).[98] The use of a reverse total shoulder implant medializes the center of rotation of the shoulder joint and improves the lever arm of the deltoid. Although long-term outcomes are unknown, early functional outcomes reported for 4 patients showed MSTS functional scores between 90% and 96.7% and active shoulder abduction averaging 175°.[98]

Allograft prosthetic composite reconstruction uses a prosthesis implanted in a sleeve of allograft bone, which is fixed distally to native bone.[94,95] This procedure allows for a more durable joint surface than osteoarticular allograft but also allows for reconstruction of the soft tissue attachments around the joint (**Fig. 6**). In 1 large series of 36 allograft prosthetic composite reconstructions of the proximal humerus, a single episode of joint instability was observed, and reported active shoulder range of motion was slightly greater than the reported range of motion for osteoarticular allograft and endoprosthetics in other studies. The predicted 10-year implant survival was 88%, compared with 100% for 1 series of endoprosthetics.[94,95]

Clavicula pro humero is a surgical procedure in which the clavicle is osteotomized near the sternoclavicular joint and turned down and stabilized to the humeral diaphysis after proximal humeral resection. The acromioclavicular joint is retained

Table 7
Outcomes of shoulder reconstruction

Technique	Reference	Number of Patients	Average Follow-Up (y)	Average MSTS Score (%)	Complications	Comments
Arthrodesis	O'Connor et al,[86] 1996	7	5.3	79	Infection (1), fracture (3), donor site (3)	Vascularized fibula autograft used in conjunction with allograft
	Probyn et al[87]	10	4.0	68.2	Infection (1), fracture (1), nonunion (2)	Allograft humerus for arthrodesis except in 3 revisions treated with vascular fibular autograft
Osteoarticular allograft	Rödl et al,[88] 2002	11	2	74 (57–90)	Fracture (3), pseudoarthrosis (1)	Axillary nerve resected in most cases
	O'Connor et al,[86] 1996	8	5.3	71	Subchondral collapse (4), fracture (1)	Revisions performed for recurrence (1) and fracture (1)
	Getty et al,[89] 1999	16	2.8	70	Infection (1), fracture (4), dislocation (8), subluxation (3)	Decline in MSTS score of 81% at 14 mo. Limitations in shoulder ROM and strength
	Potter et al,[90] 2009	17	2	71	Infection (2), fracture (9), subluxation (3), nonunion (1)	Revision rate 29%: 4 revised to APC, 1 revised to endoprosthesis
	van de Sande et al[91]	13	10	77	Subchondral collapse (6), fracture (1), nonunion (2), infection (1), subluxation (1)	Revision rate 61%
	Probyn et al[87]	11	3.8	50	Infection (2), fracture (4), subluxation (2), dislocation (1)	45% revision rate to arthrodesis
Clavicula pro humero	Rödl et al,[88] 2002	15	2	82 (67–87)	Fractures (2), infection (4), prominent acromion requiring revision (3)	Highest revision rate related to loss of fixation, clavicula pro humerus represented most stable reconstruction, axillary nerve resected in most cases
	Tsukushi et al,[92] 2006	7	2.2	69 (63–77)	Loss of fixation (1)	Higher scores for nondominant extremity. Limitation in hand positioning and lifting

	Study	n	MSTS	Complications	Comments
Endoprosthesis	Rödl et al,[88] 2002	19	2	Shoulder instability (2), tumor recurrence (2)	Axillary nerve resected in most cases
	O'Connor et al,[86] 1996	11	5.3	Instability (6), infection (1), loosening (1), implant fracture (1)	Secondary arthrodesis for instability (2) or implant failure (2)
	Potter et al,[90] 2009	16	2	Subluxation (2), dislocation (3)	No prosthesis revisions, reoperation for dislocation (3)
	Kiss et al,[78] 2007	36	4.7	Infection (1), dislocation (1)	Limited shoulder ROM
	Marulanda et al,[93] 2010	16	1.1	Infection (1 - superficial), subluxation (1)	Aortograft used to envelope and stabilize prosthesis No dislocations
	van de Sande et al[91]	14	10	Dislocation (1)	Average ROM: flexion 43°, (15°–70°); abduction 38° (15°–110°) Revision rate 7%
	Wittig et al,[94] 2002	23	10	Nerve palsy (8), loosening (1), fracture (1)	Dacron tape and muscle transfer to improve joint stability No revisions required, no joint instability
APC	Potter et al,[90] 2009	16	2	Infection (2), fracture (1), subluxation (3), nonunion (1)	Revision rate 6%: 1 revised to endoprosthesis 75% of patients had >90° of abduction
	Abdeen et al,[95] 2009	36	5	Loosening (3), delayed union (4), superior migration (5)	Revision rate 19.4% 3 for loosening, 4 for delayed union
	van de Sande et al[91]	10	10	Fracture (2), infection (2), subluxation (3), dislocation (1)	Revision rate 30%
Functional spacer	O'Connor et al,[86] 1996	18	5.3	Superior migration (7)	Limitation in hand positioning and lifting
Tikhoff-Linberg	Kiss et al,[78] 2007	5	4.7	Superior migration with skin ulceration (1)	Total scapulectomy + proximal humeral resection Prosthesis implanted as functional spacer
Autologous fibula	Kiss et al,[78] 2007	19	4.7	Fracture (5), subluxation (3), graft resorption (3)	

Abbreviations: APC, allograft prosthetic composite; ROM, range of motion.
[a] MSTS score reported as percent of mean.

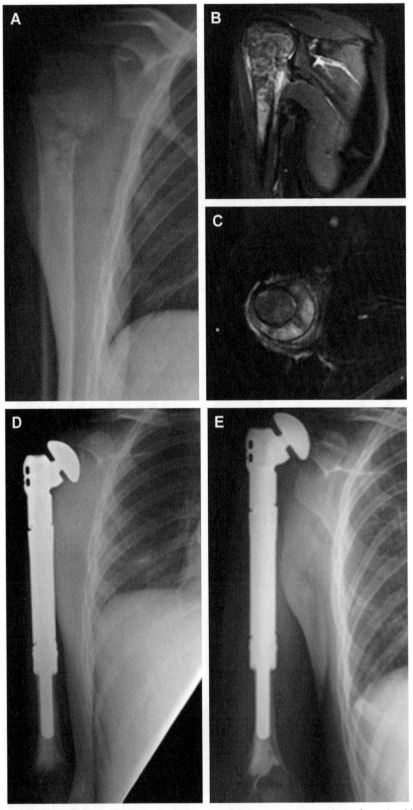

Fig. 4. Instability of shoulder endoprosthetic reconstruction. (*A*) Anteroposterior view of proximal humeral osteosarcoma. (*B*) Coronal T2 MRI of proximal humeral lesion. (*C*) Axial T2 MRI of proximal humeral lesion. (*D*) Megaprosthesis reconstruction of proximal humerus. (*E*) Postoperative dislocation of megaprosthesis. (*Courtesy of* M. Thacker, MD, Wilmington, DE.)

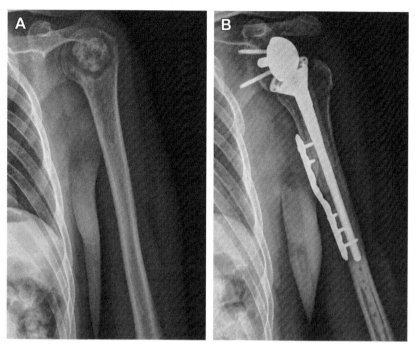

Fig. 5. Reverse total shoulder arthroplasty allograft prosthetic reconstruction. (*A*) Preoperative radiograph showing bone-forming lesion of proximal humerus. (*B*) Postoperative radiograph after reverse total shoulder arthroplasty allograft prosthetic reconstruction, after extra-articular resection of proximal humerus.

and functions as a stabilizer of the proximal arm but permits little motion. It has been proposed as an alternative to arthrodesis after shoulder resections involving the glenoid and abductor mechanism. Tsukushi and colleagues[92] detailed the results of this procedure in 7 patients and found acceptable levels of patient function when this was performed on the nondominant arm or

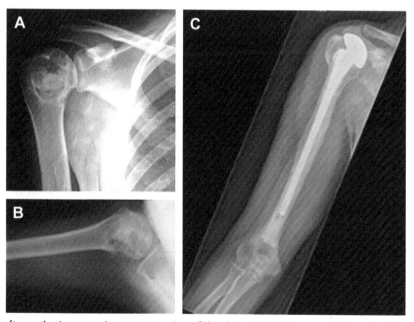

Fig. 6. Allograft prosthetic composite reconstruction of shoulder. (*A, B*) Anteroposterior and axillary radiographs of recurrent chondroblastoma. (*C*) Allograft composite reconstruction of shoulder after wide excision. (*Courtesy of* M. Thacker, MD, Wilmington, DE.)

in a young patient able to convert hand dominance to the unaffected side.

Elbow

Reconstructive options around the elbow are difficult because of the limited soft tissue envelope and proximity of traversing neurovascular structure. Only approximately 1% of bone and soft tissue sarcomas involve the elbow.[99] Reconstructive options for the elbow may include osteoarticular allografts, total elbow prosthesis, total humeral prosthesis, and allograft prosthetic composites (**Table 8**).[82,100–102] Dean and colleagues[102] described long-term outcomes of osteoarticular allografts of the elbow for primarily posttraumatic instability and observed a high rate of complications. Allograft removal was required in 26% of patients for infection, instability, or nonunion. Nerve injury may occur in 17% to 25% of these reconstructive procedures, which are often performed in the setting of previous surgeries or pathologic fracture.[100,101] Despite these complications, patients often achieve a functional range of motion and are satisfied with the outcome, particularly when faced with the alternative of amputation.[82,100,101]

Wrist

Within the upper extremity, the distal radius is a common site of primary benign and malignant bone tumors. It is the third most common site of giant cell tumors of bone and poses unique reconstructive challenges similar to the elbow, because of the limited soft tissue envelope and the proximity of neurovascular structures. Marginal resection of the distal radius is indicated in malignant tumors as well as benign but locally aggressive tumors with soft tissue extension such as grade 3 giant cell tumors. Reconstructive options include complete or partial arthrodesis, and motion-sparing procedures with osteoarticular allograft, prosthetic replacement, ulnar translocation, and vascularized or nonvascularized fibular autograft (**Table 9**).[77,103–112]

Wrist arthrodesis may be performed with a variety of sources of bone graft, such as vascularized or nonvascularized autologous fibula, distal ulna, autologous iliac crest, and autologous tibia.[109,112] Although potentially providing a more stable wrist, the loss of wrist motion associated with a complete wrist arthrodesis may not be suitable for some patients. Partial arthrodesis with sparing of the midcarpal joint by fixation of the graft to the scaphoid and lunate has been described as a means of preserving wrist motion yet providing

improved stability over proximal fibular head replacement.[106,110]

The proximal fibular head has been used either as a vascularized or nonvascularized autograft to reconstruct the distal radius with preservation of a functional range of motion in many patients.[77,105,111] The main complications related to this method of reconstruction include carpal subluxation, hardware failure, and nonunion. Carpal subluxation may be asymptomatic in some cases. The need for a vascularized graft is debated, because it requires a longer operating period and may result only in a shorter time to union than a nonvascularized graft.

Osteoarticular allograft reconstruction for reconstruction of the distal radius is an alternative to proximal fibular autograft and spares donor site morbidity (**Fig. 7**). Mixed results have been reported with this method of reconstruction.[103,104] In a series of 24 patients,[103] fracture of the allograft occurred in 25% of patients in 1 series, and revision to arthrodesis for nononcologic reasons occurred in 29.1% of patients. In the 16 surviving grafts, progressive degenerative changes and radiocarpal or radioulnar instability was observed. Despite these radiographic changes, patients retained a functional range of motion and had little pain with common activities.[103] Scoccianti and colleagues[104] reported a substantially lower complication rate in their series of 17 patients, with revision to arthrodesis being required in only 1 patient. These investigators also observed early degenerative changes of the radiocarpal joint in all of their patients, but wrist function was not compromised.

One of the largest reported series of wrist arthroplasties for oncologic reconstruction[107] used a hinged custom prosthesis in 24 patients and had an MSTS functional score of 75% at an average of 6.5 years of follow-up. Average range of motion was 45° in the flexion-extension axis and 25° in the radial to ulnar deviation. Highlighting the limited soft tissue envelope in this area, skin flap necrosis occurred in 2 (8%) patients and required wrist arthrodesis after failed soft tissue coverage. Wound infection occurred in an additional 2 patients, with 1 requiring revision to arthrodesis.

Hand

Because of the limited confines and soft tissue coverage availability in the hand, amputation may be used in addition to or as an alternative to wide local excision to achieve negative margins.[44] Low-grade malignant lesions of the distal phalanx may be best treated with amputation through the distal interphalangeal joint, whereas higher-grade

Table 8
Outcomes of elbow reconstruction

Technique	Reference	Number of Patients	Average Follow-Up (y)	Average MSTS Score (%)	Complications	Comments
Total elbow arthroplasty	Athwal et al,[100] 2005	20	2.8	—	Nonunion (2), loosening (1), fracture (2), Nerve injury (5)	90% of surgeries for pathologic fracture. 18 intralesional procedures. Two total humeral prosthesis, APC in 2 patients. Mean elbow ROM 92°. Mayo score: 75 (55–95)
	Weber et al,[101] 2003	23	2.8	77	Nerve injury (4), infection (2), UE DVT (1), graft absorption (2), Loosening (2)	Primary sarcoma (15); total humeral prosthesis (7); total humeral APC: shoulder prosthesis, OA at elbow (5). TEA (11)
	Schwab et al,[82] 2008	5	5	—	Nerve injury (1), implant failure (1)	Free/rotational flap in 7 patients. Mean elbow ROM 110° Latissimus flap for coverage and triceps reconstruction in all APC (4), prosthesis-only (1). Mean Mayo score 91 (85–95)
Osteoarticular allograft	Dean et al,[102] 1997	23	7.5	—	Nonunion (7), infection (3), instability (6), nerve injury (4)	Indications: posttraumatic instability (20), tumor resection (1), failed TEA (2) Revision rate 26%

Abbreviations: APC, allograft prosthetic composite; DVT, deep vein thrombosis; OA, osteoarticular allograft; ROM, range of motion; TEA, total elbow arthroplasty; UE, upper extremity.

Table 9
Outcomes of wrist reconstruction

Technique	Author	Number of Patients	Average Follow-Up (y)	Average MSTS Score (%)	Complications	Comments
Osteoarticular allograft	Kocher et al,[103] 1998	24	10.9	—	Fracture (6), dislocation (1), subluxation (10), ulnocarpal impaction (4), EPL rupture (2)	29.1% revision rate to arthrodesis 8.3% revised to amputation for recurrence Average flexion-extension ROM 57°; average radial-ulnar ROM 31°; average pronation-supination ROM 130°
	Scoccianti et al,[104] 2010	17	4.9	86	Nonunion (2), fracture (2)	5.8% revision rate to arthrodesis Average flexion-extension ROM 114, average pronation-supination ROM
Proximal fibular reconstruction	Maruthainar et al,[77] 2002	12	4.2	—	Subluxation (4)	Average flexion-extension ROM 38, average radial-ulnar ROM 25°; average pronation-supination ROM 118°
	Lackman et al,[105] 1987	12	—	—	Nonunion (2), fracture (3)	Nonunions treated with revision ORIF and bone grafting 2 of 3 fractures occurred after traumatic injury Average flexion-extension ROM: 49°; average pronation-supination ROM: 88°; average radial-ulnar ROM: 24°: average grip strength 49% of contralateral hand
Partial fusion	Bickert et al,[106] 2002	2	1.9	—	—	Case series, average grip strength 53% and 76% of contralateral hand. Patients reported no impairments

Abbreviations: EPL, extensor pollicis longus; ORIF, open reduction internal fixation; ROM, range of motion.

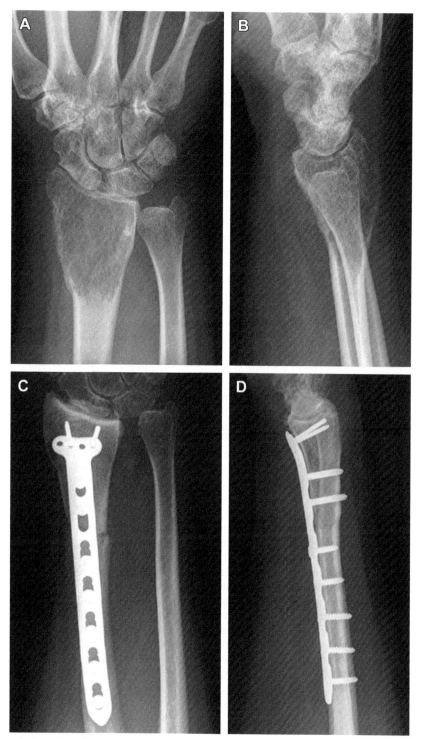

Fig. 7. Osteoarticular allograft reconstruction of distal radius. Preoperative anteroposterior (*A*) and lateral (*B*) views of distal radius giant cell tumor. Postoperative anteroposterior (*C*) and lateral (*D*) views of osteoarticular allograft reconstruction of distal radius.

lesions may require amputation through the middle phalanx or at the proximal interphalangeal joint.[113] Malignant middle phalangeal and proximal phalangeal as well as metacarpal lesions may be bested treated with ray resection because metacarpophalangeal joint disarticulation is of limited function because of the wide space left between fingers. For large tumors (>5 cm), partial hand salvage has been described, as opposed to hand amputation.[51] Indications for this salvage procedure were: (1) ability to achieve negative resection margins, (2) preservation of thumb and 1 opposable digit, and (3) preservation of median or ulnar nerve. In a series of 8 patients with large soft tissue sarcomas of the hand, local control was achieved in 87.5% of patients at an average of 69 months follow-up.[51] The average MSTS functional score was 26 in this group of patients, but lower (19 and 24) in 2 patients who received double ray resections.

Resection and replantation is a surgical technique that has been described as an alternative to forequarter amputation for a variety of Enneking stage IIB and IIIB soft tissue and primary bone malignancies, in which wide resection with full limb salvage was not believed to be feasible.[65] In 12 cases, cylindrical resections of the arm or forearm were performed outside the tumor margins.[65] If neurovascular structures were involved, vascular and nerve reconstruction was performed after determining a negative margin on frozen section. Although half of the patients died of their disease at a mean of 21.5 months, none had evidence of local recurrence. Similarly, at a follow-up of 52.2 months, there was no evidence of local recurrence in the surviving patients. In patients in whom nerve reconstruction was required, adequate sensation and motor function were restored. Hahn and colleagues[66] also reported favorable outcomes in 6 patients with malignant sarcomas or grade 3 giant cell tumors undergoing this partial limb salvage procedure. Hand function was maintained with grip and pinch strength of 66% and 72% relative to the contralateral limb. As an alternative to amputation, this procedure maintained hand function, and average MSTS functional score was 20.

SUMMARY

The upper extremity may be affected by a wide variety of neoplastic diseases. Although primary bone or soft tissue sarcomas and metastatic disease are less common than more benign processes, the clinician should be aware of the appropriate systematic evaluation in cases of suspected malignancy. Biopsy of suspected

malignancy should be well planned with consideration to not compromise definitive resection and reconstructive procedures. When feasible, this procedure is more appropriately performed by the physician who will be performing the definitive surgeries. Advances in musculoskeletal imaging, chemotherapy, radiotherapy, microsurgery, and prosthetic devices have enabled limb salvage to be performed for most malignancies. Familiarity with nerve and vessel reconstruction, tendon transfer, soft tissue coverage, and endoprosthetic reconstructions that maximize function are critical for the surgeon undertaking treatment of oncologic problems in the upper extremity.

REFERENCES

1. Howlader N, Noone AM, Krapcho M, et al, editors. SEER Cancer Statistics Review, 1975-2010. Bethesda (MD): National Cancer Institute; 2013. Available at: http://seer.cancer.gov/csr/1975_2010/. based on November 2012 SEER data submission, posted to the SEER Web site.
2. Pisters PW, Leung DH, Woodruff J, et al. Analysis of prognostic factors in 1,041 patients with localized soft tissue sarcomas of the extremities. J Clin Oncol 1996;14(5):1679–89.
3. Simon MA, Finn HA. Diagnostic strategy for bone and soft-tissue tumors. J Bone Joint Surg Am 1993;75(4):622–31.
4. Miller TT. Bone tumors and tumorlike conditions: analysis with conventional radiography. Radiology 2008;246(3):662–74.
5. Lodwick GS, Wilson AJ, Farrell C, et al. Determining growth rates of focal lesions of bone from radiographs. Radiology 1980;134:577–83.
6. McNeil BJ. Rationale for the use of bone scans in selected metastatic and primary bone tumors. Semin Nucl Med 1978;8(4):336–45.
7. Rougraff BT, Kneisl JS, Simon MA. Skeletal metastases of unknown origin. A prospective study of a diagnostic strategy. J Bone Joint Surg Am 1993; 75(9):1276–81.
8. Bastiaanet E, Groen H, Jager PL, et al. The value of FDG-PET in the detection, grading and response therapy of soft tissue and bone sarcomas; a systematic review and meta-analysis. Cancer Treat Rev 2004;30(1):83–101.
9. Mankin HJ, Lange TA, Spanier SS. The hazards of biopsy in patients with malignant primary bone and soft-tissue tumors. J Bone Joint Surg Am 1982; 64(8):1121–7.
10. Mankin HJ, Mankin CJ, Simon MA. The hazards of biopsy, revisited. Members of the Musculoskeletal Tumor Society. J Bone Joint Surg Am 1996;78(5): 656–63.

11. Styring E, Billing V, Hartman L, et al. Simple guidelines for efficient referral of soft-tissue sarcomas: a population-based evaluation of adherence to guidelines and referral patterns. J Bone Joint Surg Am 2012;94(14):1291–6.

12. Scarborough MT. The biopsy. Instr Course Lect 2004;53:639–44.

13. Enneking WF, Spanier SS, Goodman MA. A system for the surgical staging of musculoskeletal sarcoma. Clin Orthop Relat Res 1980;153:106–20.

14. Wunder JS, Healey JH, Davis AM, et al. A comparison of staging systems for localized extremity soft tissue sarcoma. Cancer 2000;88(12): 2721–30.

15. Saddegh MK, Lindholm J, Lundberg A, et al. Staging of soft-tissue sarcomas. Prognostic analysis of clinical and pathological features. J Bone Joint Surg Br 1992;74(4):495–500.

16. Fleming ID, Cooper JS, Henson DE, et al. AJCC cancer staging manual. 5th edition. Philadelphia: Lippincott-Raven; 1997.

17. Bednar MS, Weiland AJ, Light TR. Osteoid osteoma of the upper extremity. Hand Clin 1995;11(2): 211–21.

18. Soong M, Jupiter J, Rosenthal D. Radiofrequency ablation of osteoid osteoma in the upper extremity. J Hand Surg Am 2006;31(2):279–83.

19. Ambrosia JM, Wold LE, Amadio PC. Osteoid osteoma of the hand and wrist. J Hand Surg Am 1987; 12:794–800.

20. Gibbs CP, Weber K, Scarborough MT. Malignant bone tumors. J Bone Joint Surg Am 2001;83: 1728–45.

21. Okada K, Wold LE, Beabout JW, et al. Osteosarcoma of the hand. A clinicopathologic study of 12 cases. Cancer 1993;72(3):719–25.

22. Sforzo CR, Scarborough MT, Wright TW. Bone-forming tumors of the upper extremity and Ewing's sarcoma. Hand Clin 2004;20(3):303–15.

23. Anninga JK, Picci P, Flocco M, et al. Osteosarcoma of the hands and feet: a distinct clincopathological subgroup. Virchows Arch 2013; 462(1):109–20.

24. Daecke W, Bielack S, Martini AK, et al. Osteosarcoma of the hand and forearm: experience of the Cooperative Osteosarcoma Study Group. Ann Surg Oncol 2005;12(4):322–31.

25. Winkler K, Bielack SS, Delling G, et al. Treatment of osteosarcoma: experience of the Cooperative Osteosarcoma Study Group (COSS). Cancer Treat Res 1993;62:269–77.

26. Bielack SS, Kempf-Bielack B, Delling G, et al. Prognostic factors in high-grade osteosarcoma of the extremities or trunk: an analysis of 1,702 patients treated on neoadjuvant cooperative osteosarcoma study group protocols. J Clin Oncol 2002;20(3): 776–90.

27. Meyers PA, Heller G, Healey J, et al. Chemothterapy for nonmetastatic osteogenic sarcoma: the Memorial Sloan-Kettering experience. J Clin Oncol 1992;10(1):5–15.

28. Picci P, Sangiori L, Rougraff BT, et al. Relationship of chemotherapy-induced necrosis and surgical margins to local recurrence in osteosarcoma. J Clin Oncol 1994;12(12):2699–705.

29. Link MP, Goorin AM, Miser AW, et al. The effect of adjuvant chemotherapy on relapse-free survival in patients with osteosarcoma of the extremity. N Engl J Med 1986;314(25):1600–16.

30. O'Connor MI, Bancroft LW. Benign and malignant cartilage tumors of the hand. Hand Clin 2004; 20(3):317–23.

31. Unni KK, Inwards CY. Dahlin's bone tumors: general aspects and data on 10,165 cases. 6th edition. Philadelphia: Lippincott Williams & Wilkins; 2010.

32. Sassoon AA, Fitz-Gibbon PD, Harmsen WS, et al. Enchondromas of the hand: factors affecting recurrence, healing, motion and malignant transformation. J Hand Surg Am 2012;37(6):1229–34.

33. Patil S, de Silva MV, Crossan J, et al. Chondrosarcoma of small bones of the hand. J Hand Surg Br 2003;28(6):602–8.

34. Lee FY, Mankin HJ, Fondren G, et al. Chondrosarcoma of bone: an assessment of outcome. J Bone Joint Surg Am 1999;81(3):326–38.

35. Mourikis A, Mankin HJ, Hornicek FJ, et al. Treatment of proximal humeral chondrosarcoma with resection and allograft. J Shoulder Elbow Surg 2007;16(5):519–24.

36. Mittermayer F, Dominkus M, Krepler P, et al. Chondrosarcoma of the hand: is a wide surgical resection necessary? Clin Orthop Relat Res 2004;(424): 211–5.

37. Athanasian EA. Aneurysmal bone cyst and giant cell tumor of bone of the hand and distal radius. Hand Clin 2004;20(3):269–81.

38. Mankin HJ, Hornicek FJ, Ortiz-Crus E, et al. Aneurysmal bone cyst: a review of 150 patients. J Clin Oncol 2005;23(27):6756–62.

39. Gibbs CP Jr, Hefele MC, Peabody TD, et al. Aneurysmal bone cyst of the extremities. Factors related to local recurrence after curettage with a high-speed burr. J Bone Joint Surg Am 1999;81(12):1671–8.

40. Eckardt JJ, Grogan TJ. Giant cell tumor of bone. Clin Orthop Relat Res 1986;204:45–58.

41. Campanacci M, Baldini N, Boriani S, et al. Giant-cell tumor of bone. J Bone Joint Surg Am 1987; 69(1):106–14.

42. Campanacci M. Giant-cell tumor and chondrosarcomas: grading, treatment and results (studies of 209 and 131 cases). Recent Results Cancer Res 1976;(54):257–61.

43. Nijhuis PH, Schaapveld M, Otter R, et al. Epidemiological aspects of soft tissue sarcomas

(STS)–consequences for the design of clinical STS trials. Eur J Cancer 1999;35(12):1705–10.

44. Talbot SG, Mehrara BJ, Disa JJ, et al. Soft-tissue coverage of the hand following sarcoma resection. Plast Reconstr Surg 2008;121(2):534–43.

45. Murray PM. Soft tissue sarcoma of the upper extremity. Hand Clin 2004;20(3):325–33.

46. Riad S, Griffin AM, Liberman B, et al. Lymph node metastasis in soft tissue sarcoma in an extremity. Clin Orthop Relat Res 2004;426:129–34.

47. Rosenberg SA, Tepper J, Glatstein E, et al. The treatment of soft-tissue sarcomas of the extremities: prospective randomized evaluations of (1) limb-sparing surgery plus radiation therapy compared with amputation and (2) the role of adjuvant chemotherapy. Ann Surg 1982;196(3):305–15.

48. Keus RB, Rutgers EJ, Ho GH, et al. Limb-sparing therapy of extremity soft tissue sarcomas: treatment outcome and long-term functional results. Eur J Cancer 1994;30A(10):1459–63.

49. Lin PP, Guzel VB, Pisters PW, et al. Surgical management of soft tissue sarcomas of the hand and foot. Cancer 2002;95(4):852–61.

50. Pradhan A, Cheung YC, Grimer RJ, et al. Soft-tissue sarcomas of the hand: oncological outcome and prognostic factors. J Bone Joint Surg Br 2008;90(2):209–14.

51. Puhaindran ME, Steensma MR, Athanasian EA. Partial hand preservation for large soft tissue sarcomas of the hand. J Hand Surg Am 2010;35(2):291–5.

52. Puhaindran ME, Rohde RS, Chou J, et al. Clinical outcomes for patients with soft tissue sarcoma of the hand. Cancer 2011;117(1):175–9.

53. Stojadinovic A, Leung DH, Hoos A, et al. Analysis of the prognostic significance of microscopic margins in 2,084 localized primary adult soft tissue sarcomas. Ann Surg 2002;235(3):424–34.

54. Gronchi A, Casali PG, Mariani L, et al. Status of surgical margins and prognosis in adult soft tissue sarcomas of the extremities: a series of patients treated at a single institution. J Clin Oncol 2005; 23(1):96–104.

55. Gerrand CH, Wunder JS, Kandel RA, et al. Classification of positive margins after resection of soft-tissue sarcoma of the limb predicts the risk of local recurrence. J Bone Joint Surg Br 2001; 83(8):1149–55.

56. Koskinen EV, Visuri TI, Holmström T, et al. Aneurysmal bone cyst: evaluation of resection and curettage in 20 cases. Clin Orthop Relat Res 1976;118:136–46.

57. Biesecker JL, Marcove RC, Huvos AG, et al. Aneurysmal bone cysts. A clinicopathologic study of 66 cases. Cancer 1970;26(3):615–25.

58. Vergel De Deios AM, Bond JR, Shives TC, et al. Aneurysmal bone cyst. A clinicopathologic study of 238 cases. Cancer 1992;69(12):2921–31.

59. Marcove RC, Sheth DS, Takemoto S, et al. The treatment of aneurysmal bone cyst. Clin Orthop Relat Res 1995;311:157–63.

60. Peeters SP, Van der Geest IC, de Rooy JW, et al. Aneurysmal bone cyst: the role of cryosurgery as local adjuvant treatment. J Surg Oncol 2009; 100(8):719–24.

61. Puhaindran ME, Chou J, Forsberg JA, et al. Major upper-limb amputations for malignant tumors. J Hand Surg Am 2012;37(6):1235–41.

62. Malawer M, Wittig J. Overview of resections around the shoulder girdle: anatomy, surgical considerations and classification. In: Malawer M, Sugarbaker PH, editors. Musculoskeletal cancer surgery: treatment of sarcomas and allied diseases. Boston: Kluwer Academic; 2001. p. 179–202.

63. Clarkson PW, Griffin AM, Catton CN, et al. Epineural dissection is a safe technique that facilitates limb salvage surgery. Clin Orthop Relat Res 2005; 438:92–6.

64. Ferguson PC, Kulidjian AA, Jones KB, et al. Peripheral nerve considerations in the management of extremity soft tissue sarcomas. Recent Results Cancer Res 2009;179:243–56.

65. Windhager R, Millesi H, Kotz R. Resection-replantation for primary malignant tumours of the arm. An alternative to fore-quarter amputation. J Bone Joint Surg Br 1995;77(2):176–84.

66. Hahn SB, Choi YR, Kang HJ, et al. Segmental resection and replantation have a role for selected advanced sarcomas in the upper limb. Clin Orthop Relat Res 2009;467(11):2918–24.

67. Krajbich JI, Carroll NC. Van Nes rotationplasty with segmental limb resection. Clin Orthop Relat Res 1990;(256):7–13.

68. Mahendra A, Gortzak Y, Ferguson PC, et al. Management of vascular involvement in extremity of soft tissue sarcoma. Recent Results Cancer Res 2009;179:285–99.

69. Ghert MA, Davis AM, Griffin AM, et al. The surgical and functional outcome of limb-salvage surgery with vascular reconstruction for soft tissue sarcoma of the extremity. Ann Surg Oncol 2005;12(12): 1102–10.

70. Lee SK, Wolfe SW. Nerve transfers for the upper extremity: new horizons in nerve reconstruction. J Am Acad Orthop Surg 2012;20(8):506–17.

71. Ozkan T, Ozer K, Gülgönen A. Restoration of sensibility in irreparable ulnar and median nerve lesions with use of sensory nerve transfer: long-term follow-up of 20 cases. J Hand Surg Am 2001; 26(1):44–51.

72. Ratner JA, Peljovich A, Kozin SH. Update on tendon transfers for peripheral nerve injuries. J Hand Surg Am 2010;35(8):1371–81.

73. Gebert C, Hillmann A, Schwappach A, et al. Free vascularized fibular grafting for reconstruction after

tumor resection in the upper extremity. J Surg Oncol 2006;94(2):114–27.

74. Rashid S, Zia ul Islam M, Rizvi ST, et al. Limb salvage in malignant tumours of the upper limb using vascularized fibula. J Plast Reconstr Aesthet Surg 2008;61(6):648–61.

75. Murray PM. Free vascularized bone transfer in limb salvage surgery of the upper extremity. Hand Clin 2004;20(2):203–11.

76. Mack GR, Lichtman DM, MacDonald RI. Fibular autografts for distal defects of the radius. J Hand Surg Am 1979;4(6):576–83.

77. Maruthainar N, Zambakidis C, Harper G, et al. Functional outcome following excision of tumors of the distal radius and reconstruction by autologous non-vascularized osteoarticular fibula grafting. J Hand Surg Br 2002;27(2):171–4.

78. Kiss J, Sztrinkai G, Antal I, et al. Functional results and quality of life after shoulder girdle resections in musculoskeletal tumors. J Shoulder Elbow Surg 2007;16(3):273–9.

79. Hsu RW, Wood MB, Sim FH, et al. Free vascularized fibular grafting for reconstruction after tumour resection. J Bone Joint Surg Br 1997;79(1):36–42.

80. Talbot SG, Athanasian EA, Cordeiro PG, et al. Soft tissue reconstruction following tumor resection in the hand. Hand Clin 2004;20(2):181–202.

81. Lohman RF, Nabawi AS, Reece GP, et al. Soft tissue sarcoma of the upper extremity: a 5-year experience at two institutions emphasizing the role of soft tissue flap reconstruction. Cancer 2002;94(8):2256–64.

82. Schwab JH, Healey JH, Athanasian EA. Wide en bloc extra-articular excision of the elbow for sarcoma with complex reconstruction. J Bone Joint Surg Br 2008;90(1):78–83.

83. Muramatsu K, Ihara K, Taguchi T. Selection of myocutaneous flaps for reconstruction following oncologic resection of sarcoma. Ann Plast Surg 2010; 64(3):307–10.

84. Grinsell D, Di Bella C, Choong PF. Functional reconstruction of sarcoma defects using innervated free flaps. Sarcoma 2012;2012:315190.

85. Malawer MM. Tumors of the shoulder girdle. Technique of resection and description of a surgical classification. Orthop Clin North Am 1991;22(1):7–35.

86. O'Connor MI, Sim FH, Chao EY. Limb salvage for neoplasms of the shoulder girdle. Intermediate reconstructive and functional results. J Bone Joint Surg Am 1996;78(12):1872–88.

87. Probyn LJ, Wunder JS, Bell RS, et al. A comparison of outcome of osteoarticular allograft reconstruction and shoulder arthrodesis following resection of primary tumours of the proximal humerus. Sarcoma 1998;2(3-4):163–70.

88. Rödl RW, Gosheger G, Gebert C, et al. Reconstruction of the proximal humerus after wide resection of tumours. J Bone Joint Surg Br 2002;84(7):1004–8.

89. Getty PJ, Peabody TD. Complications and functional outcomes of reconstruction with an osteoarticular allograft after intra-articular resection of the proximal aspect of the humerus. J Bone Joint Surg Am 1999;81(8):1138–46.

90. Potter BK, Adams SC, Pitcher JD Jr, et al. Proximal humerus reconstructions for tumors. Clin Orthop Relat Res 2009;467(4):1035–41.

91. van de Sande MA, Dijkstra PD, Taminau AH. Proximal humerus reconstruction after tumour resection: biological versus endoprosthetic reconstruction. Int Orthop 2011;35(9):1375–80.

92. Tsukushi S, Nishida Y, Takahashi M, et al. Clavicula pro humero reconstruction after wide resection of the proximal humerus. Clin Orthop Relat Res 2006;447:132–7.

93. Marulanda GA, Henderseon E, Cheong D, et al. Proximal and total humerus reconstruction with the use of an aortograft mesh. Clin Orthop Relat Res 2010;468(11):2896–903.

94. Wittig JC, Bickels J, Kellar-Graney KL, et al. Osteosarcoma of the proximal humerus: long-term results with limb-sparing surgery. Clin Orthop Relat Res 2002;397:156–76.

95. Abdeen A, Hoang BH, Athanasian EA, et al. Allograft-prosthesis composite reconstruction of the proximal part of the humerus: functional outcome and survivorship. J Bone Joint Surg Am 2009; 91(10):2406–15.

96. Aponte-Tinao LA, Ayerza MA, Muscolo DL, et al. Allograft reconstruction for the treatment of musculoskeletal tumors of the upper extremity. Sarcoma 2013;2013:925413.

97. Gebhardt MC, Roth YF, Mankin HJ. Osteoarticular allografts for reconstruction in the proximal part of the humerus after excision of a musculoskeletal tumor. J Bone Joint Surg Am 1990;72(3):334–45.

98. De Wilde LF, Plasschaert FS, Audenaert EA, et al. Functional recovery after a reverse prosthesis for reconstruction of the proximal humerus in tumor surgery. Clin Orthop Relat Res 2005;430:156–62.

99. Pritchard DJ, Dahlin DC. Neoplasms of the elbow. In: Morrey BF, editor. The elbow and its disorders. Philadelphia: WB Saunders; 1985. p. 713–35.

100. Athwal GS, Chin PY, Adams RA, et al. Coonrad-Morrey total elbow arthroplasty for tumours of the distal humerus and elbow. J Bone Joint Surg Br 2005;87(10):1369–74.

101. Weber KL, Linn PP, Yasko AW. Complex segmental elbow reconstruction after tumor resection. Clin Orthop Relat Res 2003;415:31–44.

102. Dean GS, Holliger EH 4th, Urbaniak JR. Elbow allograft for reconstruction of the elbow with massive bone loss. Long term results. Clin Orthop Relat Res 1997;341:12–22.

103. Kocher MS, Gebhardt MC, Mankin HJ. Reconstruction of the distal aspect of the radius with use of an

osteoarticular allograft after excision of a skeletal tumor. J Bone Joint Surg Am 1998;80(3):407–19.

104. Scoccianti G, Campanacci DA, Beltrami G, et al. The use of osteo-articular allografts for reconstruction after resection of the distal radius tumour. J Bone Joint Surg Br 2010;92(12):1690–4.

105. Lackman RD, McDonald DJ, Beckenbaugh RD, et al. Fibular reconstruction for giant cell tumor of the distal radius. Clin Orthop Relat Res 1987;(218): 232–8.

106. Bickert B, Heitmann Ch, Germann G. Fibuloscapho-lunate arthrodesis as a motion-preserving procedure after tumour resection of the distal radius. J Hand Surg Br 2002;27(6):573–6.

107. Natarajan MV, Chandra Bose J, Viswanath J, et al. Custom prosthetic replacement for distal radial tumours. Int Orthop 2009;33(4):1081–4.

108. Hatano H, Morita T, Kobayashi H, et al. A ceramic prosthesis for the treatment of tumours of the distal radius. J Bone Joint Surg Br 2006;88(12):1656–8.

109. Seradge H. Distal ulnar translocation in the treatment of giant-cell tumors of the distal radius. J Bone Joint Surg Am 1982;64(1):67–73.

110. Minami A, Kato H, Iwasaki N. Vascularized fibular graft after excision of giant-cell tumor of the distal radius: wrist arthroplasty versus partial wrist arthrodesis. Plast Reconstr Surg 2002;110(1): 112–7.

111. Pho RW. Malignant giant-cell tumor of the distal end of the radius treated by a free vascularized fibular transplant. J Bone Joint Surg Am 1981; 63(6):877–84.

112. Campbell CJ, Akbarnia BA. Giant-cell tumor of the radius treated by massive resection and tibial bone graft. J Bone Joint Surg Am 1975;57(7):982–6.

113. Athanasian WA. Bone and soft tissue tumors. In: Wolfe SW, Hotchkiss RN, Pederson WC, et al, editors. Green's operative hand surgery, Vol 2, 6th edition. New York: Churchill Livingstone; 2010. p. 2142–95.

Thrower's Fracture of the Humerus

Andrew Miller, MD[a],*, Christopher C. Dodson, MD[b], Asif M. Ilyas, MD[b]

KEYWORDS

- Thrower • Throwing pitcher • Pitching • Humerus fracture • Humeral fracture • Stress fracture

KEY POINTS

- Throwing is a complex motion that involves multiple muscle groups and forces acting synergistically and antagonistically on the humerus.
- Thrower's fractures primarily occur during the cocking and acceleration phases of the throwing action.
- Thrower's fractures typically present as a mid or distal third spiral fracture of the humerus.
- Thrower's fractures may result from a preceding stress fracture of the humerus.
- Screening for a stress fracture should be considered in athletes presenting with complaints of prodromal arm pain with throwing.

INTRODUCTION

Most humeral shaft fractures are caused by a traumatic event. Nontraumatic upper extremity fractures related to throwing motions are reported less frequently in the literature, and controversy exists surrounding the cause and mechanism of injury. Throwing is a complex motion that involves multiple muscle groups and forces acting synergistically and antagonistically on the humerus. The primary movements about the shoulder include shoulder abduction, horizontal adduction, and external and internal rotation.[1] The primary movements about the elbow joint include flexion, internal and external rotation, extension, and joint compression.[2] Simultaneous kinematic changes at the shoulder and elbow contribute to the torsional forces inflicted on the humerus throughout the throwing phase.

The action of throwing can be broken down into 6 phases: wind-up, stride, arm cocking, arm acceleration, and follow-through (**Fig. 1**).[3] Historically, thrower's fractures have primarily occurred during the cocking and acceleration phases of the throwing action. The activities of various muscle groups have been cited as principal factors contributing to throwers' fractures. The antagonistic actions of the deltoid muscle and the coracobrachialis muscle during throwing were originally implicated in humeral shaft fractures in previous case studies.[4] Furthermore, Hennigan and colleagues[5] attributed the occurrence of fracture during the deceleration phase of throwing to eccentric muscular contraction. However, most thrower's fractures are spiral in nature and located distal to the insertion of these muscle groups.

During throwing, the elbow and shoulder are brought into extreme external rotation with subsequent valgus positioning of the elbow, greatest in the late cocking phase. During early acceleration there is a transition from external rotation to internal rotation at the shoulder and extension at the elbow whereby the greatest amount of torsional force in the distal humerus is experienced. Recent kinematic studies have highlighted the differential

Disclosures: The authors have not received anything any compensation for the production of this article, nor do they have any relevant financial relationships to disclose relative to the topic of the article.
^a Department of Orthopaedic Surgery, Thomas Jefferson University, 1015 Walnut Street, Suite 801, Philadelphia, PA 19107, USA; ^b Rothman Institute, Thomas Jefferson University, 925 Chestnut Street, Philadelphia, PA 19107, USA
* Corresponding author.
E-mail address: andrewmiller28@gmail.com

orthopedic.theclinics.com

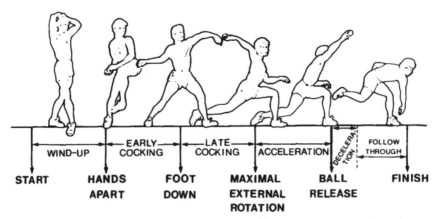

Fig. 1. Phases of throwing. Thrower's fractures primarily occur during the cocking and acceleration phases of the throwing action. (*From* Hamilton CD, Glousman RE, Jobe FW, et al. Dynamic stability of the elbow: electromyographic analysis of the flexor pronator group and the extensor group in pitchers with valgus instability. J Shoulder Elbow Surg 1996;5(5):349; with permission.)

rotational force occurring proximally and distally, resulting in a midshaft torque experienced greatest during maximal external rotation.[6] This torque occurs because the internal rotators of the shoulder and the humerus, primarily the subscapularis, latissimus dorsi, and pectoral major, initiate the internal rotation about the shoulder and proximal humerus before the distal humerus, thus allowing the distal humerus to continue to externally rotate momentarily with respect to the proximal humerus, secondary to a combination of the forearm, hand, and throwing object momentum at the transition of late cocking and early acceleration.

These rotational forces at the distal humerus are most consistent with mid to distal third spiral humerus fractures with concomitant medial butterfly fracture fragments. Kaplan and colleagues[7] also found that, in conjunction with the torsional force on the humerus, improper and uncoordinated throwing techniques, especially over time, can contribute to the likelihood of nontraumatic humeral fractures during a throwing motion, particularly during irregularly occurring athletic outings.

Radial nerve palsies associated with humeral shaft fractures occur with an overall incidence of 5% to 11%, and increase in probability with more distal and spiral patterned fractures.[8] This finding is consistent with the incidence of radial nerve palsies associated specifically with thrower's fractures reported in the literature.[9,10] Holstein-Lewis fractures are classically described as distal third spiral humerus fractures with concomitant radial nerve palsy.[11] Although some thrower's fractures overlap with Holstein-Lewis fractures with respect to fracture pattern and location, most are involved at the middle and distal third junction with a corresponding butterfly fragment.

The goal of this case report is not only to discuss and review throwers' fractures in cases seen by the authors and in the literature but also to highlight the existence of prodromal symptoms that may suggest an underlying preceding stress fracture. Early identification of these symptoms and appropriately managing and counseling patients may prevent debilitation and extension into a thrower's fracture.

CASE REPORTS
Case 1

A 27-year-old male police officer presented with acute pain and an audible pop of his right arm after pitching in his police baseball league. He related a history of many years of pitching, including as a starting pitcher for his high school baseball team. He related a prodromal history of arm pain with pitching, but no pain at rest. Postinjury radiographs showed a distal third spiral fracture of his throwing arm. Both operative and nonoperative treatment options were discussed and operative repair was selected to minimize time to recovery. Open reduction and internal fixation using plate and screw fixation through a posterior triceps-sparing approach was performed. The patient had an uneventful postoperative course that included immediate weight-bearing and range of motion under the supervision of a therapist. The patient returned to field work as a police officer by 8 weeks postoperatively and returned to a throwing rehabilitation program at 12 weeks postoperatively.

Case 2

A 25-year-old male attorney who presented with acute pain and deformity of his left arm after pitching in a club baseball league. He also experienced an acute inability to extend his fingers and wrist. He related a history of many years of pitching, including as a starting pitcher for his college and high school baseball teams. He related a prodromal history of arm pain with pitching, but no pain at rest. Physical examination findings included a radial nerve palsy. Radiographs showed a middle and distal third fracture of his throwing arm (**Fig. 2**). Both operative and nonoperative treatment options were discussed and operative repair was selected to minimize immobilization time and explore the radial nerve. Open reduction and internal fixation using plate and screw fixation through a posterior triceps-sparing approach was performed (**Fig. 3**). Radial nerve exploration identified an incarcerated radial nerve that was carefully transposed free. The patient had an uneventful postoperative course that included immediate weight-bearing and range of motion under the supervision of a therapist. Clinical radial nerve recovery began by 2 to 3 weeks postoperatively with full recovery achieved by nearly 12 weeks postoperatively.

Case 3

A 29-year-old male warehouse worker who presented with acute pain and an audible pop of his right arm after pitching in a recreational baseball league. He had participated in this league regularly since high school. He noted a history of prodromal arm pain that he experienced primarily with his

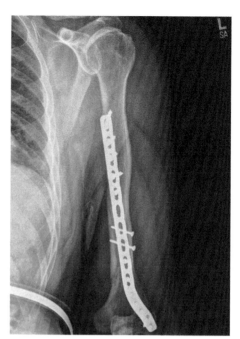

Fig. 3. Postoperative view of the humerus confirming reduction and plate fixation of the humerus.

heavy lifting responsibilities at his job. Radiographs showed a distal third spiral fracture of his throwing arm. Both operative and nonoperative treatment options were discussed and operative repair was selected to minimize his time out of work. Open reduction and internal fixation using plate and screw fixation through a posterior triceps-sparing approach was performed. The patient had an uneventful postoperative course that included immediate weight-bearing and range of motion under the supervision of a therapist. The patient returned to light duty work by 4 weeks and full duty work by 16 weeks postoperatively as a warehouse worker. Patient did not wish to return to throwing after this injury.

DISCUSSION

Several case reports have described various types of injuries to the humerus related to throwing. Baseball pitching has been cited with the greatest frequency, followed by grenade throwing, javelin throwing, and dodge ball throwing motions.[5,7,10,12–20] All of these activities are associated with similar kinematic changes about the shoulder and elbow, as previously described.

The first thrower's fracture case report was presented by Wilmoth[18] in 1930. Subsequently, others have reported a similar throwing related fracture.[5,7,10,12,14–17,19,20] Weseley and Barenfeld[14] described 6 cases of thrower's fractures with all patients between the ages of 20 and 30

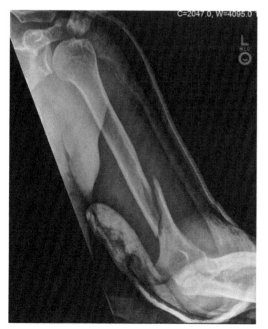

Fig. 2. Preoperative view of the humerus identifying a spiral fracture of the distal third of the humerus.

years with various levels of athletic participation, ranging from recreational to professional, who developed a similar fracture pattern during the pitching cycle.

Chao and colleagues[4] presented a large series of distal humerus spiral fractures related to grenade throwing among Chinese military recruits. All patients in this series were treated with hanging casts, and fewer than 3% had concomitant radial nerve injuries.

Ogawa and Yoshida[19] published a series of 90 patients older than 18 years who sustained distal humeral spiral fractures secondary to throwing in recreational Japanese baseball leagues. Most patients were men in their mid-20s, and the authors speculated that the fracture was more likely to occur during the acceleration phase of throwing based on self-reporting. Half of the patients in this series were treated with plate and screw fixation, whereas the other half were treated with a hanging cast. No difference in healing was observed between the groups.

The treatment for most of these injuries in the literature was a hanging cast for several weeks, with close follow-up to observe healing progression.[14,17,21] Most fractures achieved bony union between 8 and 12 weeks with appropriate activity modification in the interim. In select cases, open reduction and internal fixation with plate and screw construct was performed in patients with significant fracture displacement, delayed union or nonunion, and, in some cases, a concomitant radial nerve palsy.[7,17]

Stress fractures are related to repetitive stresses, low-grade sustained external forces, rapid and chronic application of muscular force to the bone, or an underlying disease or pathologic weakness of the bone.[22] Upper extremity stress fractures are much less common than their lower extremity counterparts. A review of stress fractures in athletes with more than 15 years of play found an incidence of total humeral involvement at a rate of approximately 0.7% to 1.2%.[23] Although not well documented in the literature, select case reports in the literature have described individuals with prodromal symptoms of mid-arm pain and soreness before sustaining a thrower's fracture.[15,20,24–26] For example, Sterling and colleagues[26] and Allen[24] reported preinjury symptoms of bone pain and deep bone aches in adolescents involved in multiple sports preceding the occurrence of the humeral injury.

Similarly, in a series of baseball pitchers 30 years of age and older with irregular pitching cycles, Branch and colleagues[15] described 12 patients with thrower's fractures and found that 9 of these experienced arm pain within a week before the fracture. These prodromal symptoms suggest an underlying stress fracture or pathologic condition predisposing the humerus to fracture through either chronic fatigue or acute stress by decreasing the threshold for fracture. Whether the presence of prodromal symptoms was absent before the injury in other case reports or was underreported is not known. The decreased incidence of thrower's fracture in more competitive athletes and sporting participants may, in contrast, be explained by graduated osseous adaptation and modeling compared with recreational participants.

The present series similarly identified recreational athletes in their third and fourth decade of life with prodromal arm pain that resulted in a thrower's fracture. Given the authors' experience and review of the literature, they recommend screening for stress fractures in both competitive and recreational athletes who complain of arm pain with throwing. Diagnostic evaluation should begin with plain radiographs. However, the gold standard for diagnosing a stress fracture remains a bone scan or magnetic resonance imaging. The mainstay of treatment of a suspected stress fracture of the humerus includes patient education and activity modification. In particular, the patient should be advised to avoid throwing, especially overhead throwing, for at least 6 to 12 weeks until symptoms subside. If a patient does present with a thrower's fracture, treatment can follow the standard algorithm of operative and nonoperative management of a humerus fracture.

SUMMARY

Throwing is a complex motion that involves multiple muscle groups and forces acting synergistically and antagonistically on the humerus. Thrower's fractures primarily occur during the cocking and acceleration phases of the throwing action. Thrower's fractures may result from a preceding stress fracture of the humerus. Screening athletes for a stress fracture and recommending activity modification to individuals who demonstrate prodromal symptoms of arm pain with throwing may help reduce the incidence throwing-related fractures of the humerus.

REFERENCES

1. Dillman CJ, Fleisig GS, Andrews JR. Biomechanics of pitching with emphasis upon shoulder kinematics. J Orthop Sports Phys Ther 1993;18(2):402–8.
2. Werner SL, Fleisig GS, Dillman CJ, et al. Biomechanics of the elbow during baseball pitching. J Orthop Sports Phys Ther 1993;17(6):274.

3. Fleisig GS, Barrentine SW, Escamilla RF, et al. Biomechanics of overhand throwing with implications for injuries. Sports Med 1996;21(6):421–37.

4. Chao SL, Miller M, Teng SW. A mechanism of spiral fracture of the humerus: a report of 129 cases following the throwing of hand grenades. J Trauma 1971;11(7):602–5.

5. Hennigan SP, Bush-Joseph CA, Kuo KN, et al. Throwing-induced humeral shaft fracture in skeletally immature adolescents. Orthopedics 1999;22(6):621–2.

6. Sabick MB, Torry MR, Kim YK, et al. Humeral torque in professional baseball pitchers. Am J Sports Med 2004;32(4):892–8.

7. Kaplan H, Kiral A, Kuskucu M, et al. Report of eight cases of humeral fracture following the throwing of hand grenades. Arch Orthop Trauma Surg 1998;117(1–2):50–2.

8. Shao YC, Harwood P, Grotz MR, et al. Radial nerve palsy associated with fractures of the shaft of the humerus: a systematic review. J Bone Joint Surg Br 2005;87(12):1647–52.

9. Brismar BO, Spangen L. Fracture of the humerus from arm wrestling. Acta Orthop Scand 1975;46(4):707–8.

10. Curtin P, Taylor C, Rice J. Thrower's fracture of the humerus with radial nerve palsy: an unfamiliar softball injury. Br J Sports Med 2005;39(11):e40.

11. Holstein A, Lewis GB. Fractures of the humerus with radial-nerve paralysis. J Bone Joint Surg Am 1963;45(7):1382–484.

12. DiCicco JD, Mehlman CT, Urse JS. Fracture of the shaft of the humerus secondary to muscular violence. J Orthop Trauma 1993;7(1):90–3.

13. Gregersen HN. Fractures of the humerus from muscular violence. Acta Orthop Scand 1971;42(6):506–12.

14. Weseley MS, Barenfeld PA. Ball throwers' fracture of the humerus: six case reports. Clin Orthop Relat Res 1969;64:153–6.

15. Branch T, Partin C, Chamberland P, et al. Spontaneous fractures of the humerus during pitching: a series of 12 cases. Am J Sports Med 1992;20(4):468–70.

16. Evans PA, Farnell RD, Moalypour S, et al. Thrower's fracture: a comparison of two presentations of a rare fracture. J Accid Emerg Med 1995;12(3):222–4.

17. Linn RM, Kriegshauser LA. Ball thrower's fracture of the humerus: a case report. Am J Sports Med 1991;19(2):194–7.

18. Wilmoth CL. Recurrent fracture of the humerus due to sudden extreme muscular action. J Bone Joint Surg 1930;12:168–9.

19. Ogawa K, Yoshida A. Throwing fracture of the humeral shaft an analysis of 90 patients. Am J Sports Med 1998;26(2):242–6.

20. Colapinto MN, Schemitsch EH, Wu L. Ball-thrower's fracture of the humerus. CMAJ 2006;175(1):31.

21. Callaghan EB, Bennett DL, El-Khoury GY, et al. Ball-thrower's fracture of the humerus. Skeletal Radiol 2004;33(6):355–8.

22. Brukner P. Stress fractures of the upper limb. Sports Med 1998;26(6):415–24.

23. Iwamoto J, Takeda T. Stress fractures in athletes: review of 196 cases. J Orthop Sci 2003;8(3):273–8.

24. Allen ME. Stress fracture of the humerus: a case study. Am J Sports Med 1984;12(3):244–5.

25. Sinha AK, Kaeding CC, Wadley GM. Upper extremity stress fractures in athletes: clinical features of 44 cases. Clin J Sport Med 1999;9(4):199–202.

26. Sterling JC, Calvo RD, Holden SC. An unusual stress fracture in a multiple sport athlete. Med Sci Sports Exerc 1991;23(3):298.

Elbow Injuries in the Throwing Athlete

Vamsi K. Kancherla, MD, Nicholas M. Caggiano, MD, Kristofer S. Matullo, MD*

KEYWORDS

- Elbow injuries • Throwing • Athlete • UCL • OCD • Neuritis • VEOS

KEY POINTS

- Overhead throwing is associated with elbow angular velocity of greater than 2300° per second and valgus torque of 64 N/m, which results in lateral-sided compression, posterior-sided shear, and medial -sided tension.
- The bony articulations, medial and lateral ligamentous stabilizers, muscle groups, and nervous structures about the elbow can undergo acute and chronic pathologic changes that result in injury.
- A thorough history, physical examination, plain radiographs, and advanced imaging (computed tomography, magnetic resonance imaging, bone scan) with or without a diagnostic arthroscopy can help determine the diagnosis.
- Failure of conservative management may require operative intervention and can lead to successful results, allowing the throwing athlete to return to play.

BACKGROUND

The elbow experiences significant forces in sports that require repeated gripping and throwing. Stability conferred by the bony articulations, ligamentous stabilizers, and muscles that envelop the elbow helps resist the large valgus forces of throwing. Over time, chronic medial tensile forces, lateral compressive forces, and posterior compressive and shear forces lead to pathologic changes and subsequent injury (**Box 1**). A thorough understanding of anatomy, biomechanics, and pathophysiology will aid in the diagnosis and treatment of elbow injuries sustained in the throwing athlete.

BIOMECHANICS OF THE THROWING ELBOW

The factors that stabilize the elbow depend on the position of the arm. In full extension, the ulnohumeral articulation, anterior joint capsule, and medial collateral ligament provide equal contributions to valgus stability.[1] As the elbow moves into 90° of flexion, the medial collateral ligament takes on 55% of the burden. Primarily, the ulnohumeral articulation, as well as the anterior joint capsule, resists varus stress. In full extension, the bony articulation provides 55% of the stabilizing force, whereas at 90° of flexion, its relative contribution increases to 75%. The radial collateral ligament provides minimal varus restraint, both in flexion (9%) and extension (14%). In extension, the anterior capsule provides 85% of the resistance to distraction. In flexion, the medial collateral ligament provides nearly 80% of resistance to distraction.

Maximum valgus force across the elbow is generated during late cocking and acceleration.[2] The elbow is flexed to 95° and the elbow is subjected to valgus forces up to 64 Nm. During acceleration, the elbow extends at more than 2300° per second. At the time of ball release, the lateral

Funding Sources: None.
Conflict of Interest: Consultant DePuy Synthes (K.S. Matullo).
Department of Orthopaedic Surgery, St. Luke's University Hospital, 801 Ostrum Street, PPHP2, Bethlehem, PA 18015, USA
* Corresponding author.
E-mail address: kristofer.matullo@sluhn.org

Orthop Clin N Am 45 (2014) 571–585
http://dx.doi.org/10.1016/j.ocl.2014.06.012

Box 1
Elbow injuries in throwing athletes

Medial

   Ulnar collateral ligament (UCL) injury

   Ulnar neuritis

   Medial epicondylar injury

   Flexor-pronator mass injury

Posterior

   Valgus extension overload syndrome (VEOS)

   Olecranon stress fracture

   Persistent olecranon physis

Lateral

   Capitellar osteochondritis dissecans

   Radiocapitellar plica

Miscellaneous

   Osteophytes and loose bodies

---

aspect of the elbow is subject to greater than 500 N of force. These extreme medial and lateral forces can cause injuries that can jeopardize the career of the throwing athlete.

MEDIAL ELBOW PAIN
Ulnar Collateral Ligament Injury

Anatomy
The ulnar collateral ligament (UCL) is composed of an anterior bundle, a posterior bundle, and a variable transverse oblique bundle, sometimes referred to as the Cooper ligament. The anterior bundle arises from the inferior-most aspect of the medial epicondyle and inserts on the sublime tubercle of the coronoid process of the ulna. The anterior bundle is composed of an anterior and a posterior band, which provide restraint against valgus stress at different degrees of flexion.[3]

The anterior bundle is the primary restraint to valgus stress of the elbow at 30° to 90° of flexion and is a coprimary restraint along with the posterior bundle at 120° of flexion.[3] The anterior band provides restraint to valgus stress from 0° to 85° of flexion, whereas the posterior band provides the most restraint from 85° to 120°. Fifty percent of the valgus torque imparted on the elbow is transmitted to the UCL. The remainder of this stress is taken up by the strong flexor-pronator muscle mass on the medial side of the elbow.[4]

Etiology
The valgus and extension forces across the elbow during throwing activities often exceed the failure strength of the UCL. Repetitive or excessive stress leads to microtrauma and potentially acute rupture of the ligament. There is a cumulative effect of this microtrauma, and athletes who do not take adequate time to heal are at increased risk for rupture.[5]

UCL injuries are seen in tennis players, football players, wrestlers, javelin throwers, and most commonly, baseball players, especially pitchers. Risk factors for UCL injury in baseball players include high-pitch velocity, inadequate warm-ups, and inadequate rest time.[6] Chronic attenuation of the UCL can lead to further injury in the elbow due to increased bony stress, including radiocapitellar arthritis and posteromedial olecranon arthritis.

History and physical
Acute injury is typically described with pain or a pop on one throwing motion. The athlete is unable to continue play and may describe a feeling of paresthesias within the ulnar nerve distribution. In contrast, patients with chronic injury to the UCL may report a loss of ball control, loss of velocity, or increased fatigability. Pain is often reported by patients to be associated with the acceleration phase of throwing.[7,8] Patients in the later stages of chronic UCL injury may report pain with terminal extension of the elbow.

Physical examination should begin with assessment of both passive and active range of motion. Any joint effusion or flexion contracture should be documented. The carrying angle of the elbow, normally 11° in men and 13° in women, may be as large as 15° in throwers. This is thought to be the result of adaptive change secondary to the repetitive stress and laxity of the UCL.[9]

The elbow should be palpated to determine sites of abnormal tenderness. Lateral pain with pronation and supination may indicate arthritic change due to overload of the lateral structures, whereas posterior discomfort in full extension suggests posteromedial olecranon arthritic change secondary to repetitive extension overload. Neurologic changes should be assessed, as laxity of the UCL can cause tension on the ulnar nerve, leading to complaints of weakness or paresthesias.

The "milking test" is used to assess for UCL laxity (**Fig. 1**). The examiner stands behind the patient while the forearm is supinated and the elbow is flexed to 90°. The examiner applies a valgus force to the elbow by pulling on the patient's thumb. Apprehension, pain on the medial side, or instability indicates laxity of the UCL.

The "moving valgus stress test" has been shown to be 100% sensitive and 75% specific for UCL laxity (**Fig. 2**).[10] The test is performed by maximally

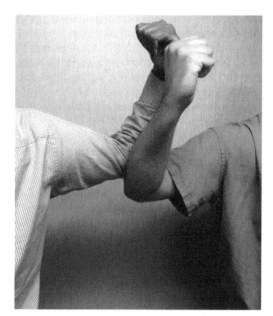

Fig. 1. Milking maneuver test: the examiner grasps onto the patient's thumb, using his elbow as a fulcrum and applies a valgus directed force to the arm.

flexing the elbow. The examiner applies a valgus torque to the elbow as it is quickly extended. Apprehension, pain, or instability, usually from 70° to 120° of flexion, signifies a positive result.

UCL disruptions are commonly seen in conjunction with other injuries of the elbow. Ulnar neuritis, medial epicondyle apophysitis, and flexor-pronator mass tendonitis must remain in the clinician's differential diagnosis. Posterior and lateral elbow pain may indicate posteromedial olecranon and radiocapitellar arthritis secondary to laxity of the medial ligaments. A thorough examination of the shoulder is also mandated, as overhead throwers may have concomitant rotator cuff and glenohumeral capsulolabral injuries.[11]

Imaging
Anteroposterior (AP), lateral, internal oblique, external oblique, and axial radiographs should be obtained. The examiner should assess for osteophytes, loose bodies, or calcification of the ligaments. In cases in which the diagnosis of UCL injury is in doubt, valgus stress views of the affected elbow in 25° of flexion should be compared with the contralateral elbow. Gapping of greater than 3 mm compared with the contralateral side indicates laxity of the UCL.[12]

Ultrasound is an inexpensive and noninvasive imaging study to assess the UCL. Sonogram of an injured UCL will exhibit heterogeneity, hypoechoic foci, thickening, and possibly calcifications. Dynamic stress ultrasonography can be a useful adjunct when static ultrasound fails to yield the diagnosis.[13,14] As with other forms of ultrasound imaging, ability to detect pathology is dependent on the skills and technique of the technician.

Advanced imaging with magnetic resonance imaging (MRI) and computed tomography (CT) arthrogram may be necessary when the diagnosis of UCL injury is in doubt, as well as for preoperative planning. For partial tears, CT arthrogram is 86% sensitive and 91% specific, whereas MRI is less sensitive (57%) and more specific (100%).[15] MR-arthrogram remains the test of choice, having the highest interobserver reliability[16] and the greatest ability to identify complete tears, with 86% sensitivity for partial tears, 95% for complete tears, and 100% specificity for both (**Fig. 3**).[17]

Treatment
Initial treatment of a partial UCL injury is typically nonoperative. The player is removed from active throwing for at least 3 months and a course of passive and active range of motion is instituted. Ice and anti-inflammatory medications are helpful for symptomatic relief. Limited data suggest that 42% of players are able to return to play nearly 6 months after institution of therapy.[18] Unfortunately, no data are available as to which findings in the history or physical examination predict successful nonoperative treatment.

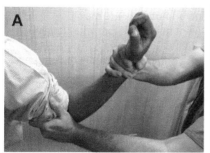
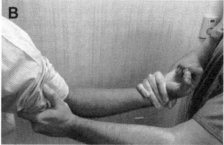

Fig. 2. Moving valgus stress test. (*A*) Examiner places valgus stress with elbow at 90° of flexion. (*B*) Elbow is quickly extended to approximately 30° with continuous valgus stress.

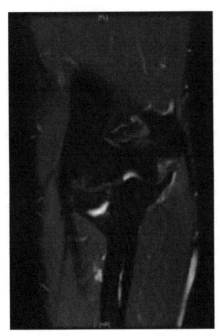

Fig. 3. MR arthrogram demonstrating a partial UCL tear.

Platelet-rich plasma (PRP) injections have shown some promise by increasing return to play rate following partial UCL tears. PRP injection for has been shown to improve Disabilities of the Arm, Shoulder, and Hand scores and decrease medial joint space gapping under stress while maintaining an 88% return to preinjury level of play.[19] Average time for return to play is 12 weeks after PRP injection. Additional studies are required to validate these results.

Surgical indications in the throwing athlete include complete ruptures of the UCL and partial tears that have failed conservative therapy. Repair of the native ligament has traditionally yielded only 50% return to play,[8] whereas early reports of reconstructive techniques showed 68%[8] rate return to play, these techniques have evolved to produce a 92% success rate.[20]

Jobe and colleagues[21] performed the first recognized UCL reconstruction in 1974. An incision over the medial epicondyle is made with identification of the medial antebrachial cutaneous nerve. The origin of the flexor-pronator mass is reflected off of the medial epicondyle. A free tendon graft (typically palmaris longus) is tunneled in a figure-of-eight fashion through bone tunnels in the medial epicondyle and the ulna. At the conclusion of the case, the ulnar nerve is transposed submuscularly. Athletes typically had a 63% return to play at preinjury levels for at least 1 year[21]; however, there were significant morbidities associated with detachment of the flexor-pronator mass as

well as ulnar nerve complications. Later modifications preserve the flexor-pronator mass with exposure of the medial epicondyle by reflecting the flexor carpi ulnaris anteriorly and without transposition of the ulnar nerve.[22] This modified Jobe reconstruction yielded excellent results in 93% of high-level athletes who had not had a previous procedure.

The "docking technique" has produced the highest statistical return to play of 92%.[20] The flexor carpi ulnaris is split to access the anterior bundle of the UCL, which is subsequently incised longitudinally to expose the joint. A single anterior humeral tunnel is created by connecting 2 smaller tunnels drilled from the posterior cortex. The graft tissue is passed through the ulna anteriorly and is "docked" to the humerus. The 2 limbs of the Krakow stitch in the graft are passed through their respective posterior tunnels and joined over a bony bridge on the dorsal aspect of the humerus. The docking procedure allows for easier placement of bone tunnels as well as greater ease of appropriate tensioning of the graft.[20]

After reconstruction of the UCL, the arm is immobilized in a posterior splint. Range of motion exercises are prescribed for the wrist and hand. After 1 week of immobilization, the elbow is placed in a hinged elbow brace that allows for 30° to 100° of flexion. At week 3, the elbow is allowed 15° to 110° and is subsequently advanced 5° of extension and 10° of flexion each week thereafter. Strengthening begins at week 4 and continues through week 9 when plyometric exercises are started. At week 12, players can begin an interval throwing program.[23] Players must be instructed that return to play can take up to a year if not longer.

Ulnar Neuritis

Etiology

The ulnar nerve arises from the medial cord of the brachial plexus, receiving major contributions from C8 and T1 and a minor contribution from C7. As the nerve courses down the medial aspect of the arm and posterior to the elbow, it is subject to multiple sites of compression leading to ulnar nerve irritation.

The most proximal site of compression exists as a thick band of fibrous tissue located 8 to 9 cm proximal to the medial epicondyle. This has historically been referred to as the "Arcade of Struthers," which in reality is neither an arcade nor did Sir John Struthers define it.[24,25] Instead, the medial intermuscular septum and the internal brachial ligament converge to form this thick band of tissue at the point where the ulnar nerve transitions from the posterior to the anterior compartments of the arm. Surgically, this can become a major site of entrapment if not released during anterior transposition of the ulnar nerve.

More distally, the medial head of the triceps, the medial intermuscular septum, and osteophytes of the medial epicondyle all potentially impinge on the ulnar nerve. As the nerve travels posterior to the medial epicondyle, it enters the cubital tunnel, the floor of which is formed by the UCL. The roof of the cubital tunnel, known as the Osborne ligament, is formed by the attachment of the humeral and ulnar heads of the flexor carpi ulnaris. As the elbow flexes, the Osborne ligament becomes taut, trapping the ulnar nerve between itself and the medial collateral ligament. The pressure inside the cubital tunnel increases 7-fold to 20-fold, causing not only deformation of the nerve but also compromising its vascular supply.[26] Osteophyte formation within the medial aspect of the elbow also may lead to narrowing of this anatomic tunnel.

The anconeus epitrochlearis is an anomalous muscle originating from the medial border of the olecranon and inserting onto the medial epicondyle. It is present in up to 34% of arms, making it the most common anomalous muscle in the upper extremity.[27] This muscle overlies the ulnar nerve posteriorly and may cause compression of the nerve with elbow flexion. As the ulnar nerve enters the forearm, it is subject to compression at the aponeuroses of both the flexor carpi ulnaris and the flexor pronator mass.

Repetitive tensile force on the ulnar nerve has been implicated as a cause of ulnar neuritis. The throwing motion subjects the elbow to significant valgus stress, which in turn causes traction on the medial structures of the elbow, including the ulnar nerve. The early acceleration phase causes an average ulnar nerve strain of 5% to 13%.[28,29] Additionally, the nerve has been noted to undergo axial translation of 12 mm as the elbow ranges from full flexion to full extension.[28]

History and examination

The diagnosis of ulnar neuritis relies heavily on clinical examination. A thorough history may reveal pain and paresthesias in the ring and small fingers and intrinsic weakness in the hand. Throwing athletes may complain of loss of ball control or coordination.

The McGowan scale is useful for preoperative grading of ulnar nerve compression. Grade I consists of purely subjective complaints of paresthesias and hypesthesia in the ulnar nerve distribution. Weakness of the hand intrinsic musculature and sensory loss define Grade II. Grade III

has the worst prognosis, with muscle atrophy, occasional clawing of the fingers, and severe sensory loss.[30]

The repetitive flexion and extension motions caused by the throwing cycle may exacerbate an ulnar nerve already prone to subluxation. The throwing athlete with ulnar nerve subluxation may describe a popping or snapping sensation at the medial elbow. This may be accompanied by pain or paresthesias both at the elbow and within the ulnar nerve distribution distally.

Physical examination may demonstrate weakness of the intrinsic musculature of the hand, the flexor digitorum profundus to the ring or small finger, or the first dorsal interosseous. Note any positive Tinel sign over a potential point of compression of the nerve. However, a Tinel sign should be interpreted within the context of the patient's complaints; 10% of the healthy population may have a positive Tinel sign at the cubital tunnel.[31] However, the negative predictive value of a Tinel at the elbow is 98%.[32]

The ulnar nerve should be palpated along its course to assess for enlargements along its course and for subluxation during flexion. The carrying angle of the elbow found to be of abnormal valgus angulation also may predispose to traction injury of the ulnar nerve. Grip strength should be recorded both as a diagnostic measure and as a tool for assessing rehabilitation.

The scratch-collapse test has an accuracy rate of 98% for compression of the ulnar nerve at the elbow (**Fig. 4**).[32] The test is performed with the elbow flexed to 90° in neutral rotation and the arm adducted. The examiner tests the patient's ability to resist internal rotation at the shoulder. The internal rotation force is removed and the arm is returned to the adducted position. The examiner gently scratches the skin over the cubital tunnel and subsequently reexamines the patient's ability to resist internal rotation. A positive result is demonstrated by significant loss of external rotation strength compared with the baseline test.

Electrodiagnostic studies are useful in cases in which the diagnosis is in doubt or where suspicion exists of multiple compression sites. The clinician should obtain electromyography as well as motor and sensory conduction studies. Motor conduction sensitivity has been reported as low as 37% for cubital tunnel syndrome.[33] Testing should be performed with the elbow in flexion, as the length of the ulnar nerve is often underestimated with the elbow extended.[26] Standardization based on the performing site and skin temperature should be included.

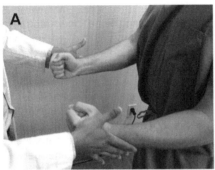
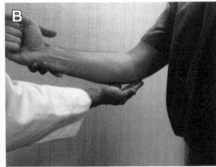
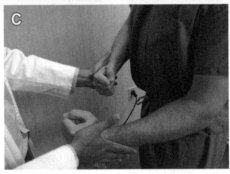

Fig. 4. Scratch collapse test of the right arm for ulnar nerve impingement at the cubital tunnel. (*A*) Patient resists internal rotation with arm adducted at the side and the elbow flexed to 90°. (*B*) Examiner scratches over the ulnar nerve at the cubital tunnel. (*C*) Positive test is an inability to resist internal rotation.

Treatment

Treatment for ulnar neuritis generally begins with a period of activity modification, anti-inflammatory medications, and physical therapy. Corticosteroid injections may cause further damage to already injured ligamentous and cartilaginous structures and should be avoided. Nocturnal extension splinting in semi-extension or elbow pads can be considered. Generally 6 weeks of abstinence from throwing is recommended. Once symptoms begin to resolve, an interval throwing program is implemented.

The role of nonoperative treatment in high-level throwing athletes is limited and consideration may be given to early operative intervention. Patients refractory to nonoperative treatment also may require operative intervention. Options include in situ decompression or anterior transposition. Decompression of the cubital tunnel[34] is a good option for stage I or II patients when the nerve does not subluxate anteriorly. However, this technique does not address intraneural tension, and may lead to anterior subluxation of the nerve.

Anterior transposition can be performed either subcutaneously or submuscularly.[35–37] Whichever method is chosen, critical importance must be placed on protecting the medial antebrachial cutaneous nerve, avoiding creation of new compression proximally or distally, and early range of motion to prevent scar formation.[38]

Subcutaneous transposition

Subcutaneous transposition is performed via a 6-cm to 8-cm incision that parallels the ulnar nerve posterior to the medial epicondyle. The incision must be long enough to allow access to the internal brachial ligament proximally and to the ulnar and humeral heads of the flexor carpi ulnaris distally. Blunt dissection is performed with protection of the medial antebrachial cutaneous nerve. Once the ulnar nerve is identified, it is mobilized while preserving the accompanying vascular structures.

All sites of compression of the nerve must be released, particularly proximally and distally. A finger is passed proximally to ensure the internal brachial ligament does not contribute to nerve compression of the nerve and should be released. The same technique distally evaluates the fascia of the flexor carpi ulnaris. The first motor branch of the ulnar nerve to the flexor carpi ulnaris may need to be mobilized to allow for untethered anterior transposition.

At the elbow, the surgeon must identify and release the anconeus epitrochlearis, if present, and the cubital retinacular ligament.[39] A segment of the intermuscular septum is resected and a judicious pocket is created in the subcutaneous tissue into which the nerve is placed. The nerve is checked once more to ensure smooth gliding with flexion and extension of the elbow. The patient may be placed in a sling until the first postoperative visit when early range-of-motion exercises are begun.

Submuscular transposition

Submuscular transposition begins with a slightly larger incision than its subcutaneous counterpart. After the nerve is mobilized as described previously, a z-plasty incision is made in the tendon of the flexor-pronator origin. The musculofascial flaps are elevated, taking care not to disrupt the first motor branch to the flexor carpi ulnaris. The nerve is laid deep to the flexor-pronator mass next to the median nerve. The nerve is inspected throughout its course to ensure that no proximal or distal site of compression exists with elbow range of motion. The flexor-pronator origin is repaired in a slightly lengthened position with nonabsorbable suture. The wound is irrigated and closed and a posterior splint is applied with the elbow at 90° of flexion for 2 weeks. Passive range-of-motion exercises and formal therapy are begun at the first postoperative visit.

Little League Elbow

Little league elbow is a term used to describe a multitude of injuries affecting the adolescent throwing athlete. These injuries are caused by tension forces on the medial elbow, compression forces on the lateral elbow, and shear forces on the posterior elbow. As single-sport participation and year-round training become more popular, so does the incidence of injury. Elbow injuries in young pitchers are directly correlated to increased innings played and increasing pitch count without appropriate rest.[5,40]

Medial epicondylar injury

Medial epicondyle apophysitis is the most common cause of little league elbow and probably exists on a spectrum with damage to the apophyseal plate or avulsion injury of the medial epicondyle in adolescent throwing athletes and young pitchers.[41]

Adolescent throwing athletes with medial elbow pain will commonly describe an insidious onset of pain accompanied by a steady decrease in velocity and accuracy. An acute onset of pain, although rare, should prompt the examiner to look for signs of apophyseal avulsion injury. A thorough history will include any change in training schedule, pitch count, and innings pitched.

The patient will demonstrate point tenderness over the medial epicondyle as well as medial elbow pain with resisted wrist flexion and pronation. More advanced cases may exhibit decreased range of motion of the elbow. Medial epicondylar fractures will present with swelling, often accompanied by a flexion contracture.

AP, lateral, and axial radiographs of both elbows for comparison should be obtained. In the case of normal films, a stress view may be necessary to determine physeal versus ligamentous injury. Widening of the epiphyseal lines or hypertrophy of the medial epicondyle suggests chronic and advanced injury.

Medial epicondylar apophysitis is treated by complete cessation of throwing injuries. Ice, massage, and oral analgesia may be used as adjuncts. Splinting may be required for refractory cases or patients with pain at rest. Pediatric athletes with stable avulsion fractures of the medial epicondyle and minimal displacement can be treated in a long-arm cast for 3 to 4 weeks with excellent results.[42] Open fractures and fractures with incarcerated fragments are absolute indications for surgery. Although the degree of fracture displacement has long been used as a threshold for surgical intervention, recent literature has shown that interobserver reliability on plain radiographs is poor.[43] CT scan, although exposing the athlete to increased radiation, may help in determining the true fracture displacement and better guiding treatment.[44] Although surgical indications based on fragment displacement vary from 5 to 15 mm,[45–47] the ultimate decision for surgical intervention should be based on mechanism of injury, degree of elbow instability, and patient expectations. The surgeon should remain aware that avulsion fractures can occur in association with UCL injury and the medial ligaments may require treatment as well.

Prevention of medial epicondylar injury in pitchers through limiting pitch counts and innings pitched should be performed.[5,40] Contrary to popular thought, pitch count is more important than type of pitch thrown.[48] Additionally, consideration must be given for the child's skeletal age, especially when playing in an age-determined league.[34]

Flexor-pronator mass injury

The valgus forces across the elbow during late-cocking and early acceleration phases of throwing often exceed the failure strength of the UCL. The flexor-pronator muscles act as dynamic stabilizers of the elbow against valgus stress and help to prevent injury to the medial ligamentous complex. Laboratory studies suggest that the flexor carpi ulnaris and the flexor digitorum superficialis contribute to the greatest stability during throwing activities.[4]

The tendinous origins of these medial-sided muscles are predisposed to injury because of their dynamic function. Repetitive throwing can cause a spectrum of injury from inflammation and tendinitis to acute tears. Athletes will complain of pain over the origin of the flexor-pronator mass. The location of tenderness elicited by palpation on examination should be carefully recorded; flexor-pronator mass injury will exhibit pain just distal to the medial epicondyle, whereas the location of pain in medial ligamentous injury is more distal and posterior, corresponding to the anterior band of the UCL location.

Flexor-pronator mass injuries respond well to conservative treatment. The athlete should cease throwing activities but can continue with active range-of-motion exercises accompanied by ice and anti-inflammatory agents. Once the patient's pain has resolved, an interval throwing program is instituted with anticipated return to preinjury level of play. Athletes who fail initial conservative therapy may benefit from a well-placed corticosteroid injection. However, care must be taken to avoid introduction of steroid into the UCL complex.

Recalcitrant cases should prompt the clinician to investigate other causes of medial elbow pain, particularly UCL injury. In the absence of concomitant injury, the athlete may benefit from open debridement and repair of the flexor-pronator mass to the medial epicondyle. Passive range-of-motion therapy is instituted early in the postoperative period and full return to play can be expected within 10 to 12 weeks after regaining motion and strength.

POSTERIOR ELBOW PAIN
Valgus Extension Overload Syndrome with Posterior Olecranon Impingement

Valgus extension overload syndrome (VEOS) can occur in up to 65% of overhead throwing athletes. During ball release, the elbow reaches full extension, providing an opportunity for osteophytes on the medial and less commonly posterior aspects of the olecranon to impinge within the olecranon fossa. Patients may report locking, catching, pain, and/or crepitus in the posterior compartment. Posteromedial impingement can be confirmed by a positive valgus extension overload test. Physical examination also should include assessment of neighboring ligamentous (UCL), muscular (flexor pronator mass), bony (radiocapitellar articulation), and nervous (ulnar nerve subluxation vs impingement by medial osteophytes) structures.[49] In addition, imaging with plain radiographs and CT scans may identify loose bodies and osteophyte fragmentation.[49]

An injured UCL can be concomitantly present in a patient with VEOS. The UCL relies on the articulation of the olecranon within its fossa to dampen the significant valgus forces of the medial elbow. This articulation serves as an important secondary stabilizer to a lax UCL. As stress transfer occurs to the posteromedial olecranon, osteophyte formation can occur and exacerbate symptoms by shear mass effect. Conservative management with rest and throwing restrictions for 2 to 6 weeks followed by an interval throwing program is first-line treatment. Dynamic stabilization and strengthening exercises often focus on improving eccentric strength of the flexor pronator mass and the elbow flexors.[50] When no further improvement can be obtained with conservative management, surgical intervention with open or arthroscopic resection of the osteophyte(s) is often successful.

Open arthrotomy with excision of osteophytes has been noted to be successful in pitchers with return to play for at least 1 season at 9 to 20 months of follow-up.[51,52] With the more recent arthroscopic approach, results have shown 85% of professional athletes returning to their previous level of competition.[53] Both approaches allow for thorough evaluation of the anterior, posterior, and lateral elbow compartments. In addition to removal of osteophytes, loose bodies can be removed and all chondral surfaces can be evaluated for damage. It is important to note that significant posteromedial olecranon resection can lead to increased elbow valgus[54,55] and subsequent increased strain on the UCL. Hence, goals of surgical intervention are osteophyte removal with preservation of normal bone. If a valgus stress test is positive, suggesting UCL insufficiency, reconstruction can be performed at the same time.

Olecranon Stress Fracture

A transverse or oblique olecranon stress fracture is typically a result of increased stress on the olecranon as the elbow undergoes a valgus extension load, which is similar in mechanism to VEOS. Both repetitive microtrauma caused by olecranon impingement or excessive triceps tensile stress have also been implicated as etiologies.[9] The transverse-type fracture occurs when triceps traction and extension forces predominate, whereas the oblique type occurs with increased valgus and extension forces.

Athletes may present with decreased elbow extension, pain with forced elbow extension and/or resisted triceps muscle testing, or tenderness over the physis (if present) or posterior/posteromedial/posterolateral olecranon. Plain radiographs of the affected elbow are useful for detecting fracture remodeling, whereas that of the contralateral elbow may help with determining physeal widening (if present). If early radiographs are inconclusive, advanced imaging with CT, bone scan, or MRI is often diagnostic.[9]

Conservative management in the form of rest, temporary splinting, and return to an interval-throwing program[56] after symptom resolution has been successful. Some data suggest early surgical treatment to reduce the time to resumption of throwing.[57] Orava and Hulkko have recommended tension band fixation for transverse fractures and cannulated compression screw (6.5 or 7.3 mm) for oblique fractures (**Fig. 5**).[58] Using both methods of fixation also has yielded acceptable outcomes.[54,58] Furthermore, arthroscopically assisted procedures can allow for additional diagnosis of associated lesions (loose bodies, osteophytes, ligament injury, and chondral damage) and direct visualization of the intra-articular portion of the olecranon stress fracture.[9] In cases of persistent fracture, bone grafting has been shown to be effective.[59,60]

Persistent Olecranon Physis

The olecranon physis has 2 ossification centers, a posterior center responsible for the longitudinal axis of the ulna and an anterior center at the olecranon tip that contributes to the joint surface. These 2 centers fuse and create a single physis that persists until age 16 in boys and age 14 in girls. A persistent olecranon physis, although similar to an olecranon stress fracture, is a result of repetitive elbow stress leading to sclerotic changes during physeal closing. Adolescents typically present with posterior elbow pain at terminal elbow extension in the follow-through phase of throwing. Plain radiographs of the bilateral elbows may show a sclerotic physis, widened as high as

5 mm on the affected side. A T2-weighted MRI may show physeal edema.

Initial management consists of rest, cessation of throwing, nonsteroidal anti-inflammatory drugs (NSAIDs), and ice, with success in most patients. However, resolution of symptoms can take as long as 4 months.[61–63] Surgical treatment may be beneficial after failing conservative management. In a recent study looking at the utility of radiographic criteria for guiding nonoperative versus operative treatment, sclerotic change was found to be a highly predictive variable for requiring operative intervention.[62]

The highest rates of successful union have been shown in patients undergoing bone grafting with or without fixation.[61,63] Both a tension-band wire construct and a single lag screw have been described as successful fixation options.[64–66] Charlton and Chandler[61] found that operative stabilization with internal fixation and autogenous iliac crest bone grafting can resolve symptoms and allow a skeletally mature overhead athlete to return to previous throwing performance. Fixation alone, however, may lead to a 66% failure rate.[61,63]

LATERAL ELBOW PAIN
Capitellar Osteochondritis Dissecans

Radiocapitellar compression can lead to capitellar osteochondritis dissecans (OCD), also known as Panner disease or little league elbow, in preadolescent, adolescent, or young adults.[67] It occurs most frequently in young male throwing athletes and female gymnasts. OCD is a noninflammatory degeneration of subchondral bone of the capitellum that has been reported to be due to ischemia, trauma, and genetic factors.[68] Specifically, large valgus stresses during throwing or axial loads from activities like gymnastics can disrupt the tenuous blood flow to the capitellum. Either repetitive microtrauma or a single traumatic event can

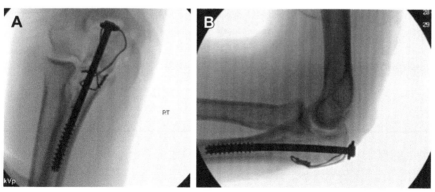

Fig. 5. Tension band fixation of a transverse olecranon fracture using a 7.3-mm cannulated screw and 18-gauge wire. (*A*) AP. (*B*) Lateral.

injure the 2 end arteries that course from posterior to anterior.[69]

Patients typically present with activity-related pain, mild effusion, elbow stiffness, and/or mechanical symptoms of locking or catching if loose bodies are present. On physical examination, tenderness over the radiocapitellar joint laterally, as well as a 15° to 20° flexion contracture may be present. Pain can be reproduced via an active radiocapitellar compression test, which is positive when pain is elicited in the lateral compartment of an extended elbow with forearm pronation and supination.

Initial imaging with AP films of the elbow in full extension and 45° flexion, as well as a lateral view, may be negative early. As progression occurs, capitellar flattening and sclerosis on the anterolateral aspect will become apparent. Areas of lucency and loose bodies also may be identified. The radiographic classification by Minami and colleagues[70] is used to describe such lesions. Grade I is a translucent cystic shadow, Grade II is a lesion with a clear split line between the lesion and its subchondral bone, and Grade III is a lesion with loose bodies present. All patients with this diagnosis should obtain an MRI for evaluating lesion size, location, and stability (**Fig. 6**). Unstable lesions typically demonstrate fluid under the articular surface. The addition of arthrography can further reveal separation of a detached or partially detached fragment.

Management of OCD lesions should take into account features of the lesion (size, location, chronicity, and stability), demands of the patient, and findings from imaging and arthroscopy. The staging system by Ahmad and colleagues[67] can be helpful in deciding when to operate and for determining prognosis (**Table 1**). There is sufficient evidence to suggest that stage I, stable lesions can heal nonoperatively,[67,71,72] particularly with an open capitellar physes, localized flattening, or radiolucency of the subchondral bone, and good elbow motion.[67] Contained, stable lesions involving less than 50% of the capitellar surface may require debridement after failing nonoperative management.[9,67]

Surgical management is usually warranted for unstable lesions, mechanical symptoms, loose bodies, or if nonsurgical treatment has failed. The decision for open arthrotomy versus arthroscopy is dependent on surgeon preference, although evidence does suggest arthroscopy to be associated with less operative morbidity, earlier return to play, and the ability to visualize the entire elbow joint for identifying other unexpected lesions.[9]

Nonoperative treatment consists of 6 months of elbow rest without throwing, initiation of NSAIDs, and a hinged elbow brace, with progressive strengthening when pain resolves. Six-week interval radiographs can be obtained to follow healing. When in doubt, repeat MRIs at 3-month intervals can be obtained to determine the presence of healing. If motion is found to be improving in the absence of symptoms with no deterioration on imaging, an interval throwing program can be initiated at 6 months.

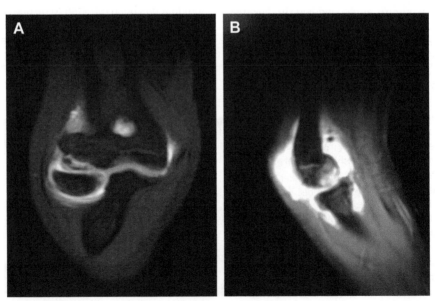

Fig. 6. MRI of the elbow demonstrating a capitellar OCD lesion with fluid behind the fragment. (*A*) AP. (*B*) Lateral.

Table 1
Osteochondritis dissecans staging

Stability	Stage	Radiographic Findings	Arthroscopic Findings
Stable	I	Normal x-rays T1 MRI: abnormal, T2 MRI: normal	• Intact cartilage • Subchondral bone edema
Unstable	II	Abnormal x-rays T1/T2 MRI: abnormal Contrast shows lesion margins	• Partial detached fragment • Cartilage fracture • Subchondral bone collapse • Lateral buttress involvement portends poor prognosis
	III	Loose bodies Associated radial head deformity	• Completely detached fragment Any of the above

Abbreviation: MRI, magnetic resonance imaging.

Most OCD lesions are diagnosed at stage II and are by definition unstable because of some combination of partial fragment detachment, cartilage fracture, subchondral bone collapse, or lateral buttress involvement. Surgical strategies, performed open or arthroscopic, include debridement, fragment fixation with or without cancellous bone graft, microfracture or drilling with a Kirschner wire after fragment excision and bed preparation, and osteochondral grafting (autograft, allograft, or synthetic). The use of humeral osteotomy or capitellar arthroplasty for end-stage OCD of the capitellum is supported by limited evidence, but may be promising.[9,73]

Stage II lesions can be addressed based on size, acuity, and location. Small stage II lesions can be treated with debridement; however, early arthritis has been associated with the long-term natural history of the disease.[67] Acute lesions that are relatively large and unfragmented may be amenable to fixation via bioabsorbable or headless compression screws; however, healing potential and clinical results are often variable.[74,75] Lesions involving the lateral column of the capitellum (>6–7 mm) are less likely to tolerate the compressive forces of a valgus or axially loaded elbow. Hence, such lesions should not be treated with microfracture or drilling. Instead, the loose fragment should be removed and the void can be treated with mosaicplasty or osteochondral replacement.[76]

Stage III lesions also are unstable detached loose bodies. Like stage II lesions, acute detachment can be primarily fixed, but have inconsistent results. Otherwise, treatment should again be guided by lateral column involvement with less than 6 to 7 mm involvement addressed by microfracture drilling and more than 6 to 7 mm involvement treated with cartilage replacement with mosaicplasty or osteochondral transplantation.[76] Of note, degenerative changes of the radial head

with greater than 30% involvement limits OCD treatment for lesions of any stage to debridement, drilling, and microfracture. Ahmad and colleagues[67] have concluded that such severe radiocapitellar arthritis is a relative contraindication to mosaicplasty.

With open or arthroscopic treatment, the elbow should be protected for 2 to 3 weeks with a hinged elbow brace with immediate initiation of passive and active range of motion exercises to avoid stiffness. This can be followed with progressive strengthening at 3 months, a formal throwing program at 5 months, and return to play at 6 months. Athletes treated with debridement or microfracture can return to sports 1 to 2 months sooner.[67]

Radiocapitellar Plica

Impingement at the posterolateral elbow can be due to a thickened, hypertrophic radiocapitellar plica. Repetitive microtrauma is related to the thickening and fibrosis of the plica, which represents a congenitally originated fold.[77] The plica can occur in association with capitellar OCD and often presents with painful clicking, catching, effusions, and snapping with pronated elbow flexion greater than 90°.[78,79] The physical examination is largely normal, although the patient may have tenderness posterior to the lateral epicondyle and centered over the joint. Imaging with plain radiographs and MRI are often negative. Other findings include chondromalacia of the anterolateral radial head and capitellum.[78] Conditions that may mimic symptomatic plicae include lateral epicondylitis, proximal radial head dislocation, and radial tunnel syndrome.[64]

Conservative management with rest, NSAIDs, and gentle motion with the addition of an intra-articular steroid injection can diminish symptoms and reduce inflammation. When such measures have failed, arthroscopy can be diagnostic and allow resection of the plica with good to excellent results.[67,78,80] During arthroscopy, after debridement of the synovitis surrounding the radial neck and the anterior capsule, the lateral plica can be seen as a fibrous band folding over the radial head, which can snap over the radial neck and head during elbow flexion/extension. This band is typically resected to the normal annular ligament and a repeat physical examination is performed to ensure adequate release. Kim and colleagues,[80] in a series of 12 athletes, found return to competitive play to average 4.8 months.

Postoperative management consists of early range of motion, progressive strengthening, and the initiation of an interval throwing program at 8 weeks until resolution of symptoms.

MISCELLANEOUS
Osteophytes and Loose Bodies

Loose bodies found in the elbow joint can result from arthrosis of the radiocapitellar joint, advanced osteochondritis dissecans, or from chondrosis of the posterior medial ulnohumeral articulation that occurs as a result of repetitive shear.[68] The throwing athlete typically has osteophytes overlying the posteromedial olecranon or at the olecranon tip. As osteophytes develop in response to elbow stress, they can fracture and subsequently dislodge into the elbow joint to become loose bodies. Pain during full extension, occurring during ball release and follow-through, is often reproduced and exacerbated with hyperextension and valgus stress.

Although plain radiographs are only 27% sensitive,[81] MRI can provide additional bone and soft tissue detail for identifying the source(s) of pain (**Fig. 7**). Arthroscopy is often diagnostic and can provide sufficient therapeutic value via debridement and removal of loose bodies. Additionally, although a small posterior medial arthrotomy is often warranted in cases in which significant disease is present, attention must be paid to protecting the ulnar nerve.[68] Barnes and Tullos, in a report of 100 professional and collegiate baseball players, found that the throwing athlete can return to play for an average of 3.6 seasons.[82] Despite resolution of symptoms, recurrence is appreciable and often necessitates repeat treatment.[9,68]

SUMMARY

Thorough evaluation of a throwing athlete's elbow will often detect some combination of medial-based, lateral-based, and posterior-based pathology. Although history and physical examination will aid in the diagnosis, plain radiographs and advanced imaging can be confirmatory. Most elbow injuries can be initially managed conservatively. Failing a nonoperative course, surgical intervention and postoperative rehabilitation can successfully return the throwing athlete to competitive play.

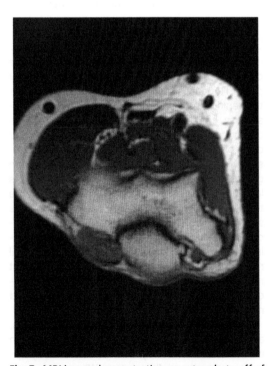

Fig. 7. MRI image demonstrating an osteophyte off of the olecranon process.

REFERENCES

1. Morrey BF, An KN. Articular and ligamentous contributions to the stability of the elbow joint. Am J Sports Med 1983;11(5):315–9.
2. Fleisig GS, Andrews JR, Dillman CJ, et al. Kinetics of baseball pitching with implications about injury mechanisms. Am J Sports Med 1995;23(2):233–9.
3. Callaway GH, Field LD, Deng XH, et al. Biomechanical evaluation of the medial collateral ligament of the elbow. J Bone Joint Surg Am 1997; 79(8):1223–31.
4. Park MC, Ahmad CS. Dynamic contributions of the flexor-pronator mass to elbow valgus stability. J Bone Joint Surg Am 2004;86-A(10):2268–74.
5. Lyman S, Fleisig GS, Andrews JR, et al. Effect of pitch type, pitch count, and pitching mechanics on risk of elbow and shoulder pain in youth baseball pitchers. Am J Sports Med 2002;30(4):463–8.
6. Petty DH, Andrews JR, Fleisig GS, et al. Ulnar collateral ligament reconstruction in high school baseball players: clinical results and injury risk factors. Am J Sports Med 2004;32(5):1158–64.

7. Chen FS, Rokito AS, Jobe FW. Medial elbow problems in the overhead-throwing athlete. J Am Acad Orthop Surg 2001;9(2):99–113.

8. Conway JE, Jobe FW, Glousman RE, et al. Medial instability of the elbow in throwing athletes. Treatment by repair or reconstruction of the ulnar collateral ligament. J Bone Joint Surg Am 1992;74(1):67–83.

9. Cain EL Jr, Dugas JR, Wolf RS, et al. Elbow injuries in throwing athletes: a current concepts review. Am J Sports Med 2003;31(4):621–35.

10. O'Driscoll SW, Lawton RL, Smith AM. The "moving valgus stress test" for medial collateral ligament tears of the elbow. Am J Sports Med 2005;33(2):231–9.

11. Burkhart SS, Morgan CD, Kibler WB. Shoulder injuries in overhead athletes. The "dead arm" revisited. Clin Sports Med 2000;19(1):125–58.

12. Murthi AM, Keener JD, Armstrong AD, et al. The recurrent unstable elbow: diagnosis and treatment. Instr Course Lect 2011;60:215–26.

13. Nazarian LN, McShane JM, Ciccotti MG, et al. Dynamic US of the anterior band of the ulnar collateral ligament of the elbow in asymptomatic major league baseball pitchers. Radiology 2003;227(1):149–54.

14. Sasaki J, Takahara M, Ogino T, et al. Ultrasonographic assessment of the ulnar collateral ligament and medial elbow laxity in college baseball players. J Bone Joint Surg Am 2002;84-A(4):525–31.

15. Timmerman LA, Schwartz ML, Andrews JR. Preoperative evaluation of the ulnar collateral ligament by magnetic resonance imaging and computed tomography arthrography. Evaluation in 25 baseball players with surgical confirmation. Am J Sports Med 1994;22(1):26–31 [discussion: 32].

16. Carrino JA, Morrison WB, Zou KH, et al. Noncontrast MR imaging and MR arthrography of the ulnar collateral ligament of the elbow: prospective evaluation of two-dimensional pulse sequences for detection of complete tears. Skeletal Radiol 2001;30(11):625–32.

17. Schwartz ML, al-Zahrani S, Morwessel RM, et al. Ulnar collateral ligament injury in the throwing athlete: evaluation with saline-enhanced MR arthrography. Radiology 1995;197(1):297–9.

18. Rettig AC, Sherrill C, Snead DS, et al. Nonoperative treatment of ulnar collateral ligament injuries in throwing athletes. Am J Sports Med 2001;29(1):15–7.

19. Podesta L, Crow SA, Volkmer D, et al. Treatment of partial ulnar collateral ligament tears in the elbow with platelet-rich plasma. Am J Sports Med 2013;41(7):1689–94.

20. Rohrbough JT, Altchek DW, Hyman J, et al. Medial collateral ligament reconstruction of the elbow using the docking technique. Am J Sports Med 2002;30(4):541–8.

21. Jobe FW, Stark H, Lombardo SJ. Reconstruction of the ulnar collateral ligament in athletes. J Bone Joint Surg Am 1986;68(8):1158–63.

22. Thompson WH, Jobe FW, Yocum LA, et al. Ulnar collateral ligament reconstruction in athletes: muscle-splitting approach without transposition of the ulnar nerve. J Shoulder Elbow Surg 2001;10(2):152–7.

23. Azar FM, Andrews JR, Wilk KE, et al. Operative treatment of ulnar collateral ligament injuries of the elbow in athletes. Am J Sports Med 2000;28(1):16–23.

24. Bartels RH. Redefining the "arcade of Struthers". J Hand Surg 2004;29(2):335 [author reply: 335].

25. von Schroeder HP, Scheker LR. Redefining the "arcade of Struthers". J Hand Surg 2003;28(6):1018–21.

26. Posner MA. Compressive ulnar neuropathies at the elbow: I. Etiology and diagnosis. J Am Acad Orthop Surg 1998;6(5):282–8.

27. Masear VR, Hill JJ Jr, Cohen SM. Ulnar compression neuropathy secondary to the anconeus epitrochlearis muscle. J Hand Surg 1988;13(5):720–4.

28. Aoki M, Takasaki H, Muraki T, et al. Strain on the ulnar nerve at the elbow and wrist during throwing motion. J Bone Joint Surg Am 2005;87(11):2508–14.

29. Toby EB, Hanesworth D. Ulnar nerve strains at the elbow. J Hand Surg 1998;23(6):992–7.

30. McGowan AJ. The results of transposition of the ulnar nerve for traumatic ulnar neuritis. J Bone Joint Surg Br 1950;32-B(3):293–301.

31. Rayan GM, Jensen C, Duke J. Elbow flexion test in the normal population. J Hand Surg 1992;17(1):86–9.

32. Cheng CJ, Mackinnon-Patterson B, Beck JL, et al. Scratch collapse test for evaluation of carpal and cubital tunnel syndrome. J Hand Surg 2008;33(9):1518–24.

33. Landau ME, Campbell WW. Clinical features and electrodiagnosis of ulnar neuropathies. Phys Med Rehabil Clin N Am 2013;24(1):49–66.

34. DeLee J, Drez D, Miller MD. DeLee & Drez's orthopaedic sports medicine: principles and practice. 3rd edition. Philadelphia: Saunders/Elsevier; 2010.

35. Charles YP, Coulet B, Rouzaud JC, et al. Comparative clinical outcomes of submuscular and subcutaneous transposition of the ulnar nerve for cubital tunnel syndrome. J Hand Surg 2009;34(5):866–74.

36. Chung KC. Treatment of ulnar nerve compression at the elbow. J Hand Surg 2008;33(9):1625–7.

37. Macadam SA, Gandhi R, Bezuhly M, et al. Simple decompression versus anterior subcutaneous and submuscular transposition of the ulnar nerve for cubital tunnel syndrome: a meta-analysis. J Hand Surg 2008;33(8):1314.e1–12.

38. Mackinnon SE. Comparative clinical outcomes of submuscular and subcutaneous transposition of the ulnar nerve for cubital tunnel syndrome. J Hand Surg 2009;34(8):1574–5 [author reply: 1575].

39. O'Driscoll SW, Horii E, Carmichael SW, et al. The cubital tunnel and ulnar neuropathy. J Bone Joint Surg Br 1991;73(4):613–7.

40. Olsen SJ 2nd, Fleisig GS, Dun S, et al. Risk factors for shoulder and elbow injuries in adolescent baseball pitchers. Am J Sports Med 2006;34(6): 905–12.

41. Torg JS, Pollack H, Sweterlitsch P. The effect of competitive pitching on the shoulders and elbows of preadolescent baseball players. Pediatrics 1972;49(2):267–72.

42. Lawrence JT, Patel NM, Macknin J, et al. Return to competitive sports after medial epicondyle fractures in adolescent athletes: results of operative and nonoperative treatment. Am J Sports Med 2013;41(5):1152–7.

43. Pappas N, Lawrence JT, Donegan D, et al. Intraobserver and interobserver agreement in the measurement of displaced humeral medial epicondyle fractures in children. J Bone Joint Surg Am 2010; 92(2):322–7.

44. Edmonds EW. How displaced are "nondisplaced" fractures of the medial humeral epicondyle in children? Results of a three-dimensional computed tomography analysis. J Bone Joint Surg Am 2010; 92(17):2785–91.

45. Case SL, Hennrikus WL. Surgical treatment of displaced medial epicondyle fractures in adolescent athletes. Am J Sports Med 1997;25(5):682–6.

46. Farsetti P, Potenza V, Caterini R, et al. Long-term results of treatment of fractures of the medial humeral epicondyle in children. J Bone Joint Surg Am 2001; 83-A(9):1299–305.

47. Woods GW, Tullos HS. Elbow instability and medial epicondyle fractures. Am J Sports Med 1977;5(1): 23–30.

48. Dun S, Loftice J, Fleisig GS, et al. A biomechanical comparison of youth baseball pitches: is the curveball potentially harmful? Am J Sports Med 2008; 36(4):686–92.

49. Ahmad CS, Conway JE. Elbow arthroscopy: valgus extension overload. Instr Course Lect 2011;60: 191–7.

50. Wilk KE, Reinold MM, Andrews JR. Rehabilitation of the thrower's elbow. Clin Sports Med 2004;23(4): 765–801, xii.

51. Bennett GE. Elbow and shoulder lesions of baseball players. Am J Surg 1959;98:484–92.

52. Wilson FD, Andrews JR, Blackburn TA, et al. Valgus extension overload in the pitching elbow. Am J Sports Med 1983;11(2):83–8.

53. Reddy AS, Kvitne RS, Yocum LA, et al. Arthroscopy of the elbow: a long-term clinical review. Arthroscopy 2000;16(6):588–94.

54. Ahmad CS, El Attrache NS. Valgus extension overload syndrome and stress injury of the olecranon. Clin Sports Med 2004;23(4):665–76, x.

55. Kamineni S, Hirahara H, Pomianowski S, et al. Partial posteromedial olecranon resection: a kinematic study. J Bone Joint Surg Am 2003;85-A(6):1005–11.

56. Nuber GW, Diment MT. Olecranon stress fractures in throwers. A report of two cases and a review of the literature. Clin Orthop Relat Res 1992;(278): 58–61.

57. Suzuki K, Minami A, Suenaga N, et al. Oblique stress fracture of the olecranon in baseball pitchers. J Shoulder Elbow Surg 1997;6(5):491–4.

58. Orava S, Hulkko A. Delayed unions and nonunions of stress fractures in athletes. Am J Sports Med 1988;16(4):378–82.

59. Stephenson DR, Love S, Garcia GG, et al. Recurrence of an olecranon stress fracture in an elite pitcher after percutaneous internal fixation: a case report. Am J Sports Med 2012;40(1):218–21.

60. Tullos HS, Erwin WD, Woods GW, et al. Unusual lesions of the pitching arm. Clin Orthop Relat Res 1972;88:169–82.

61. Charlton WP, Chandler RW. Persistence of the olecranon physis in baseball players: results following operative management. J Shoulder Elbow Surg 2003;12(1):59–62.

62. Matsuura T, Kashiwaguchi S, Iwase T, et al. The value of using radiographic criteria for the treatment of persistent symptomatic olecranon physis in adolescent throwing athletes. Am J Sports Med 2010;38(1):141–5.

63. Skak SV. Fracture of the olecranon through a persistent physis in an adult. A case report. J Bone Joint Surg Am 1993;75(2):272–5.

64. Lowery WD Jr, Kurzweil PR, Forman SK, et al. Persistence of the olecranon physis: a cause of "little league elbow". J Shoulder Elbow Surg 1995; 4(2):143–7.

65. Maffulli N, Chan D, Aldridge MJ. Overuse injuries of the olecranon in young gymnasts. J Bone Joint Surg Br 1992;74(2):305–8.

66. Rettig AC, Wurth TR, Mieling P. Nonunion of olecranon stress fractures in adolescent baseball pitchers: a case series of 5 athletes. Am J Sports Med 2006;34(4):653–6.

67. Ahmad CS, Vitale MA, ElAttrache NS. Elbow arthroscopy: capitellar osteochondritis dissecans and radiocapitellar plica. Instr Course Lect 2011; 60:181–90.

68. Schickendantz MS. Diagnosis and treatment of elbow disorders in the overhead athlete. Hand Clin 2002;18(1):65–75.

69. Haraldsson S. On osteochondrosis deformas juvenilis capituli humeri including investigation of intraosseous vasculature in distal humerus. Acta Orthop Scand Suppl 1959;38:1–232.

70. Minami M, Nakashita K, Ishii S, et al. Twenty-five cases of osteochondritis dissecans of the elbow. Rinsho Seikei Geka 1979;14:805–10.

71. Takahara M, Mura N, Sasaki J, et al. Classification, treatment, and outcome of osteochondritis dissecans of the humeral capitellum. J Bone Joint Surg Am 2007;89(6):1205–14.

72. Takahara M, Mura N, Sasaki J, et al. Classification, treatment, and outcome of osteochondritis dissecans of the humeral capitellum. Surgical technique. J Bone Joint Surg Am 2008;90(Suppl 2 Pt 1): 47–62.

73. Nakagawa Y, Matsusue Y, Ikeda N, et al. Osteochondral grafting and arthroplasty for end-stage osteochondritis dissecans of the capitellum. A case report and review of the literature. Am J Sports Med 2001;29(5):650–5.

74. Kuwahata Y, Inoue G. Osteochondritis dissecans of the elbow managed by Herbert screw fixation. Orthopedics 1998;21(4):449–51.

75. Larsen MW, Pietrzak WS, DeLee JC. Fixation of osteochondritis dissecans lesions using poly(l-lactic acid)/poly(glycolic acid) copolymer bioabsorbable screws. Am J Sports Med 2005; 33(1):68–76.

76. Chappell JD, ElAttrache NS. Clinical outcome of arthroscopic treatment of OCD lesions of the capitellum. Orlando (FL): American Orthopaedic Society for Sports Medicine; 2008.

77. Ruch DS, Papadonikolakis A, Campolattaro RM. The posterolateral plica: a cause of refractory lateral elbow pain. J Shoulder Elbow Surg 2006; 15(3):367–70.

78. Antuna SA, O'Driscoll SW. Snapping plicae associated with radiocapitellar chondromalacia. Arthroscopy 2001;17(5):491–5.

79. Steinert AF, Goebel S, Rucker A, et al. Snapping elbow caused by hypertrophic synovial plica in the radiohumeral joint: a report of three cases and review of literature. Arch Orthop Trauma Surg 2010;130(3):347–51.

80. Kim DH, Gambardella RA, Elattrache NS, et al. Arthroscopic treatment of posterolateral elbow impingement from lateral synovial plicae in throwing athletes and golfers. Am J Sports Med 2006;34(3):438–44.

81. Andrews JR, Timmerman LA. Outcome of elbow surgery in professional baseball players. Am J Sports Med 1995;23(4):407–13.

82. Barnes DA, Tullos HS. An analysis of 100 symptomatic baseball players. Am J Sports Med 1978;6(2):62–7.

Index

Note: Page numbers of article titles are in **boldface** type.

http://dx.doi.org/10.1016/S0030-5898(14)00127-8

United States Postal Service

Statement of Ownership, Management, and Circulation
(All Periodicals Publications Except Requestor Publications)

1. Publication Title	2. Publication Number	3. Filing Date
Orthopedic Clinics of North America	9 5 0 - 9 2 0	9/14/14

4. Issue Frequency	5. Number of Issues Published Annually	6. Annual Subscription Price
Jan, Apr, Jul, Oct	4	$310.00

7. Complete Mailing Address of Known Office of Publication (Not printer) (Street, city, county, state, and ZIP+4®)

Elsevier Inc.
360 Park Avenue South
New York, NY 10010-1710

Contact Person
Stephen R. Bushing
Telephone: (Include area code)
215-239-3688

8. Complete Mailing Address of Headquarters or General Business Office of Publisher (Not printer)

Elsevier Inc., 360 Park Avenue South, New York, NY 10010-1710

9. Full Names and Complete Mailing Addresses of Publisher, Editor, and Managing Editor (Do not leave blank)

Publisher (Name and complete mailing address)

Linda Belfus, Elsevier Inc., 1600 John F. Kennedy Blvd., Suite 1800, Philadelphia, PA 19103-2899

Editor (Name and complete mailing address)

Jennifer Flynn-Briggs, Elsevier Inc., 1600 John F. Kennedy Blvd., Suite 1800, Philadelphia, PA 19103-2899

Managing Editor (Name and complete mailing address)

Adrianne Brigido, Elsevier Inc., 1600 John F. Kennedy Blvd., Suite 1800, Philadelphia, PA 19103-2899

10. Owner (Do not leave blank. If the publication is owned by a corporation, give the name and address of the corporation immediately followed by the names and addresses of all stockholders owning or holding 1 percent or more of the total amount of stock. If not owned by a corporation, give the names and addresses of the individual owners. If owned by a partnership or other unincorporated firm, give its name and address as well as those of each individual owner. If the publication is published by a nonprofit organization, give its name and address.)

Full Name	Complete Mailing Address
Wholly owned subsidiary of	1600 John F. Kennedy Blvd, Ste. 1800
Reed/Elsevier, US holdings	Philadelphia, PA 19103-2899

11. Known Bondholders, Mortgagees, and Other Security Holders Owning or Holding 1 Percent or More of Total Amount of Bonds, Mortgages, or Other Securities. If none, check box ☐ None

Full Name	Complete Mailing Address
N/A	

12. Tax Status (For completion by nonprofit organizations authorized to mail at nonprofit rates) (Check one)
The purpose, function, and nonprofit status of this organization and the exempt status for federal income tax purposes:
☐ Has Not Changed During Preceding 12 Months
☐ Has Changed During Preceding 12 Months (Publisher must submit explanation of change with this statement)

PS Form 3526, August 2012 (Page 1 of 3 (Instructions Page 3)) PSN 7530-01-000-9931 PRIVACY NOTICE: See our Privacy policy in www.usps.com

---

13. Publication Title	14. Issue Date for Circulation Data Below
Orthopedic Clinics of North America	July 2014

15. Extent and Nature of Circulation			Average No. Copies Each Issue During Preceding 12 Months	No. Copies of Single Issue Published Nearest to Filing Date
a. Total Number of Copies (Net press run)			1,205	1,251
b. Paid Circulation (By Mail and Outside the Mail)	(1)	Mailed Outside-County Paid Subscriptions Stated on PS Form 3541. (Include paid distribution above nominal rate, advertiser's proof copies, and exchange copies)	440	481
	(2)	Mailed In-County Paid Subscriptions Stated on PS Form 3541 (Include paid distribution above nominal rate, advertiser's proof copies, and exchange copies)		
	(3)	Paid Distribution Outside the Mails Including Sales Through Dealers and Carriers, Street Vendors, Counter Sales, and Other Paid Distribution Outside USPS®	296	331
	(4)	Paid Distribution by Other Classes Mailed Through the USPS (e.g. First-Class Mail®)		
c. Total Paid Distribution (Sum of 15b (1), (2), (3), and (4))			736	812
d. Free or Nominal Rate Distribution (By Mail and Outside the Mail)	(1)	Free or Nominal Rate Outside-County Copies Included on PS Form 3541	123	174
	(2)	Free or Nominal Rate In-County Copies Included on PS Form 3541		
	(3)	Free or Nominal Rate Copies Mailed at Other Classes Through the USPS (e.g. First-Class Mail)		
	(4)	Free or Nominal Rate Distribution Outside the Mail (Carriers or other means)		
e. Total Free or Nominal Rate Distribution (Sum of 15d (1), (2), (3) and (4))			123	174
f. Total Distribution (Sum of 15c and 15e)			859	986
g. Copies not Distributed (See instructions to publishers #4 (page #3))			346	265
h. Total (Sum of 15f and g)			1,205	1,251
i. Percent Paid (15c divided by 15f times 100)			85.68%	82.35%

16 Total circulation includes electronic copies. Report circulation on PS Form 3526-X worksheet.

17. Publication of Statement of Ownership
If the publication is a general publication, publication of this statement is required. Will be printed in the October 2014 issue of this publication.

18. Signature and Title of Editor, Publisher, Business Manager, or Owner

Stephen R. Bushing — Inventory Distribution Coordinator

Date September 14, 2014

I certify that all information furnished on this form is true and complete. I understand that anyone who furnishes false or misleading information on this form or who omits material or information requested on the form may be subject to criminal sanctions (including fines and imprisonment) and/or civil sanctions (including civil penalties).

PS Form 3526, August 2012 (Page 2 of 3)

Moving?

Make sure your subscription moves with you!

To notify us of your new address, find your **Clinics Account Number** (located on your mailing label above your name), and contact customer service at:

Email: journalscustomerservice-usa@elsevier.com

800-654-2452 (subscribers in the U.S. & Canada)
314-447-8871 (subscribers outside of the U.S. & Canada)

Fax number: 314-447-8029

Elsevier Health Sciences Division
Subscription Customer Service
3251 Riverport Lane
Maryland Heights, MO 63043

*To ensure uninterrupted delivery of your subscription, please notify us at least 4 weeks in advance of move.

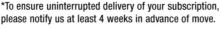

Printed and bound by CPI Group (UK) Ltd, Croydon, CR0 4YY

03/10/2024

01040377-0017